# Device Therapy for Congestive Heart Failure

# Device Therapy for Congestive Heart Failure

Edited by

Kenneth A. Ellenbogen, M.D.
Kontos Professor of Medicine and Director
Electrophysiology Laboratory and Pacing
Medical College of Virginia, Richmond

G. Neal Kay, M.D.
Professor of Medicine
Director, Clinical Cardiac Electrophysiology
University of Alabama at Birmingham

Bruce L. Wilkoff, M.D.
Associate Professor of Internal Medicine
Director, Cardiac Pacing and Tachyarrhythmia Devices
Director, Clinical Electrophysiology Research
The Cleveland Clinic Foundation
Cleveland, Ohio

*With ten contributing authors*

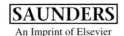

**SAUNDERS**
An Imprint of Elsevier

SAUNDERS

An Imprint of Elsevier

The Curtis Center
Independence Square West
Philadelphia, Pennsylvania 19106

Device Therapy for Congestive Heart Failure                    ISBN   0-7216-0279-7

---

**NOTICE**

Cardiac resynchronization therapy is an ever-changing field. Standard safety precautions must be followed, but as new research and clinical experience broaden our knowledge, changes in treatment and drug therapy may become necessary or appropriate. Readers are advised to check the most current product information provided by the manufacturer of each drug to be administered to verify the recommended dose, the method and duration of administration, and contraindications. It is the responsibility of the licensed prescriber, relying on experience and knowledge of the patient, to determine dosages and the best treatment for each individual patient. Neither the publisher nor the author assumes any liability for any injury and/or damage to persons or property arising from this publication.

---

**Library of Congress Cataloging-in-Publication Data**

Device therapy for congestive heart failure / [edited by] Kenneth A. Ellenbogen, Bruce L. Wilkoff, G. Neal Kay.–1st ed.
     p. ; cm
     ISBN 0-7216-0279-7
     1. Congestive heart failure–Treatment. 2. Cardiac pacing. I. Ellenbogen, Kenneth A. II. Wilkoff, Bruce L. III. Kay, G. Neal.
     [DNLM: 1. Heart Failure, Congestive–therapy. 2. Cardiac Pacing, Artificial. 3. Pacemaker, Artificial. WG 370 D492 2004]
     RC685.C53D48 2004
     616.1′290645–dc22                                                    2003055942

*Acquisitions Editor:* Anne Lenehan
*Editorial Assistant:* Vera Ginsburgs

Printed in the United States of America

Last digit is the print number: 9   8   7   6   5   4   3   2   1

To my family and parents for their infinite patience, understanding and love
Phyllis, Michael, Amy
Roslyn and Leon

KAE

To our patients who place their hopes in us. May we learn from each of them so that we help others with ever more compassion and skill.

GNK

To my parents, Glenna and Harvey, who taught me to thirst after knowledge, truth and wisdom; to my sons, Jacob, Benjamin and Ephram, for whom my prayer is that they never stop seeking the same; and to my wife, Ellyn, who has given me love and the opportunity to explore new ideas and much more. Finally, to my Lord, Yeshua the Messiah, who has given me life and health, hope and love, and a plan for my life.

BLW

# Contributors

Alfred E. Buxton, M.D.
Professor of Medicine, Cardiovascular Division, Department of Medicine, Brown Medical School; Director of Arrythmia Services and Electrophysiology Laboratory, Department of Cardiology, Rhode Island Hospital and Miriam Hospital, Providence, Rhode Island.

Michael R. Gold, M.D., Ph.D.
Michael E. Assey Professor of Medicine, Department of Medicine, Division of Cardiology; Chief, Division of Cardiology; Medical Director, Heart and Vascular Center, Medical University of South Carolina, Charleston, South Carolina.

Richard A. Grimm, D.O.
Program Director, Cardiovascular Imaging Fellowship, Department of Cardiovascular Medicine, Cleveland Clinic Foundation, Cleveland, Ohio.

David A. Kass, M.D.
Professor of Medicine; Professor of Biomedical Engineering, Division of Cardiology, Department of Medicine, Johns Hopkins Medical Institutions, Baltimore, Maryland.

Angel R. Leon, M.D.
Associate Professor of Medicine, Department of Medicine–Cardiology, Emory University School of Medicine; Chief of Cardiology, Emory Crawford Long Hospital, Atlanta, Georgia.

Leslie A. Saxon, M.D.
Professor, Cardiac Electrophysiology, Division of Cardiovascular Medicine, USC Keck School of Medicine, University Hospital; Section Chief, Cardiac Electrophysiology, USC University Hospital, Section Chief, Cardiac Electrophysiology, Los Angeles County/USC General Hospital, Los Angeles, California.

Lynne Warner Stevenson, M.D.
Associate Professor of Medicine, Harvard Medical School; Co-Director, Cardiomyopathy and Heart Failure Program, Brigham and Women's Hospital, Boston, Massachusetts.

J. Marcus Wharton, M.D.
Professor of Medicine, Division of Cardiology; Director, Cardiac Electrophysiology, Medical University of South Carolina, Charleston, South Carolina.

Seth J. Worley, M.D.
Director of Pacing and Electrophysiology, The Heart Center, Lancaster General Hospital; Medical Director, Lancaster Heart Foundation, Lancaster, Pennsylvania.

Paul C. Zei, M.D., Ph.D.
Fellow, Department of Cardiology, Brigham and Women's Hospital, Boston, Massachusetts.

# Preface

Cardiac resynchronization therapy represents a major advance for the treatment of some of the millions of patients with congestive heart failure. Resynchronization therapy has become an area of intense interest to clinicians, patients, and researchers. Its impact on the care of patients with congestive heart failure has not yet been fully realized. However, the current devices are challenging to implant and to follow. It is therefore important that clinicians thoroughly understand the indications, fundamental physiologic principles, and electrical characteristics of cardiac resynchronization devices if optimal patient outcomes are to be achieved. This book aims to provide, in one volume, the fundamental principles and clinical pearls necessary to rationally apply cardiac resynchronization device implantation and follow-up, as well as general management of implantable devices in the patient with congestive heart failure. The information included in this volume should be useful to cardiologists, cardiac surgeons, pacemaker and implantable cardioverter defibrillator technicians, and clinical engineers. We have attempted to provide information that is critically important in the daily care of patients with heart failure and implantable devices. The authors of each chapter are internationally recognized experts in this new field and have done a spectacular job of sharing new and important information in this evolving field. We hope that we have achieved these goals, and dedicate this book to our patients, students, and colleagues, who on a daily basis remind us of the importance of advancing the clinical practice of medicine.

*Kenneth A. Ellenbogen, M.D.*
Richmond, Virginia

*G. Neal Kay, M.D.*
Birmingham, Alabama

*Bruce L. Wilkoff, M.D.*
Cleveland, Ohio

# Contents

# Epidemiology and Prognosis of Heart Failure

## Paul C. Zei • Lynne W. Stevenson

## Heart Failure Incidence, Morbidity, and Mortality

The terms *heart failure* and *cardiomyopathy* refer to a spectrum of diseases that encompass several different clinical entities, with a common underlying pathophysiology of inadequate function of one or both ventricles. In chronic heart failure, this process begins with injury or stress to the myocardium, resulting in impairment of either systolic contraction or diastolic relaxation. In response, the heart remodels, leading to changes in the myocardial structure and the neurohormonal milieu of the entire cardiovascular system. These changes occur in response to increased wall stresses in the failing heart, and they lead to alterations in the geometry of the heart as the ventricle(s) hypertrophy or dilate. These changes generally precede clinical symptoms for some time.

Heart failure is a major health problem that continues to increase in prevalence. By recent estimates, heart failure affects 5 million people in the United States, with an estimated incidence of 500,000 per year.[1] This patient population accounts for up to 15 million office visits, more than 2 million hospitalizations, and more than 6 million hospital days each year. Treatment of heart failure accounts for between 2% and 3% of the national health care budget. Moreover, heart failure is increasingly becoming a disease of the elderly, affecting between 6% and 10% of people older than 65 years; up to 80% of patients hospitalized for heart failure are in this age group[2,3] (Figure 1–1). The prevalence of heart failure is likely to increase in the future as the general population ages and as therapies continue to improve for coronary artery disease, the major cause of heart failure in this country.

In the overall population of patients with heart failure, there is a wide spectrum of disease severity and prognosis. Clinical data gathered over the past 20 years have provided significant insights into some of the factors that govern these outcomes. Determining the relative impact of these factors on clinical outcomes becomes increasingly important when one is considering therapies and management strategies that entail significant cost and potentially significant morbidity. It is

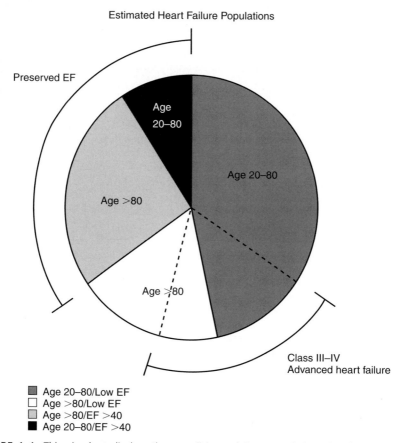

Estimated Heart Failure Populations

**FIGURE 1–1.** This pie chart displays the overall heart failure population, classified into several subcategories. The subgroups of patients older than 80 years versus those between 20 and 80 years of age are shown. The subgroups of patients with preserved versus reduced left ventricular ejection fraction (LVEF) are also shown. In addition, the proportions of patients with reduced LVEF and class III-IV advanced symptoms are shown. The majority of patients with heart failure are younger than 80 years, but among those older than 80 years, a larger proportion have preserved LVEF.

therefore critically important to understand the defining characteristics of the subgroups of patients who will benefit most from these therapies, specifically which patients will benefit from devices that augment systolic function, and which patients will benefit from therapies that reduce the risks of arrhythmias and sudden death.

## Subpopulations

Several subcategories of patients with heart failure are commonly described. These categorizations are often useful in delineating management strategies and the prognosis for individual patients.

### Systolic Versus Diastolic Heart Failure

Between 30% and 50% of patients with heart failure have preserved left ventricular ejection fraction (LVEF). They are often assumed to have abnormal diastolic relaxation as the primary mechanism of heart failure; however, diastolic dysfunction is variably identified and diagnosed.[4] The underlying pathophysiologic mechanisms may include left ventricular (LV) hypertrophy resulting from long-standing systemic hypertension or valvular heart disease, infiltrative diseases, or the spectrum of diseases that encompass the hypertrophic cardiomyopathies. Few definitive clinical trials have been performed to guide the management of these cases. Rehospitalization rates among patients with heart failure are similar regardless of LVEF, and the survival rates among patients with heart failure and preserved LVEF vary from slightly better than to the same as rates among those with reduced LVEF.[5]

### Ischemic Versus Nonischemic Heart Failure

In the United States, coronary artery disease and myocardial infarctions account for most heart failure (approximately 50% to 70% of cases).[6,7] Various nonischemic etiologies account for the remainder, including presumed viral, other infectious causes, hypertension, alcohol, valvular disease, idiopathic, inherited, drug-induced, autoimmune-mediated, and pregnancy-induced cardiomyopathies. The distinction between ischemic and nonischemic mechanisms of heart failure is essential for both management and prognostic implications. The presence of coronary artery disease portends a worse prognosis, even when the degree of systolic dysfunction and ventricular dilation are matched, although it has been proposed that this difference may be due to a higher incidence of diabetes in this population.[6,8] In addition, the specific risk of sudden death is worse for patients with ischemic heart failure.[9] The predictive value of tests to stratify risk for patients with nonischemic forms of heart failure is less than for patients with ischemic heart failure.[10,11] Moreover, the majority of clinical trials examining medical therapies and therapies for prevention of sudden death in the heart failure population have focused on patients with ischemic heart failure.[12,13]

## Race and Gender

The effects of gender and race on the prognosis for heart failure are not well understood. African Americans have probably been best studied. Heart failure is attributed to hypertension in a high proportion of African Americans (60%), whereas coronary artery disease accounts for only 30% of cases in this population.[14] It appears that socioeconomic factors do not account for these differences. The clinical severity of disease is worse in African Americans as well. Potential differences in clinical features among other racial groups within the United States and even across nations have not been studied in great detail. Differences in the clinical features of heart failure also appear to exist between genders. Because of the higher incidence of coronary artery disease and cardiomyopathy among them, men have accounted for 70% to 80% of most heart failure populations. However, at least among older patients, heart failure with preserved LVEF is slightly more common in women than in men.[15,16] These intriguing differences raise questions that warrant future investigation.

## Right-Sided Heart Failure

Patients with right ventricular (RV) dysfunction usually present with symptoms and signs that include peripheral edema, hepatic congestion, anorexia, and nausea. This may result from intrinsic disorders of the RV myocardium or from RV failure secondary to chronic pressure or volume overload from left-sided cardiac disease, chronic pulmonary disease, or pulmonary vascular disease. The most common etiology of right-sided heart failure remains left-sided heart failure. The prognosis of isolated right-sided heart failure is primarily determined by the underlying disease etiology. However, in patients with primarily left-sided heart failure, the additional presence of RV dysfunction predicts a worse outcome.[17]

## Specific Etiologies

Several particular etiologies of heart failure warrant a brief overview, because they have quite specific natural histories and, in many cases, therapies. A detailed discussion is beyond the scope of this text, and other sources should be examined for additional information. *Inherited genetic factors* account for a significant portion (approximately 20% to 30%) of patients with dilated cardiomyopathy of unclear etiology. Most of these cases (approximately 75%) have an autosomal dominant inheritance pattern, and most of the remaining cases have an X-linked pattern. Mutations in multiple molecular components of the myocyte structural and contractile apparatus, particularly the cytoskeletal proteins, have been identified as the root cause in many of these cases.[18,19] The dystrophin mutations specifically cause the Duchenne and Becker X-linked muscular dystrophies. Mutations in the emerin protein result in the X-linked Emery-Dreifuss muscular dystrophy (EDMD). Mutations in the lamin protein result in dilated cardiomyopathy in some family members, atrial fibrillation (AF) in others, and conduction block in other family members with or without clinically apparent cardiomyopathy. Mutations in mitochondrial elements are implicated in the Kearns-Sayre syndrome with cardiomyopathy, ophthalmoplegia, retinopathy, and cerebellar ataxia. The role of genetic factors in heart failure becomes more complex when considering inherited abnormalities in cardiovascular regulatory mechanisms that may lead to heart failure as a secondary response. For instance, genetic defects in the renin-angiotensin axis may result in an abnormal response to hypertension, leading to heart failure. Likewise, mutations in elements of the immune response may affect susceptibility to infectious agents implicated in viral cardiomyopathies. Overall outcomes in these patients are not well characterized.

Patients with *hypertrophic cardiomyopathy* develop abnormal hypertrophy of the left ventricle, particularly those in the minority of cases with severe LV outflow obstruction and its particular hemodynamic and arrhythmic consequences. Until the end-stages of the disease, systolic function is generally preserved. Genetic mutations in both structural and contractile elements of myocytes appear to be the molecular basis for most cases.[20] Therapeutic strategies differ significantly from strategies for patients with systolic dysfunction. Despite a good ejection fraction, these patients have a significant, albeit variable, risk of mortality and sudden death, and therapies to reduce these risks are warranted in appropriate cases. In the 1960s and 1970s, surgical procedures to repair many forms of *congenital heart disease* were developed and refined, resulting in a rapidly growing cohort of adult patients with corrected or partially corrected congenital heart disease.[21,22] Despite good ejection fractions, these patients often develop heart failure well into adulthood with dilated ventricular chamber(s) and reduced systolic contractile function. They can also develop both supraventricular and ventricular arrhythmias, and they likely have a significant risk of sudden death.[23]

Because experience with this population is still growing, there are few clinical data to guide therapy to reduce morbidity, mortality, and the risk of sudden death for these patients. An increasingly recognized etiology of heart failure is *cardiomyopathy induced by prolonged periods of tachyarrhythmia.*[24] Control of the underlying tachyarrhythmia is the mainstay of therapy. In *right ventricular dysplasia (RVD),* there is progressive fatty and fibrous tissue infiltration into the myocardium, predominantly within the right ventricle, although the left ventricle can also be involved.[25] Patients can develop right-sided systolic dysfunction, ventricular tachyarrhythmias, or both. Diagnosis can be difficult, but possible findings include electrocardiographic abnormalities (epsilon waves and ventricular premature beats originating from diseased myocardium), nonsustained or sustained ventricular tachycardia (VT), and RV dilation and systolic dysfunction on noninvasive testing (echocardiography or magnetic resonance imaging [MRI]). Prognosis and severity of disease are quite variable in RVD. As a result, the management of arrhythmias and means of preventing sudden death in this population are still evolving, though the implantable cardioverter-defibrillator (ICD) has an important role.

## Outcomes in Heart Failure

### Signs and Symptoms

The underlying pathophysiology and disease mechanisms in heart failure may be quite variable, but the resulting signs and symptoms are for the most part similar across the spectrum of heart failure populations. Signs and symptoms of heart failure generally result from the effects of one of three mechanisms: congestion from elevated filling pressures, pump failure from inadequate forward cardiac output, and arrhythmias. Left-sided congestion can cause dyspnea upon exertion, coughing or dyspnea upon lying down (orthopnea), or dyspnea at rest. Right-sided congestion can result in edema, abdominal bloating, nausea, anorexia, and ascites. Signs and symptoms of pump failure include hypotension, lack of energy, fatigue, and decreased mental acuity. Arrhythmias can lead to palpitations, paroxysms of dizziness, syncope, or sudden death. Only a modest correlation appears to exist between the degree of cardiac dysfunction and the severity of symptoms. Recent studies suggest that noncardiac factors, including changes in peripheral vascular function, skeletal muscle physiology, pulmonary hemodynamics, and neurohormonal activity, play a significant role in producing symptoms.[13] As heart failure advances, changes in resting symptoms correlate increasingly with changes in parameters that reflect intracardiac filling pressures. The contribution of symptoms and signs of heart failure to limitation of activity and quality of life is highly variable. The degree to which these symptoms limit a patient's functional capacity and quality of life is usually quantified according to the scheme developed by the New York Heart Association (NYHA classes I–IV).[12] Functional class remains one of the most reliable predictors of prognosis in heart failure, and perhaps more important, it quantifies the impact of heart failure on each patient's day-to-day life. Quality-of-life tools for heart failure include the Minnesota and Kansas City questionnaires, which are increasingly being employed to better understand the effects of interventions.

### Causes of Death

Death in the chronic heart failure population may occur suddenly or be related to pump failure, with a significant contribution also from cardiovascular events such as recurrent infarction. Sudden deaths are caused primarily by arrhythmias, including supraventricular and ventricular tachyarrhythmias, bradyarrhythmias, and unexplained syncope, which in turn is likely due to arrhythmias in the majority of cases. However, because sudden death by nature is often unobserved, particularly outside of the hospital setting, it also encompasses noncardiac etiologies, including thromboembolic phenomena, neurologic events, respiratory events, and metabolic catastrophes. In contrast, systolic pump failure is usually a relentless and progressive process, involving progressive end-organ hypoperfusion and its consequences, hypotension, and in the end-stages, mechanical-electrical dissociation. It is crucial to distinguish between the risks of pump failure and those of sudden death, because potential therapeutic options to reduce mortality may differ between the two.

## Specific Predictors of Mortality

In addition to overall functional class, multiple physiologic parameters have been shown to correlate with prognosis for patients with heart failure. These parameters can be categorized as measures of hemodynamic function and cardiac structural changes, measures of the degree of altered neurohormonal and metabolic regulation, and integrated measures of functional limitation. Although these parameters serve as markers of the severity of cardiac dysfunction and its clinical impact, they should not be considered surrogate endpoints for therapies, because some therapies may alter these parameters without changing outcome, whereas others may change outcome without changing these recognized predictors. Although most of these markers predict sudden death as well as heart failure–related death, efforts continue to identify electrophysiologic predictors of sudden death.

### Ventricular Ejection Fraction, Dilation, and Hemodynamics

Morphologic markers of disease severity that can be easily measured have been extensively sought. LVEF predicts outcome when populations with a broad range of LV dysfunction are included. Once class III or IV symptoms have developed in patients with LVEF (of <30%), other parameters become more useful. LV dimension is a strong predictor of death. In a study of patients referred with class IV symptoms and LVEF of less than 25%, 2-year survival was 60% if the LV diastolic dimension was less than 70 mm but only 20% if greater than 85 mm.[26] Increased LV size and decreased systolic function likely reflect a greater extent of dysfunctional myocardium, increased proarrhythmic substrate, increased likelihood of pump failure, and increased neurohormonal activation. RV function has also been shown to correlate with outcome in cases of advanced heart failure; increased severity of RV dysfunction is associated with increased mortality.[17] The severity of mitral regurgitation, independent of LV dimension, also correlates with outcome.[27] The same is true of the degree of tricuspid regurgitation. Hemodynamic values provide information beyond ejection fraction, because stroke volume may be preserved despite low LVEF if the chamber volume is large and valvular regurgitation is limited. Cardiac output and ventricular filling pressures and patterns can be assessed both invasively and echocardiographically; the value of bioimpedance measurements is still under investigation. Parameters reflecting right- or left-sided filling pressures correlate with outcome: increased right atrial pressure, pulmonary artery pressure, and pulmonary wedge pressure measured by pulmonary artery catheterization predict poor outcome. Restrictive filling patterns and elevated pulmonary artery pressures determined on the basis of Doppler flow patterns also identify patients with higher risk of death.[28,29] Although a normal cardiac index is associated with a more favorable prognosis than a low cardiac index, there is a more robust continuous relation between filling pressures or their correlates and outcome once heart failure is advanced.

## Neurohormonal Predictors

Endogenous neurohormonal pathways are activated in chronic heart failure.[13,30] Studies have shown elevated serum levels of various mediators of these neurohormonal pathways, including norepinephrine, endothelin, angiotensin II, and naturetic peptides (ANP, BNP, and their prohormones) in patients with chronic heart failure.[31-35] Moreover, increased serum levels of cytokines, including tumor necrosis factor (TNF) and homocysteine, have been noted in patients with chronic heart failure.[36,37] Average values of these hormones have been shown to correlate with general clinical status and to diminish with effective therapy in trial populations.[38] However, interpretation in individual patients is confounded by wide interpatient variability and the complex interactions between these hormones during therapy. These neurohormonal markers therefore should not be considered surrogate endpoints for therapies.

## Renal Homeostasis

Renal function is a powerful predictor of outcome of asymptomatic though advanced heart failure in every subpopulation. Even minor elevations in serum creatinine concentration predict more hospitalizations and higher mortality rates. Renal insufficiency and diabetes worsen the prognosis for patients across all functional classes.[39,40] Serum sodium concentration is a robust predictor of outcome in all studies of symptomatic heart failure. Once it is below 140 mmol/L, a decreasing serum sodium concentration parallels worsening disease severity. Hyponatremia consistently predicts higher total mortality rates and often correlates more strongly with heart failure deaths (pump failure) than with unexpected deaths attributed to arrhythmias.[41]

## Functional Predictors

In addition to the cardiac parameters and neurohormonal markers described previously, integrated functional parameters commonly measured in patients with heart failure correlate with outcome. Clinical class is the most simple and most commonly used. When assessed after optimization of therapy among patients with reduced LV systolic function, annual mortality is 10% to 15% among patients with stable NYHA class I and II symptoms, 15% to 20% for patients with class III symptoms, and 20% to 50% for patients with class IV symptoms.[42] Mortality is higher when clinical class is combined with more specific prognostic factors such as renal dysfunction and hyponatremia.[39,41] Likewise, the risk of sudden death increases with increasing NYHA class.[42] Of parameters measured during exercise testing, peak oxygen consumption, anaerobic threshold, and ventilatory parameters require gas exchange analysis. Peak oxygen consumption and/or anaerobic threshold measured during exercise testing has long been used to assist in timing of cardiac transplantation in patients with advanced heart failure, because a decline in these parameters to below critical values predicts severe disease, poor prognosis, and therefore potential candidacy for transplantation.[43,44] The distance walked in 6 minutes is easy to measure, is reproducible, and correlates broadly with outcome in populations, but it is less sensitive to change than more objective measurements.[40,45,46] Subjective functional-status questionnaires have been utilized as tools to help predict outcome in cases of heart failure, but they are more commonly utilized as tools to assess quality of life and subjective changes in symptoms.[47]

## Electrophysiologic Predictors

As discussed earlier, sudden death accounts for an important fraction of deaths in the heart failure population. Sudden deaths are attributable to arrhythmias in the majority of cases. In some cases, severe bradycardia is implicated. However, the most common cause remains ventricular tachyarrhythmia.[9,48] One or more electrophysiologic markers might therefore be expected to predict sudden death. However, despite significant effort and evaluation, there are currently no individual electrophysiologic markers with sufficient sensitivity or specificity to reliably predict the risk of sudden death. Furthermore, the prognostic accuracy of these electrophysiologic predictors differs between patients with ischemic versus nonischemic heart failure. This distinction is quite important because etiology influences decisions regarding potential interventions to decrease risk of fatal arrhythmias. It has been well established that ambient ventricular premature beats (VPBs) and nonsustained VT (NSVT) recorded during ambulatory electrocardiographic monitoring are seen more frequently in patients with LV dysfunction—from 30% to 80%, depending on the definitions of NSVT used, the populations studied, and monitoring techniques.[11,49] The incidence of ectopy also increases with worsening heart failure severity.[50,51] In some clinical trials of medical therapy for heart failure, the presence of ventricular ectopic rhythms during ambulatory monitoring predicts increased total mortality rates but does not predict death adjudicated as sudden.[52,53] Despite this inconclusive evidence, monitoring for the presence of ambient ventricular ectopy is a simple and inexpensive test that has been performed to satisfy inclusion criteria in many recent trials of therapy with ICDs.[54,55] Exercise testing to detect increased frequency of ventricular arrhythmias during exercise and recovery has been evaluated in other populations but not specifically in heart failure populations.[56,57] T-wave alternans analysis during exercise testing is another marker under evaluation.[58]

A prolonged QRS duration during resting electrocardiography, another proposed electrophysiologic marker of sudden death, predicts worse outcome for patients with nonischemic heart failure but not those with ischemic heart failure.[59] Signal-averaged electrocardiography (SAECG) is influenced by underlying heterogeneity in ventricular repolarization and therefore potentially reflects the risk of ventricular arrhythmias and sudden death.[59] However, the strength of the SAECG in predicting sudden death risk is moderate at best. For the Coronary Artery Bypass Graft Patch (CABG-Patch) trial,[60] investigators used abnormal SAECG findings as an entry criterion for enrollment in a randomized study examining the effect of ICD implantation at the time of CABG surgery. There was no improvement in mortality rate in the ICD therapy group, perhaps in part because SAECG was imperfect for screening patients for increased risk of sudden death. Similarly, the degree of QT dispersion during resting electrocardiography, another potential measure of the heterogeneity of ventricular repolarization, is not sufficiently accurate to identify either high-risk or low-risk patients with underlying heart failure.[61]

Programmed stimulation during invasive electrophysiologic testing is the strongest available predictor of risk of sudden death. However, the predictive value of electrophysiologic testing differs for patients with ischemic versus nonischemic cardiomyopathies. Among patients with coronary artery disease, reduced LVEF, and NSVT on ambulatory monitoring, monomorphic VT can be induced in 20% to 45% of patients.[62-64] Patients whose studies are positive have a significantly greater risk of cardiac arrest or sudden death than do patients in whom monomorphic VT is noninducible. Conversely, in patients with nonischemic heart failure with reduced LVEF, programmed stimulation during electrophysiologic study has poor negative predictive value. For patients with nonischemic heart failure who have no inducible VT during electrophysiologic studies, the mortality rate at 6 months is still up to 30%.[11,65]

None of these electrophysiologic markers reliably predict either low or high risk of sudden death. Even invasive electrophysiologic testing is unreliable in nonischemic cardiomyopathy. Furthermore, the importance of electrophysiologic markers in guiding potential therapies may in fact wane as investigators in clinical trials increasingly forgo these markers as inclusion criteria and as the boundaries of appropriate indications for device therapies expand.

## Effects of Medical Therapies on Morbidity and Mortality

Almost 100,000 patients have been enrolled in heart failure trials thus far. Slightly fewer than half of these trials have demonstrated their tested therapies to be beneficial. Furthermore, outcomes in these trial populations may be better because of younger age, strict entry criteria, and the meticulous follow-up provided. One-year mortality rates in these multicenter trials generally range between 10% and 30%.[66-70] In contrast, a study of a large group ($N = 66,547$) of consecutive patients discharged after hospitalization for heart failure demonstrated a mortality rate of 44.5% at 1 year, despite reasonable, modern medical therapies initiated for most of these patients.[71] Nonetheless, the therapies validated by these trials have been translated to general heart failure populations, in which there has been a major impact on disease progression and survival when they are integrated into heart failure management programs.

### Medications

The fundamental components of current medical therapy for heart failure are inhibitors of the renin-angiotensin system, β-adrenergic blocking agents, and diuretics for fluid retention. Because these therapies for heart failure will continue to reduce morbidity and mortality as they gain widespread use earlier in the course of disease, life expectancy will likely continue to extend beyond the expectations described earlier.

Angiotensin-converting enzyme (ACE) inhibitors block the renin-angiotensin axis through inhibition of the enzyme that converts angiotensin I to angiotensin II. Experimental models suggest that the beneficial effects of ACE inhibitors in heart failure are mediated primarily via inhibition of the myocardial remodeling process seen in the failing heart rather than through pure afterload reduction.[13,72] Vascular remodeling and effects on the extracellular matrix may also be important.[73] In several large-scale, randomized, double-blinded, placebo-controlled trials, ACE inhibitors conferred both significant symptomatic relief and significant mortality reduction, between 16% and 28%.[74-76] ACE inhibitors also decrease the rates of new diuretic requirements and hospitalization for heart failure, and in some studies they have improved exercise tolerance.[77,78] Direct angiotensin receptor antagonists improve outcome after myocardial infarction and decrease heart failure–related hospitalizations, but these benefits appear less pronounced than with ACE inhibitors.[79,80] These differences will be further clarified with ongoing studies.[81,82]

The combination of aldosterone antagonists and ACE inhibitors decreases mortality and hospitalizations for patients with evidence of heart failure after myocardial infarction and for patients with class IV heart failure.[83] The concordance of beneficial effects from therapies targeting different levels of the renin-angiotensin-aldosterone axis suggests that this system plays a critical role in the progression of heart failure. Improved outcome from the use of vasodilators other than ACE inhibitors, in comparison with placebo, was demonstrated in the V-HeFT I trial,[84] although these agents were shown to be less beneficial than ACE inhibitors in V-HeFT II.[85] As heart failure advances, the renin-angiotensin axis may become more crucial in supporting blood pressure and renal function, because the 1-year mortality rate among those patients who develop late intolerance to ACE inhibitors due to circulatory-related renal limitations is more than 50%.[86]

β-Adrenergic receptor antagonists decrease the potentially detrimental impact of sympathetic nervous system overstimulation. Several clinical trials have shown that beta-blockers indeed improve mortality in the heart failure population (see later discussion). Their benefit appears to be greatest in those patients with high resting heart rates and elevated catecholamine levels, but it is not known to what degree decreasing heart rate itself contributes to the overall benefit.[87] Many mechanisms have been proposed for the beneficial effects seen in both selective and nonselective beta-blocking agents.[67,69,70] Although antagonism of the sympathetic system is in some ways analogous to inhibition of the renin-angiotensin system, there are key differences. The greater dependence on the sympathetic system for baseline hemodynamic support is suggested by greater intolerance to beta-blockers than to ACE inhibitors in advanced heart failure.[88,89] The route of inhibition is critical, because reduction of circulating catecholamines with moxonidine has been associated with increased mortality. Given the significant benefits of beta-blocking agents in heart failure, intensive efforts are warranted to introduce and titrate these agents in heart failure. In practice, a significant minority of patients cannot tolerate beta-blockers because of fatigue, pre-existing pulmonary disease, or other side effects. However, benefit is conferred even by doses well below target doses, particularly if further titration is limited by bradycardia.[90]

Digoxin has been shown in smaller trials to improve exercise tolerance, symptoms, and functional capacity in patients with mild to moderate heart failure independent of underlying rhythm (AF versus sinus rhythm).[13] However, the large, placebo-controlled Digitalis Investigation Group (DIG) trial demonstrated no significant mortality benefit from the administration of digoxin to patients with heart failure. It did demonstrate a significant reduction in hospitalization for heart failure with digoxin use (28%), as well as a trend toward improved survival rates among patients with more severe heart failure at baseline.[68] In most programs, digoxin is added for moderate to severe heart failure.

Although no large randomized clinical trials have demonstrated a mortality benefit from the use of diuretics in cases of heart failure, these medications are well accepted as therapy in the management of heart failure for relief of congestion, particularly in combination with other drugs, including beta-blockers and ACE inhibitors. There is no indication for diuretics in the absence of fluid retention or hypertension. A unique role has been demonstrated for the aldosterone antagonists. These mild diuretics confer a significant mortality benefit in cases of heart failure, a benefit attributed to their inhibition of the renin-angiotensin axis rather than their diuretic effects.[91] These components of the medical regimen should be tailored to individual profiles of heart failure and in a stepwise fashion (Figure 1–2).[92] Benefit appears to be greatest in the context of a disease management program that includes extensive patient education, exercise prescriptions, and regular phone contact to identify and treat decompensation early.[92] In both historically controlled trials and prospective randomized trials, heart failure management programs have been shown to significantly decrease hospitalizations by 25% to 75%.[93-95] Systematic considera-tion should be provided for additional interventions, including screening for sleep-disorder–associated breathing problems and depression.[96]

### Therapies for Advanced Heart Failure

The subpopulation of patients with *advanced* heart failure has limiting symptoms that persist despite adequate therapy with agents with proven efficacy. However, reasonable functional status can often be recovered with individualized therapy, even for these patients.[92] In some cases, tailoring to specific hemodynamic goals with use of invasive hemodynamic monitoring (with inpatient short-term indwelling right-side heart catheterization) rather than clinical assessment may improve the ability to optimize loading conditions and maintain freedom from congestion when empirical attempts have been unsuccessful.[92] In addition to medical therapy, a limited number of options are available for assisting the systolic function of the failing heart with mechanical and other artificial means. Given these current limitations, biventricular pacing strategies will likely become an increasingly attractive option in appropriate patient populations.

Cardiac transplantation is a well-established therapeutic option that provides a clear survival benefit for patients with refractory symptoms and severely impaired functional status.[12] However, despite its popularity and perceived success in the lay community and even within the general medical community, transplantation is a therapeutic option with miniscule epidemiologic impact,[97] because the extremely limited availability of donor hearts limits transplantation as a viable therapeutic option for most patients (Figure 1–3). The totally artificial heart continues to hold great theoretical promise, but it is still in active development and will not likely see

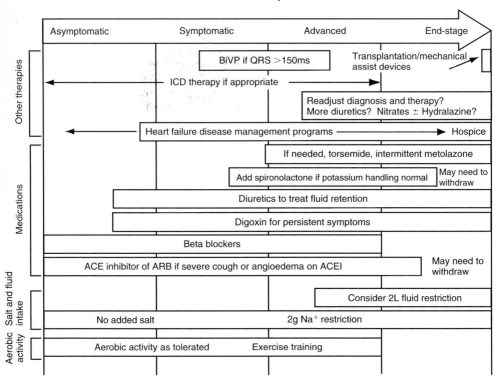

Disease Severity

FIGURE 1–2. This figure displays recommended therapies for patients with heart failure and reduced left ventricular ejection fraction (LVEF) as a function of disease severity. The horizontal axis represents disease severity, from asymptomatic through end-stage disease, and the vertical axis represents therapy options. Among medications, angiotensin-converting enzyme (ACE) inhibitors (or, alternatively, angiotensin receptor blockers [ARBs], if ACE inhibitors [ACEI] lead to intolerable side effects) should be used in all stages of disease. For some end-stage patients, ACE inhibitors may need to be withdrawn because of hypotension, hyperkalemia, and/or worsening renal function. Beta-blockers should be administered to all patients except those with advanced or end-stage disease. Digoxin and diuretics should be given for symptomatic relief. Spironolactone should be added to the regimen for patients with more advanced symptoms if potassium-handling and renal function are adequate. In advanced disease, the medical regimen should be frequently reassessed. Therapy with implantable cardioverter-defibrillators (ICDs) should be utilized if appropriate. Biventricular pacing has a role in patients with significant symptoms and for patients who satisfy current inclusion criteria. Transplantation and mechanical assist devices are reserved for a small fraction of patients with end-stage disease. Salt and fluid intake management should become more strict as disease progresses. Exercise is recommended for all patients except those with symptoms at rest. Comprehensive management programs are cost-effective. Benefits are most obvious in recently hospitalized patients. BiVP = biventricular pacing. *(Adapted from Nohria A, Lewis E, Stevenson LW: Medical management of advanced heart failure. JAMA 2002;287(5):628-640.)*

widespread use for some time. Implantation of an LV, RV, or biventricular assist device is well accepted as bridge therapy to cardiac transplantation, but recent data demonstrate that these devices can improve survival rates and may be useful for so-called *destination therapy*.[98,99] Noninvasive extracorporeal counterpulsation devices are under active investigation. Gene therapy for myocardial tissue

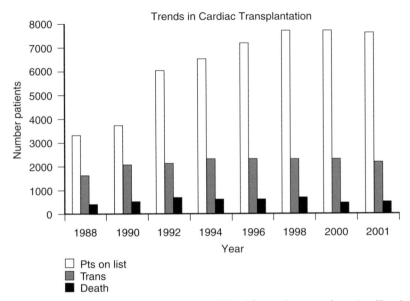

**FIGURE 1–3.** The absolute numbers of patients (*Pts*) listed for cardiac transplantation (*Trans*), who have undergone transplantation, and who have died after transplantation in the United States are plotted as a function of year from 1988 through 2001. The number of patients listed for transplantation has more than doubled over this period, from just over 3000 patients in 1988 to over 7000 patients in 2001. This number has leveled off over the past several years. Despite this trend, the number of transplantations performed has remained constant over this period, almost exclusively because of the limited number of available donor organs. *(Adapted from Hlatky MA, Bigger JT. Cost-effectiveness of the implantable cardioverter defibrillator. Lancet 2001;357: 1817-1818.)*

replacement or for neoangiogenesis is also an active area of basic research, but its clinical impact is not imminent.[100]

## Rhythm Disturbances in Heart Failure

Abnormal rhythms, including both bradyarrhythmias and tachyarrhythmias, occur commonly in heart failure. They can lead to significant morbidity in the form of palpitations, presyncope or syncope, and sudden death.

### Atrial Fibrillation and Flutter

AF and flutter are common in the heart failure population, occurring in 10% to 30% of patients, with incidence proportional to the degree of heart failure severity.[101,102] AF confers an increased risk of mortality in most studies.[103,104] However, it remains unclear whether AF in heart failure directly leads to increased mortality or is merely a marker for more severe disease. Physiologic consequences of AF that may lead to worse outcomes include increased risk of thromboembolic phenomenon, the adverse hemodynamic effects of rapid ventricular rate, impaired diastolic filling, loss of atrial contraction, and the potentially adverse effects of antiarrhythmic therapy. Furthermore, the rapid ventricular response of poorly controlled AF may lead to ventricular systolic impairment, which then begets further cardiac chamber dilation and an increased AF substrate, leading to a vicious cycle.

Guidelines for management of AF in heart failure are not well established. Despite its presumed significant impact, recent data suggest that in the general population, there is no benefit to a strategy of maintaining sinus rhythm as opposed to a strategy of rate control and anticoagulation.[105] There is in fact worse outcome due to an increased rate of stroke, likely because anticoagulation was often discontinued in the sinus rhythm maintenance group. If a strategy of maintaining sinus rhythm is undertaken, there are probably safe therapeutic options. Dofetilide has not worsened mortality rates in published trials, but it increases the risk of torsades de pointes (TdP).[106] Amiodarone is well accepted in practice for antiarrhythmic therapy in the heart failure population and specifically for AF.[13] However, no large-scale randomized trials have evaluated whether a strategy of maintaining sinus rhythm is beneficial specifically in the heart failure population, where the impact of AF is likely significant. An ongoing clinical trial is evaluating this question.

### Ventricular Tachyarrhythmias

## Incidence and Prognosis

Sudden death attributable to ventricular tachyarrhythmias, particularly VT or ventricular fibrillation (VF), is a significantly common occurrence in the heart failure population. In the general population, approximately 200,000 to 400,000 sudden deaths occur annually. Among those with heart failure, the rate of sudden death is increased by approximately ninefold, according to the Framingham Heart Study.[107] Despite implementation of multiple medical therapies that reduce mortality, the overall mortality rate in the symptomatic heart failure population (NYHA class II-IV) is still in the range of 20% to 25% per year.[84,108,109] Sudden death accounts for approximately 50% of these deaths. As heart failure severity increases, the absolute number of sudden deaths increases, but the fraction of total deaths due to sudden death actually decreases. Most sudden deaths are attributable to VT or VF, but bradycardias and electromechanical dissociation occur as well, both as primary events and as a result of terminal vascular events.

As alluded to previously (Electrophysiologic Markers), the nature of VT and VF in patients with heart failure with ischemic versus nonischemic cardiomyopathy may differ significantly. Even the pathophysiologic mechanisms of VT and VF in these two populations may be somewhat disparate. In ischemic cardiomyopathy, VT results primarily from re-entry associated with infarct-induced myocardial scarring. In nonischemic cardiomyopathy, fibrosis is more diffuse, and scar-related re-entry may be less common. Macroreentry via bundle branches or fascicles and focal automaticity account for a significant portion of VT and VF occurrences in nonischemic cardiomyopathy.[110,111] The predictive accuracy of electrophysiologic markers such as NSVT noted on ambulatory monitoring or even inducible VT in electrophysiologic studies is therefore quite poor for these patients.[11,112] The portion of deaths attributable to sudden cardiac death may be higher in the ischemic heart failure population.[9] Despite these differences, sudden death remains the primary mode of premature death in the overall heart failure population, and there has been great effort over the past several years to find effective therapies to prevent sudden death.

## Effect of Antiarrhythmic Medications on Mortality

Several classes of antiarrhythmics have been studied for their potential ability to prevent sudden death and malignant ventricular tachyarrhythmias. The results of trials focusing on class I agents (flecainide, encainide, and moricizine in the Cardiac Arrhythmia Suppression Trial [CAST][113] and propafenone in the Cardiac Arrest Study of Hamburg [CASH][114]) and class III agents (D-sotalol in the Survival With Oral D-Sotalol [SWORD] Study[115] and dofetilide in the Danish Investigators of Arrhythmia and Mortality on Dofetilide: Congestive Heart Failure [DIAMOND-CHF] Study[106]) have been disappointing, demonstrating either harm or lack of benefit. The increased mortality seen in the CAST and SWORD studies was likely due to the proarrhythmic effects of the medications used and was correlated with worsening LV systolic function. Beta-blockers, on the other hand, have a clearly beneficial impact on total mortality in the heart failure population and have been associated with mortality reductions between 32% and 65% in several trials.[67,69,70,89] As a result, they have been included in standard therapy (see Figure 1–2). Reductions in sudden death accounted for much of the observed benefit. In the heart failure population, the most commonly used antiarrhythmic agent is amiodarone, which acts through primarily class III effects as well as class I, II, and IV effects. The Cardiac Arrest in Seattle Conventional Versus Amiodarone Drug Evaluation (CASCADE) study demonstrated that amiodarone conferred better outcomes than conventional antiarrhythmics in secondary prevention of sudden death for survivors of cardiac arrest with depressed LVEF.[116] However, because there was no placebo group, it is unclear if this mortality benefit was due to elimination of the increased risk of sudden death associated with conventional antiarrhythmic therapy. Several studies have examined the effects of amiodarone on the primary prevention of sudden death in the heart failure population, including the European Myocardial Infarct Amiodarone Trial (EMIAT), Canadian Amiodarone Myocardial Infarction Arrhythmia Trial (CAMIAT), Survival Trial of Antiarrhythmic Therapy in Congestive Heart Failure (STAT-CHF), and the Grupo de Estudio de la Sobrevida en la Insuficiencia Cardiaca en Argentina (GESICA) trial.[109,112,117,118] Results of these trials were mixed. In both the EMIAT and the CAMIAT, sudden deaths were reduced by 35% to 49% by amiodarone, but there was no beneficial effect on overall mortality rates. In the STAT-CHF, there was no difference in rates of overall mortality or sudden death between the amiodarone and placebo groups. The GESICA trial demonstrated a significant reduction (28%) in overall mortality, with statistically nonsignificant reductions in sudden deaths (27%) and progressive heart failure–related deaths (23%). The disparate results in the GESICA trial are likely attributable to the unique profile of the involved heart failure cases: 61% were nonischemic, including 32% that were alcohol-related, 21% that were idiopathic, and 9% that were due to Chagas disease. Overall, beta-blockers clearly provide a significant mortality benefit in the heart failure population; class I agents are harmful, whereas the pure class III agent dofetilide provides no survival advantage but does not appear to be harmful for most patients (although dosing is complex); and amiodarone is safe for administration to patients with heart failure but confers no significant mortality benefit.

## Ventricular Tachyarrhythmias: Implantable Cardioverter-Defibrillators

With the advent of ICDs, much attention has been focused on the potential impact of ICD therapy on mortality in the heart failure population. Because coronary artery disease accounts for the majority of heart failure cases in this country and the risk of sudden death and mortality overall is significantly higher for these patients (see earlier discussion), this population accounts for most patients studied in trials of ICD therapy. Most conclusions drawn from these trials therefore apply primarily to the population with coronary artery disease and heart failure with low LVEF; few data are available to guide the management of nonischemic cardiomyopathies.

### Secondary Prevention: Survivors of Cardiac Arrest, Near Sudden Death, and Unexplained Syncope

Three large trials compared ICD therapy to medications for patients who survived an episode of near sudden death: the Antiarrhythmic Versus Implantable Defibrillator (AVID) trial,[119] the Canadian Implantable Defibrillator Study (CIDS),[120] and CASH.[114] These trials each enrolled slightly different patient populations, with variable reductions of LVEF, coronary disease prevalence, and randomization protocols. Reduction in total mortality was significant in all three studies, ranging from 19.7% to 37%, demonstrating a significant benefit of ICD therapy over medications. However, the number of patients who fit these criteria is relatively small. A special situation encountered is the patient with heart failure who presents with unexplained syncope. In retrospective analyses, the syncope is most often attributed to ventricular arrhythmias.[121] There is a significantly increased risk of subsequent sudden death in such patients, even if no etiology is found for their syncope, with 1-year mortality as high as 45%.[121] With this degree of risk, the performance of randomized trials comparing ICD therapy with a control group is not likely.

### ICD Therapy as Primary Prevention

The first wave of trials that evaluated the role of ICD therapy for primary prevention of sudden death all utilized noninvasive or invasive electrocardiographic markers of NSVT or abnormal SAECG as part of their inclusion criteria. Three major trials have compared ICD therapy to medical therapy: the Multicenter Unsustained Tachycardia Trial (MUSTT),[55] the Multicenter Automatic Defibrillator Trial (MADIT I),[54] and the CABG-Patch trial.[60] Most enrolled patients had reduced LVEF, most had coronary artery disease, and all three trials utilized electrophysiologic markers as entry criteria. The MUSTT and MADIT I demonstrated significantly lower mortality rates with ICD than with medical therapy, but the CABG-Patch trial demonstrated no improvement with ICD therapy. This lack of benefit is attributed primarily to elimination of the underlying proarrhythmic substrate through surgical revascularization in enrollees, as well as the imperfect inclusion criteria of an abnormal SAECG (see earlier discussion). The follow-up study, MADIT II, progressed to the next logical step, eliminating any electrophysiologic inclusion criteria during the trial.[122] In this study, among patients with coronary disease and reduced LVEF (<30%), those who underwent prophylactic ICD therapy had significantly lower mortality (relative risk reduction of 31%) than those treated with conventional medicine therapy. Arrhythmia-related deaths were decreased in the ICD-treated group as well (3.6% versus 9.4%). These results have significant implications for heart failure management, although only 10% of patients in these trials had class III or IV symptoms of heart failure.

## Bradyarrhythmias

Bradyarrhythmias, manifesting as heart block and sinus node dysfunction, are a significant cause of morbidity and death in the heart failure population. Patients with heart failure attributable to sarcoidosis or Chagas disease are at particular risk for bradyarrhythmias due to conduction system disease.[112,123] Accurate quantification of the contribution of bradyarrhythmias to out-of-hospital sudden cardiac death is difficult because of the lack of monitoring. Among patients hospitalized for intensive heart failure management or transplantation evaluation, sudden bradyarrhythmias have accounted for 62% of cardiac arrests.[124] However, a primary cause of the bradyarrhythmia (myocardial infarction, pulmonary embolism, or electrolyte imbalance) was found for approximately half of these patients. Transient heart block has been shown to be an independent risk factor for sudden death in cases of nonischemic cardiomyopathy. First- or second-degree heart block was noted during ambulatory monitoring for 28% of patients with nonischemic heart failure in one study and was associated with a fourfold increase in the risk of sudden death.[125] The presence of significant bradyarrhythmia and its resultant risks should be considered when a patient is being assessed for device therapies, because standard ICDs can provide back-up pacing, whereas biventricular pacing depends on ventricular pacing 100% of the time.

## Intraventricular Conduction Defects (Desynchronization)

Infrahisian conduction disease in the form of bundle branch or fascicular block is quite common in the heart failure population. This likely reflects the presence of large, diseased left ventricles in these patients. Intraventricular conduction disease, most commonly left bundle branch block (LBBB), is present in 40% of patients with heart failure and dilated cardiomyopathy (both ischemic and nonischemic).[126] Intraventricular conduction disease is also present in a significant portion of patients who present with complete heart block,[127] a circumstance suggesting that at least some sudden deaths result from a progression to complete heart block and subsequent ventricular asystole. The presence of bundle branch block may be more important for hemodynamic consequences than for any association with arrhythmias; recent meta-analysis data suggest that the reduction in mortality imparted by biventricular pacing results from the prevention of pump-failure-related death rather than the prevention of sudden death.[128]

Approximately 15% of the heart failure population and 30% of patients with moderate to severe symptoms of congestive heart failure will have interventricular and intraventricular conduction delays with QRS durations greater than or equal to 120 milliseconds. Prolonged QRS duration has been associated with increased risk of adverse outcome. In a review of the Italian Network on Congestive Heart Failure Registry, which includes 5517 patients with heart failure, the relationship between QRS and mortality was determined. The presence of an LBBB (QRS duration >140 milliseconds) was associated with an increased 1-year mortality rate (hazard ratio, 1.70; 95% confidence interval, 1.41–2.05) and an increased 1-year rate of sudden death (hazard ratio, 1.58; 95% confidence interval, 1.21–2.06). In multivariate analyses, QRS duration was associated with a significant increase in deaths, even after adjustment for other variables such as age, underlying cardiac disease, and use of beta-blockers and ACE inhibitors.[129]

## Implications of Device Therapy: New Directions

### ICD Therapy

As new evidence has increased the number of recommended medications and therapies available to patients with heart failure, the potential for further decreasing the mortality rate has increased (Figure 1–4). As baseline mortality declines, the absolute benefit of new interventions will be smaller, such that larger studies will be required to demonstrate significant mortality reduction. As ICD therapy provides further reductions in mortality, many practitioners are already advocating ICD therapy for patients who satisfy the enrollment criteria for MADIT II (history of myocardial infarction and an LVEF <30%). However, several caveats should be emphasized. The clinical severity of heart failure in the ICD therapy trials was mild to moderate. Although this severity is similar to that seen in the large ACE inhibitor trials, the role of ICD therapy for patients with more symptomatic heart failure (class III) is not as well defined. However, the COMPANION trial suggests a mortality benefit for patients with class III congestive heart failure. ICD therapy may actually worsen heart failure; recently it has been assumed that this detriment relates to dual-chamber defibrillating device (DDD) pacing modes used.[130] Furthermore, there may be no benefit to preventing sudden death if protracted hemodynamic decline will result from advanced heart failure. Overall mortality rates observed in ICD trials are in general higher than seen previously for patients with heart failure with similar clinical characteristics, likely reflecting additional arrhythmic risks inherent in these

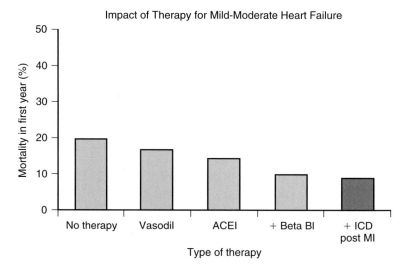

FIGURE 1–4. Displayed is the mortality (%) observed within the first year with various available therapies for heart failure, as a function of the type of therapy. Quantities are derived from data reported from clinical trials of each listed therapy. Mortality over the first observed year approaches 20% without any therapy (natural course of disease), whereas mortality progressively decreases with administration of vasodilators (Vasodil), angiotensin-converting enzyme inhibitors (ACEI), and the combination of ACEI and beta-blockers (Beta BI). Among patients receiving both ACEI and beta-blockers, as the patients in the trials of therapy with implantable cardioverter-defibrillators (ICDs) generally are, mortality is further reduced by ICD therapy following myocardial infarction (post MI).

patients, possibly in part due to residual coronary ischemia. Finally, most patients enrolled in the ICD therapy trials had ischemic heart failure; there are no data on the basis of which to recommend ICD therapy for patients with nonischemic cardio-myopathies. We await the results of the Sudden Cardiac Death in Heart Failure Trial (SCD-HeFT), an ongoing trial comparing ICD therapy to administration of amio-darone and placebo in cases of mild to moderate heart failure, involving a significant number of patients with nonischemic heart failure.

Whereas most medical therapies aim to decrease heart failure progression and improve survival rates, with ICD therapy these two goals may actually conflict: improvement of quality of life versus prolongation of life. ICD therapy may confer a survival benefit but at a cost of potentially painful and traumatic shock therapies, associated psychologic trauma, and perhaps even worsening heart failure. In partic-ular, if backup pacing is used a significant portion of the time, the detrimental hemo-dynamic effects of conventional pacing from the RV apex should be considered.[130] At the very end-stages of advanced heart failure, these complex considerations are highlighted as the goal of improving quality of life increases in importance, while prolonging life diminishes in importance. In fact, guidelines from the American College of Cardiology/American Heart Association indicate that placement of ICDs in patients with class IV heart failure is contraindicated.[12] However, mild to moderate heart failure noted at the time of evaluation often progresses toward more severe disease. As death becomes imminent, VT and VF often become increasingly frequent, which can result in an increased rate of ICD firings. At that point, concerns about the quality of life impaired by multiple ICD firings need to be counterbalanced with the likely diminishing mortality benefit of ICD therapy while pump failure–related death is imminent. An appropriate question to ask at this stage is whether the ICD should be turned off. These competing factors should be weighed when determining the course of therapy for each patient.

### Resynchronization Therapy

Biventricular pacing, also termed *resynchronization therapy,* has shown promise for symptomatic heart failure in recent trials. Heart failure symptoms diminish and objective measures of functional status improve with biventricular pacing.[131] A recent meta-analysis suggests a significant reduction in mortality rates, primarily due to prevention of pump failure deaths. The companion trial has demonstrated that cardiac resynchronization with ICD junction may further improve the survival in congestive heart failure with a prolonged QRS duration. Biventricular pacing therefore has the potential to be one of the few heart failure therapies that addresses both symptomatic relief and mortality reduction. The details of implementation and a review of the currently published trials examining efficacy is discussed in subsequent chapters. As operator skill at implantation improves and as the heart failure popula-tion continues to grow, guidelines are needed for the selection of patients most likely to benefit from this type of therapy. Hopefully, this therapy will find its place among the long list of therapies that have demonstrated benefit for heart failure.

### Additional Questions

The population with advanced heart failure faces an interesting crossroads in device therapy. By current definitions, most patients who qualify under current indications for biventricular pacing also qualify for ICD therapy according to MADIT II criteria, because these are significantly overlapping population groups. Should all of these patients therefore undergo both therapies? The answer is not clear at this point, particularly because the indications for ICD therapy continue to evolve. However, the COMPANION trial suggests that CRT-D may be superior to CRT alone. Beyond antiarrhythmic medications, ICD therapy, and resynchronization therapy, the role of additional treatment modalities is not clearly defined. Radiofrequency catheter ablation of ventricular (as well as supraventricular) tachyarrhythmias is potentially curative in the appropriate patient population, but its effects on sudden death risk and symptomatic relief are not well studied. Therefore it is appropriate to consider this and other alternative therapies on an individual basis.

The heart failure population will continue to grow in the next several years, as the result of several factors: (1) an aging population, (2) improved therapies for treatment of underlying etiologies (particularly coronary artery disease), and (3) improved therapies for patients with heart failure. Moreover, the indications for ICD therapy continue to increase, resulting in a potentially tremendous population of patients who qualify for therapy. The cost-effectiveness of these therapies will therefore become an increasingly prominent issue. On the one hand, as manufacturing techniques and operator skills improve, particularly for biventricular device implantation, costs will diminish. On the other hand, as highlighted in cases of end-stage heart failure, appropriate selection of patients for therapy will always be crucial. Moreover, initial estimates of standard cost-effectiveness measures demonstrate mixed results.[132,133]

## Conclusions

Patients with heart failure are a heterogeneous population, with significant variability in clinical severity, mortality, and therapies with proven efficacy. Rhythm disturbances are common in this population and cause significant morbidity and mortality. The clinical markers that are available to help elucidate the subpopulation of patients at higher risk of poor outcome remain inadequate. The available therapeutic options for heart failure continue to expand and already exceed what is feasible and prudent to implement for each individual patient. The statistical benefits in morbidity and mortality demonstrated in large clinical trials need to be judiciously applied to each patient through individualized therapeutic regimens. As the heart failure population expands, issues affecting the overall heart failure population, not to mention society at large, become increasingly important. At the end stages of disease, these complex issues are highlighted.[134] A distinction must be made between using these effective therapies to prolong a life with reasonable quality and inappropriately prolonging the dying process. The role of device therapy in heart failure within this context continues to evolve, and difficult decisions in determining both overall policy and individual treatment regimens will likely be encountered.

## REFERENCES

1. O'Connell JB, Bristow MR: Economic impact of heart failure in the United States: Time for a different approach. *J Heart Lung Transplant* 1994;13(4):S107–S112.
2. Haldeman G, Croft JB, Giles WH, Rashidee A: Hospitalization of patients with heart failure: National Hospital Discharge Survey 1985 to 1995. *Am Heart J* 1999;137:352–360.

3. Kannel WB, Ho K, Thom T: Changing epidemiological features of cardiac failure. *Br Heart J* 1994;72(2 Suppl):S3–9.
4. Adams KF, Zannad F: Clinical definition and epidemiology of advanced heart failure. *Am Heart J* 1998;135(6):S204–S215.
5. Zile MR, Nappi J: Diastolic heart failure. *Curr Treat Options Cardiovasc Med* 2000;2(5):439–450.
6. Stevenson WG, Stevenson LW, Middlekauff HR, et al: Improving survival for patients with advanced heart failure: A study of 737 consecutive patients. *J Am Coll Cardiol* 1995;26(6):1417–1423.
7. Gheorghiade M, Bonow RO: Chronic heart failure in the United States: A manifestation of coronary artery disease. *Circulation* 1998;97:282–289.
8. Dries DL, Sweitzer NK, Drazner MH, et al: Prognostic impact of diabetes mellitus in patients with heart failure according to the etiology of left ventricular systolic dysfunction. *J Am Coll Cardiol* 2001;38(2):421–428.
9. Stevenson WG, Stevenson LW, Middlekauff HR, Saxon LA: Sudden death prevention in patients with advanced ventricular dysfunction. *Circulation* 1993;88(6):2953–2961.
10. Poll DS, et al: Usefulness of programmed stimulation in idiopathic dilated cardiomyopathy. *Am J Cardiol* 1986;58:992–997.
11. Stevenson WG, Stevenson LW, Weiss J, Tillisch JH: Inducible ventricular arrhythmias and sudden death during vasodilator therapy of severe heart failure. *Am Heart J* 1988;116:1447–1454.
12. Hunt JA, Baker DW, Chin MH, et al: ACC/AHA guidelines for the evaluation and management of chronic heart failure in the adult: Executive summary. A report of the American College of Cardiology/American Heart Association Task Force on Practice Guidelines (Committee to Revise the 1995 Guidelines for the Evaluation and Management of Heart Failure), developed in collaboration with the International Society for Heart and Lung Transplantation; endorsed by the Heart Failure Society of America. *Circulation* 2001;104(24):2996–3007.
13. Packer M, Cohn JN: Consensus recommendations for the management of chronic heart failure. *Am J Cardiol* 1999;83(2A):1A–38A.
14. Yancy CW: Heart failure in blacks: etiologic and epidemiologic differences. *Curr Cardiol Rep* 2001;3(3):191–197.
15. Olivetti G, Gambert SR, Ariversa P, et al: Gender differences and aging: Effects on the human heart. *J Am Coll Cardiol* 1995;26:1068–1079.
16. Chen HH, Lainchbury JG, Senni M, et al: Diastolic heart failure in the community: Clinical profile, natural history, therapy, and impact of proposed diagnostic criteria. *J Card Fail* 2002;8(5):279–287.
17. Di Salvo TG, Mathier M, Semigran MJ, Dec GW: Preserved right ventricular ejection fraction predicts exercise capacity and survival in advanced heart failure. *J Am Coll Cardiol* 1995;5(5):1143–1153.
18. Grunig E, Tasman JA, Kücherer H, et al: Frequency and phenotypes of familial dilated cardiomyopathy. *J Am Coll Cardiol* 1998;31:186–194.
19. Towbin JA, Bowles NE: The failing heart. *Nature* 2002;415(6868):227–233.
20. Spirito P, Seidman CE, McKenna WJ, Maron BJ: The management of hypertrophic cardiomyopathy. *N Engl J Med* 1997;336(11):775–785.
21. Therrien J, Dore A, Gersony W, et al: Canadian Cardiovascular Society Consensus Conference 2001 update: Recommendations for the management of adults with congenital heart disease. Part I. *Can J Cardiol* 2001;17(9):940–959.
22. Therrien J, Gatzoulis M, Graham T, et al: Canadian Cardiovascular Society Consensus Conference 2001 update: Recommendations for the Management of Adults with Congenital Heart Disease– Part II. *Can J Cardiol* 2001;17(10):1029–1050.
23. McNamara DG: The adult with congenital heart disease. *Curr Probl Cardiol* 1989;14(2):57–114.
24. Shinbane JS, Wood MA, Jensen DN, et al: Tachycardia-induced cardiomyopathy. *J Am Coll Cardiol* 1997;29:709–715.
25. Gemayel C, Pelliccia A, Thompson PD: Arrhythmogenic right ventricular cardiomyopathy. *J Am Coll Cardiol* 2001;38(7):1773–1781.
26. Stevenson LW, Couper, G, Natterson B, et al: Target heart failure populations for newer therapies. *Circulation* 1995;92(9 Suppl II):174–181.
27. Bolling SF, Smolens IA, Pagani FD: Surgical alternatives for heart failure. *J Heart Lung Transplant* 2001;20(7):729–733.
28. Stevenson LW, Tillisch JH, Hamilton M, et al: Importance of hemodynamic response to therapy in predicting survival with ejection fraction less than or equal to 20% secondary to ischemic or nonischemic dilated cardiomyopathy. *Am J Cardiol* 1990;66(19):1348–1354.
29. Pierpont GL, Cohn JN, Franciosa JA: Combined oral hydralazine-nitrate therapy in left ventricular failure: Hemodynamic equivalency to sodium nitroprusside. *Chest* 1978;73(1):8–13.

30. Francis GS, Goldsmith SR, Levine TB, et al: The neurohormonal axis in congestive heart failure. *Ann Intern Med* 1984;10:370–377.
31. Mulder P, Richard V, Derumeaux G, et al: Role of endogenous endothelin in chronic heart failure: effect of long-term treatment with an endothelin antagonist on survival, hemodynamics, and cardiac remodeling. *Circulation* 1997;96(6):1976–1982.
32. Pfeffer MA, Lamas GA, Vaughan DE, et al: Effect of captopril on progressive ventricular dilatation after anterior myocardial infarction. *N Engl J Med* 1988;319(2):80–86.
33. McDonald KM, Garr M, Carlyle PF, et al: Relative effects of alpha 1-adrenoceptor blockade, converting enzyme inhibitor therapy, and angiotensin II subtype 1 receptor blockade on ventricular remodeling in the dog. *Circulation* 1994;90(6):3034–3046.
34. Weber KT, Villarreal D: Aldosterone and antialdosterone therapy in congestive heart failure. *Am J Cardiol* 1993;71(3):3A–11A.
35. Hillege HL, Girbes ARJ, de Kam PJ, et al: Renal function, neurohormonal activation, and survival in patients with chronic heart failure. *Circulation* 2000;102(2):203–210.
36. Levine B, Kalman J, Mayer L, et al: Elevated circulating levels of tumor necrosis factor in severe chronic heart failure. *N Engl J Med* 1990;323(4):236–241.
37. Ramachandran SV, Beiser A, D'Agostino, et al: Plasma homocysteine and risk for congestive heart failure in adults without prior myocardial infarction. *JAMA* 2003;289(10):1251–1257.
38. Maisel AS, Koon J, Krishnaswamy P, et al: Utility of B-natriuretic peptide as a rapid, point-of-care test for screening patients undergoing echocardiography to determine left ventricular dysfunction. *Am Heart J* 2001;141(3):367–374.
39. Dries DL, Exner DV, Domanski MJ, et al: The prognostic implications of renal insufficiency in asymptomatic and symptomatic patients with left ventricular systolic dysfunction. *J Am Coll Cardiol* 2000;35(3):681–689.
40. Lucas C, Johnson W, Hamilton MA, et al: Freedom from congestion predicts good survival despite previous class IV symptoms of heart failure. *Am Heart J* 2000;140(6):840–847.
41. Lee WH, Packer M. Prognostic importance of serum sodium concentration and its modification by converting-enzyme inhibition in patients with severe chronic heart failure. *Circulation* 1986;73(2):257–267.
42. Uretsky BF, Sheahan RG. Primary prevention of sudden cardiac death in heart failure: will the solution be shocking? *J Am Coll Cardiol* 1997;30(7):1589–1597.
43. Myers J, Gullestad L, Vagelos R, et al: Cardiopulmonary exercise testing and prognosis in severe heart failure: 14 mL/kg/min revisited. *Am Heart J* 2000;139(1 Pt 1):78–84.
44. Osada N, Chaitman BR, Miller LW, et al: Cardiopulmonary exercise testing identifies low risk patients with heart failure and severely impaired exercise capacity considered for heart transplantation [see comments]. *J Am Coll Cardiol* 1998;31(3):577–582.
45. Bittner V, Weiner DH, Yusuf S, et al: Prediction of mortality and morbidity with a 6-minute walk test in patients with left ventricular dysfunction. SOLVD Investigators [see comments]. *JAMA* 1993;270(14):1702–1707.
46. Lucas C, Stevenson LW, Johnson W, et al: The 6-min walk and peak oxygen consumption in advanced heart failure: aerobic capacity and survival [see comments]. *Am Heart J* 1999;138(4 Pt 1):618–624.
47. Rector TS, Tschumperlin LK, Kubo SH, et al: Use of the Living With Heart Failure questionnaire to ascertain patients' perspectives on improvement in quality of life versus risk of drug-induced death. *J Card Fail* 1995;1(3):201–206.
48. Pratt CM, Greenway PS, Schoenfeld MH, et al: Exploration of the precision of classifying sudden cardiac death: Implications for the interpretation of clinical trials. *Circulation* 1996;93(3):519–524.
49. Sweeney MO: Sudden death in heart failure associated with reduced left ventricular function: Substrates, mechanisms, and evidenced-based management, part I. *J Pacing Clin Electrophysiol* 2000;24(5):871–888.
50. Packer M: Sudden unexpected death in patients with congestive heart failure: A second frontier. *Circulation* 1985;72(4):681–685.
51. Kjekshus J: Arrhythmias and mortality in congestive heart failure. *Am J Cardiol* 1990;65 (19):421–481.
52. Goldman S, Johnson G, Gohn JN, et al: Mechanism of death in heart failure: The Vasodilator-Heart Failure Trials. The V-HeFT VA Cooperative Studies Group. *Circulation* 1993;87:V124–V131.
53. Bigger JT, Fleiss JL, Kleiger R, et al: The relationships among ventricular arrhythmias, left ventricular dysfunction, and mortality in the 2 years after myocardial infarction. *Circulation* 1984;69(2):250–258.
54. Moss AJ, Hall WJ, Cannom DS, et al: Improved survival with an implanted defibrillator in patients with coronary disease at high risk for ventricular arrhythmia. Multicenter Automatic Defibrillator Implantation Trial Investigators. *N Engl J Med* 1996;335(26):1933–1940.

55. Buxton AE, Lee KL, Fisher JD, et al: A randomized study of the prevention of sudden death in patients with coronary artery disease. Multicenter Unsustained Tachycardia Trial Investigators. *N Engl J Med* 1999;341(25):1882–1890.
56. Jouven X, Zureik M, Desnos M, et al: Long-term outcome in asymptomatic men with exercise-induced premature ventricular depolarizations. *N Engl J Med* 2000;343:826–833.
57. Frolkis JP, Pothier CE, Blackstone EH, Lauer MS: Frequent ventricular ectopy after exercise as a predictor of death. *N Engl J Med* 2003;348:781–790.
58. Armoundas AA, Tomaselli GF, Esperer HD: Pathophysiological basis and clinical application of T-wave alternans. *J Am Coll Cardiol* 2002;40(2):207–217.
59. Silverman ME, Pressel MD, Brackett JC, et al: Prognostic value of the signal-averaged electrocardiogram and a prolonged QRS in ischemic and nonischemic cardiomyopathy. *Am J Cardiol* 1995;75(7):460–464.
60. Bigger JT, et al: Prophylactic use of implanted cardiac defibrillators in patients at high risk for ventricular arrhythmias after coronary-artery bypass graft surgery. The Coronary Artery Bypass Graft (CABG) Patch Trial Investigators. *N Engl J Med* 1997;337:1569–1575.
61. Somberg JC, Molnar J: Usefulness of QT dispersion as an electrocardiographically derived index. *Am J Cardiol* 2002;89(3):291–294.
62. Wilber DJ, Olshansky B, Moran JF, Scanlon PJ: Electrophysiological testing and nonsustained ventricular tachycardia: Use and limitations in patients with coronary artery disease and impaired ventricular function. *Circulation* 1990;82(2):350–358.
63. Buxton AE, Marchlinski FE, Flores BT, et al: Nonsustained ventricular tachycardia in patients with coronary artery disease: Role of electrophysiologic study. *Circulation* 1987;75(6):1178–1185.
64. Klein RC, Machell C: Use of electrophysiological testing among patients with nonsustained ventricular tachycardia: Prognostic and therapeutic implications. *J Am Coll Cardiol* 1989;14:155–161.
65. Sing SN, Carson PE, Fisher SG: Nonsustained ventricular tachycardia in severe heart failure: Independent marker of increased mortality due to sudden death. GESICA-GEMA Investigators [comment]. *J Am Coll Cardiol* 1996;94:3198–3203.
66. Massie BM, Shah NB: Evolving trends in the epidemiologic factors of heart failure: rationale for preventive strategies and comprehensive disease management. *Am Heart J* 1997;133:703–712.
67. Packer M, Bristow MR, Cohn JN, et al: The effect of carvedilol on morbidity and mortality in patients with chronic heart failure. U.S. Carvedilol Heart Failure Study Group [see comments]. *N Engl J Med* 1996;334(21):1349–1355.
68. The Digitalis Investigation Group: The effect of digoxin on mortality and morbidity in patients with heart failure. *N Engl J Med* 1997;336(8):525–533.
69. The Cardiac Insufficiency Bisoprolol Study II (CIBIS-II): A randomised trial. *Lancet* 1999;353 (9146):9–13.
70. Effect of metoprolol CR/XL in chronic heart failure: Metoprolol CR/XL Randomised Intervention Trial in Congestive Heart Failure (MERIT-HF). *Lancet* 1999;353(9169):2001–2007.
71. MacIntyre K, Capwell S, Stewart S, et al: Evidence of improving prognosis in heart failure. *Circulation* 2000;102:1126–1131.
72. Pfeffer MA, Braunwald E, Moye LA, et al: Effect of captopril on mortality and morbidity in patients with left ventricular dysfunction after myocardial infarction: Results of the survival and ventricular enlargement trial. The SAVE Investigators [see comments]. *N Engl J Med* 1992;327(10):669–677.
73. Drexler H, Banhardt U, Meinertz T, et al: Contrasting peripheral short-term and long-term effects of converting enzyme inhibition in patients with congestive heart failure: A double-blind, placebo-controlled trial. *Circulation* 1989;79(3):491–502.
74. The SOLVD Investigators: Effect of enalapril on survival in patients with reduced left ventricular ejection fractions and congestive heart failure [see comments]. *N Engl J Med* 1991;325(5): 293–302.
75. The CONSENSUS Trial Study Group: Effects of enalapril on mortality in severe congestive heart failure: Results of the Cooperative North Scandinavian Enalapril Survival Study (CONSENSUS). *N Engl J Med* 1987;316(23):1429–1435.
76. Garg R, Yusuf S: Overview of randomized trials of angiotensin-converting enzyme inhibitors on mortality and morbidity in patients with heart failure. Collaborative Group on ACE Inhibitor Trials [erratum appears in JAMA 1995;274(6):462]. *JAMA* 1995;273(18):1450–1456.
77. The Captopril-Digoxin Multicenter Research Group: Comparative effects of therapy with captopril and digoxin in patients with mild to moderate heart failure. *JAMA* 1988;259:539–544.
78. Pacher R, Stanek B, Globits S, et al: Effects of two different enalapril dosages on clinical, haemodynamic and neurohumoral response of patients with severe congestive heart failure. *Eur Heart J* 1996;17(8):1223–1232.

79. Pitt B, Segal R, Martinez FA, et al: Randomised trial of losartan versus captopril in patients over 65 with heart failure (Evaluation of Losartan in the Elderly Study, ELITE) [see comments]. *Lancet* 1997;349(9054):747–752.

80. McKelvie RS, Yusuf S, Pericak D, et al: Comparison of candesartan, enalapril, and their combination in congestive heart failure: Randomized evaluation of strategies for left ventricular dysfunction (RESOLVD) pilot study. The RESOLVD Pilot Study Investigators. *Circulation* 1999;100 (10):1056–1064.

81. Cohn JN, Tagnoni G, Glazer RD, et al: Rationale and design of the Valsartan Heart Failure Trial: a large multinational trial to assess the effects of valsartan, an angiotensin- receptor blocker, on morbidity and mortality in chronic congestive heart failure [see comments]. *J Card Fail* 1999;5(2):155–160.

82. Pitt B, Poole-Wilson PA, Segal R, et al: Effect of losartan compared with captopril on mortality in patients with symptomatic heart failure: randomised trial. The Losartan Heart Failure Survival Study ELITE II. *Lancet* 2000;355(9215):1582–1587.

83. Pitt B, Remme W, Zannad F, et al: Eplerenone, a selective aldosterone blocker, in patients with left ventricular dysfunction after myocardial infarction. *N Engl J Med* 2003;348(14):1309–1321.

84. Cohn JN, Archibald DG, Ziesche S, et al: Effect of vasodilator therapy on mortality in chronic congestive heart failure. Results of a Veterans Administration Cooperative Study. *N Engl J Med* 1986;314(24):1547–1552.

85. Cohn JN, Johnson G, Ziesche S, et al: A comparison of enalapril with hydralazine-isosorbide dinitrate in the treatment of chronic congestive heart failure [see comments]. *N Engl J Med* 1991;325(5):303–310.

86. Pinto M, Stevenson LW, Shah MR, et al: Development of ACE inhibitor intolerance identifies patients with high early mortality (abstract). *Circulation* 2002;106:II,472.

87. Schleman KA, Lindenfeld J, Lowes BD, et al: Predicting response to carvedilol for the treatment of heart failure: A multivariate retrospective analysis. *J Card Fail* 2001;7(1):4–12.

88. Packer M, Poole-Wilson PA, Armstrong PW, et al: Comparative effects of low and high doses of the angiotensin-converting enzyme inhibitor, lisinopril, on morbidity and mortality in chronic heart failure. ATLAS Study Group. *Circulation* 1999;100(23):2312–2318.

89. Packer M, Coats A, Fowler MB, et al: Effect of carvedilol on survival in severe chronic heart failure. *N Engl J Med* 2001;344(22):1651–1658.

90. Bristow MR, Gilbert EM, Abraham WT, et al: Carvedilol produces dose-related improvements in left ventricular function and survival in subjects with chronic heart failure. MOCHA Investigators [see comments]. *Circulation* 1996;94(11):2807–2816.

91. Effectiveness of spironolactone added to an angiotensin-converting enzyme inhibitor and a loop diuretic for severe chronic congestive heart failure: The Randomized Aldactone Evaluation Study (RALES). *Am J Cardiol* 1996;78(8):902–907.

92. Nohria A, Lewis E, Stevenson LW: Medical management of advanced heart failure. *JAMA* 2002;287(5):628–640.

93. Hanumanthu S, Butler J, Chomsky D, et al: Effect of a heart failure program on hospitalization frequency and exercise tolerance [see comments]. *Circulation* 1997;96(9):2842–2848.

94. Rich MW, Beckham V, Wittenberg C, et al: A multidisciplinary intervention to prevent the readmission of elderly patients with congestive heart failure. *N Engl J Med* 1995;333(18):1190–1195.

95. McAlister FA, Lawson FME, Teo KK, Armstrong PW: A systematic review of randomized trials of disease management programs in heart failure. *Am J Med* 2001;110(5):378–384.

96. Skotzko CE, Krichten C, Zietowski G, et al: Depression is common and precludes accurate assessment of functional status in elderly patients with congestive heart failure. *J Card Fail* 2000;6(4):300–305.

97. Hosenpud JD, Bennett LE, Keck BM, et al: The Registry of the International Society for Heart and Lung Transplantation: Seventeenth official report, 2000. *J Heart Lung Transplant* 2000;19 (10):909–931.

98. Rose EA, Moskowitz AJ, Packer M, et al: The REMATCH trial: Rationale, design, and end points. Randomized evaluation of mechanical assistance for the treatment of congestive heart failure. *Ann Thorac Surg* 1999;67(3):723–730.

99. Rose EA, Gelijns AC, Moskowitz AJ, et al: Long-term use of a left ventricular assist device for end-stage heart failure. *N Engl J Med* 2001;345(20):1435–1443.

100. Hajjar RJ, del Monte F, Rosenzweig A: Prospects for gene therapy for heart failure. *Circ Res* 2000;86:616–621.

101. Stevenson WG, Stevenson LW, Middlekauff HR, et al: Improving survival for patients with atrial fibrillation and advanced heart failure. *J Am Coll Cardiol* 1996;28(6):1458–1463.

102. Maisel WH, Stevenson LW: Atrial fibrillation in heart failure: Epidemiology, pathophysiology, and rationale for therapy. 2003;in press.
103. Dries DL, Exner DV, Gersh, et al: Atrial fibrillation is associated with an increased risk for mortality and heart failure progression in patients with asymptomatic and symptomatic left ventricular systolic dysfunction: A retrospective analysis of the SOLVD trials. Studies of left ventricular dysfunction. *J Am Coll Cardiol* 1998;32(3):695–703.
104. Middlekauff HR, Stevenson WG, Stevenson LW: Prognostic significance of atrial fibrillation in advanced heart failure: A study of 390 patients. *Circulation* 1991;84(1):40–48.
105. The Atrial Fibrillation Follow-up Investigation of Rhythm Management (AFFIRM) Investigators : A comparison of rate control and rhythm control in patients with atrial fibrillation. *N Engl J Med* 2002;347:1825–1833.
106. Torp-Pedersen C, Møller M, Bloch-Thomsen PE, et al: Dofetilide in patients with congestive heart failure and left ventricular dysfunction [see comments]. Danish Investigations of Arrhythmia and Mortality on Dofetilide Study Group. *N Engl J Med* 1999;341(12):857–865.
107. Kannel WB, Plehn JF, Cupples A: Cardiac failure and sudden death in the Framingham study. *Am Heart J* 1988;115:869–875.
108. The SOLVD Investigators: Effect of enalapril on mortality and the development of heart failure in asymptomatic patients with reduced left ventricular ejection fractions [see comments] [erratum appears in N Engl J Med 1992;327(24):1768]. *N Engl J Med* 1992;327(10):685–691.
109. Singh SN, Fletcher RD, Fisher SG, et al: Amiodarone in patients with congestive heart failure and asymptomatic ventricular arrhythmia: Survival trial of antiarrhythmic therapy in congestive heart failure [see comments]. *N Engl J Med* 1995;333(2):77–82.
110. Pogwizd SM, McKenzie JP, Cain ME: Mechanisms underlying spontaneous and induced ventricular arrhythmias in patients with idiopathic dilated cardiomyopathy. *Circulation* 1998;98:2404–2414.
111. Delacretaz E, Stevenson WG, Ellison KE, et al: Mapping and radiofrequency catheter ablation of the three types of sustained monomorphic ventricular tachycardia in nonischemic heart disease. *J Cardiovasc Electrophysiol* 2000;11(1):11–17.
112. Doval HC, Nul DR, Grancelli HO, et al: Randomised trial of low-dose amiodarone in severe congestive heart failure [see comments]. Grupo de Estudio de la Sobrevida en la Insuficiencia Cardiaca en Argentina (GESICA). *Lancet* 1994;344(8921):493–498.
113. The Cardiac Arrhythmia Suppression Trial (CAST) Investigators: Effect of encainide and flecainide on mortality in a randomized trial of arrhythmia suppression after myocardial infarction. *N Engl J Med* 1989;321:406–412.
114. Kuck KH, Cappato R, Siebels J, Ruppel R: Randomized comparison of antiarrhythmic drug therapy with implantable defibrillators in patients resuscitated from cardiac arrest: The Cardiac Arrest Study Hamburg (CASH). *Circulation* 2000;102(7):748–754.
115. Waldo AL, Camm AJ, de Ruyter H, et al: Effect of d-sotalol on mortality in patients with left ventricular dysfunction after recent and remote myocardial infarction: Survival with oral d-sotalol [see comments] [erratum appears in Lancet 1996;348(9024):416]. The SWORD investigators. *Lancet* 1996;348(9019):7–12.
116. Greene HL: The CASCADE Study: Randomized antiarrhythmic drug therapy in survivors of cardiac arrest in Seattle. *Am J Cardiol* 1993;72:70F–74F.
117. Cairns J, ftC Investigators: Randomized trial of outcome after myocardial infarction among patients with frequent or repetitive ventricular premature depolarizations: CAMIAT. *Lancet* 1997; 349:675–682.
118. Julian DG, ftE Investigators: Randomized trial of effect of amiodarone on mortality among patients with left ventricular dysfunction after recent myocardial infarction. *Lancet* 1997;349:667–674.
119. The Antiarrhythmics Versus Implantable Defibrillators (AVID) Investigators: A comparison of antiarrhythmic-drug therapy with implantable defibrillators in patients resuscitated from near-fatal ventricular arrhythmias. *N Engl J Med* 1997;337(22):1576–1583.
120. Connolly SJ, Gent M, Roberts RS, et al: Canadian implantable defibrillator study (CIDS): A randomized trial of the implantable cardioverter defibrillator against amiodarone. *Circulation* 2000;101:1297–1302.
121. Middlekauff HR, Stevenson WG, Stevenson LW, et al: Syncope in advanced heart failure: High risk of sudden death regardless of origin of syncope. *J Am Coll Cardiol* 1993;21(1):110–116.
122. Moss AJ, Zareba W, Hall WJ, et al: Prophylactic implantation of a defibrillator in patients with myocardial infarction and reduced ejection fraction. *N Engl J Med* 2002;346:877–883.
123. Sekiguchi M, Yazak Y, Isobe M, et al: Cardiac sarcoidosis: diagnostic, prognostic, and therapeutic considerations. *Cardiovasc Drugs Ther* 1996;10(5):495–510.

124. Luu M, Stevenson WG, Stevenson LW, et al: Diverse mechanisms of unexpected cardiac arrest in advanced heart failure. *Circulation* 1989;80:1675–1680.

125. Schoeller R, Andersen D, Buttner P, et al: First- or second-degree atrioventricular block as a risk factor in idiopathic dilated cardiomyopathy. *Am J Cardiol* 1993;71(8):720–726.

126. Leclerq C, Kass D, Retiming the failing heart: principles and current clinical status of cardiac resynchronization. *J Am Coll Cardiol* 2002;39:194–201.

127. Lasser RP, Haft JI, Frediberg CK. Relationship of right bundle branch block and marked left axis deviation (with left parietal or peri-infarction block) to complete heart block and Adams-Stokes syndrome. *Circulation* 1968;37:429–437.

128. Bradley DJ, Bradley EA, Baughman KL, et al: Cardiac resynchronization and death from progressive heart failure: A meta-analysis of randomized controlled trials. *JAMA* 2003;289(6):730–740.

129. Baldasseroni S, Opasich C, Gorini M, et al. Left bundle-branch block is associated with increased 1-year sudden and total mortality rate in 5517 outpatients with congestive heart failure: A report from the Italian Network on Congestive Heart Failure. *Am Heart J* 2002;143:398–405.

130. Wilkoff BL, Cook JR, Epstein AE, et al: Dual-chamber pacing or ventricular backup pacing in patients with an implantable defibrillator: The Dual Chamber and VVI Implantable Defibrillator (DAVID) Trial. *JAMA* 2003;288(24):3115–3123.

131. Abraham WT, Fisher WG, Smith AL, et al: Cardiac resynchronization in chronic heart failure. *N Engl J Med* 2002;346(24):1845–1853.

132. Larsen G, Hallstrom A, McAnulty J, et al: Cost-effectiveness of the implantable cardioverter-defibrillator versus antiarrhythmic drugs in survivors of serious ventricular tachyarrhythmias: Results of the Antiarrhythmics Versus Implantable Defibrillators (AVID) Economic Analysis Substudy. *Circulation* 2002;105(17):2049–2057.

133. Hlatky MA, Bigger JT. Cost-effectiveness of the implantable cardioverter defibrillator. *Lancet* 2001;357:1817–1818.

134. Bennett LE, Keck BM, Hertz MI, et al: Worldwide thoracic organ transplantation: a report from the UNOS/ISHLT international registry for thoracic organ transplantation. *Clinical Transplants* 2001:25–40.

# 2

# Pathophysiology of Cardiac Dyssynchrony and Resynchronization

### David A. Kass

Dilated cardiomyopathy (DCM) combines primary abnormalities of the heart muscle with altered chamber loading, neurohormonal activation, and molecular maladaptations triggered by elevated wall stress and hypertrophy. In addition to these changes, which affect the myocardium diffusely, electrical conduction disease can develop that can alter atrioventricular (AV) timing or delay activation of one portion of the left ventricle relative to another, generating contractile dyssynchrony. The latter is often observed in patients with a widened QRS complex and left bundle branch block (LBBB)–pattern intraventricular conduction delay. In patients with DCM, such delays pose an independent risk for worsened morbidity and mortality.[1-4] In a recent analysis of more than 5000 patients, LBB delay was associated with a 60% to 70% higher risk of sudden death and mortality and was an independent risk factor after adjustment for age, underlying cardiac disease, the severity of heart failure, and concomitant drug therapies.[5] Unilateral loss of normal rapid stimulation of the myocardium effectively results in polarization of the heart into two regions: early activated and late-activated territories. When this condition is superimposed on a dilated heart with generalized slowed conduction and weak muscle contraction, such delays result in marked dyssynchrony, with the net consequence being substantial compromise of systolic function and reduced energetic efficiency.

Over the past decade, investigators have established that ventricular stimulation of right and left ventricles together (biventricular pacing), or just the left ventricular (LV) free wall itself, can improve the mechanics and energetics of the failing heart with discoordinate contraction. This therapy, most commonly referred to as cardiac resynchronization therapy (CRT), has been the focus of recent reviews.[6-8] Trials of long-term therapy have confirmed that CRT improved clinical symptoms, increased exercise capacity, and led to cessation or even reversal of chronic chamber remodeling.[9-12] As with all heart failure therapies, the individual response to CRT has varied, but most reported series have shown a 20% to 30% nonresponse rate. Improvements in the methods of identification of likely responsive patients are needed, but these appear to be evolving on the basis of more direct analysis of mechanical dyssynchrony. This review discusses the pathophysiology of conduction abnormalities in cardiac failure, focusing principally on distal delay with ventricular dyssynchrony and the impact of CRT on this substrate.

## Conduction Abnormalities of the Atrium or AV Node

To understand factors associated with the clinical efficacy of CRT, it is important to review the primary pathophysiology of altered electrical conduction. The normal cardiac conduction system modulates contraction rate, the mechanical impact of atrial systole, and contractile coordination of ventricular chambers. Disease of any of these components can lead to suboptimal cardiac performance.

Sinus node disease results in chronotropic incompetence, which can be problematic in individuals with little preload or contractile reserve. This has become more common in patients with DCM because of the increasing use of adrenergic blockade, which can slow too greatly the rate and/or rate response in a heart with limited Frank-Starling reserve. Chronotropic disease is also associated with the use of amiodarone and calcium channel blockers, although the latter are less often used in the setting of DCM. This problem can be treated with a dual-chamber rate-responsive pacemaker (DDDR). However, as is discussed later in this chapter, pacing the ventricle itself induces dyssynchrony of contraction and can exacerbate underlying chamber dysfunction. Thus, although potential benefits of maintaining adequate heart rate response are evident, efforts should be made to ensure that only atrial stimulation is employed as much as possible, even if this means setting an unusually long AV delay or accepting somewhat slower basal heart rates.

AV nodal disease can take several forms: diseases in which AV delay is shortened, usually because of a bypass tract, and those in which the AV delay is lengthened. When the AV delay exceeds 250 msec, atrial contraction no longer occurs near the onset of LV systolic contraction but rather is superimposed on early passive filling. This effectively eliminates its value as a booster pump for enhancing late diastolic filling.[13,14] Figure 2–1 displays results of a study examining the net effect of varying AV delay on cardiac filling. In dogs with complete AV-nodal block, the AV delay was varied while net LV chamber filling was measured by integration of the flow signal measured by an in-line mitral annular flow probe.[13] Increasing the delay from zero (simultaneous AV contraction) to the physiologic value of ~120 msec enhanced net chamber filling, as would be expected. However, at longer delays, particularly those exceeding 275 msec, net filling gradually declined, eventually falling below that observed with no AV delay. The fall in net filling at long delays relates to two factors. One, as atrial contraction occurs further from the initiation of LV systole, its hemodynamic benefit as a booster pump is also lost because both atrial and passive filling effectively occur during the same period. In addition, the long delay can enhance mitral regurgitation, particularly during the early systolic (pre-ejection) period. With too much delay, the mitral valve leaflets remain open in a mid-plane position at the start of systole. Valve closure is therefore entirely dependent on the rising pressure within the ventricle, and while this occurs but before the valve fully closes, mitral regurgitation (MR) is more likely. This behavior was highlighted by the study of Brecker et al. involving patients with DCM and prolonged AV delay.[15] Shortening the AV delay, often to quite short values (i.e., 50–75 msec), by means of a pacing lead placed in the right ventricular (RV)

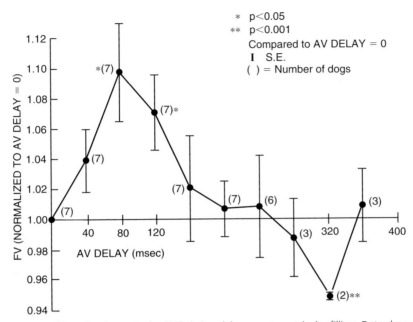

FIGURE 2–1. Effect of atrioventricular (AV) timing delay on net ventricular filling. Data shown are net left ventricular (LV) filling volume (FV) values, normalized to the value measured at a zero AV delay (S.E. = standard error). Canine hearts had complete AV block, and atrial contraction was induced at varying delays. Net filling of the heart is enhanced as AV delay is increased from zero (i.e., synchronous atrial and ventricular contraction) to the more physiologic range of 100–120 msec. At this delay time, atrial systole is just completed as LV pressure is beginning to rise, so closure of the mitral valve occurs as both pressures meet each other. With longer delay times, atrial systole is superimposed with early rapid filling, and closure of the mitral valve is dependent purely on the LV pressure rise. This generates presystolic regurgitation, and net LV filling declines. *(Used with permission from Meisner JS, McQueen DM, Ishida Y, et al: Effects of timing of atrial systole on LV filling and mitral valve closure: computer and dog studies. Am J Physiol 1985;249:H604–H619.)*

apex reduced pre-ejection regurgitation, enhanced net diastolic filling, and lengthened the period for diastolic filling. Indeed, the field of cardiac stimulation therapy for DCM first focused on these factors and manipulation of the AV delay as a primary therapeutic goal. However, as subsequent studies demonstrated, this effect was more often quite modest, even in patients with long AV delays; thus other factors were sought that might benefit more from cardiac stimulation. The answer came from targeting infranodal conduction abnormalities.

## Infranodal Conduction Delay: Dyssynchrony

Infranodal conduction delay, which most commonly occurs with a LBBB pattern, induces discoordinate LV contraction.[16,17] Studies performed more than 15 years ago revealed hemodynamic deterioration from inhomogeneous temporal activation in the normal heart.[18,19] Although the effects of dyssynchrony were noticeable, they generally were not dramatic and certainly did not attract much clinical attention. Recently, however, studies have been performed in which this pathophysiology has been applied to the DCM heart, and the net effect appears to be more substantial. This may be related in part to the enlarged size of the failing ventricle, which renders greater geographic separation between early activated and late-activated regions, worsening their impact on net systolic function. In addition, factors such as slowed or weakened contraction and delayed cell-to-cell conduction in the failing heart can worsen dyssynchrony. Although differences in the impact of dyssynchrony on normal versus failing dilated hearts remain somewhat speculative, the clinical impact does appear greater and therefore has garnered far more attention recently.

LBBB-type conduction delay involves initial wall motion in the septal region, often accompanied by reciprocal lateral wall prestretch. Much of this early septal shortening occurs prior to closure of the mitral valve,[20] blurring the distinction between end-diastole and early systole. The reason for this is that the early activated myocardium cannot generate sufficient chamber pressure to close the valve, as most of the energy is transferred to prestretching the opposing yet-to-be activated wall. The mitral valve remains open, and diastolic filling can still potentially occur as long as the LV pressure remains below mean left atrial pressure. Thus, from the standpoint of mitral valve closure and initiation of isovolumic contraction, diastole is prolonged and systole initiated later by contractile dyssynchrony.

The second phase of systole starts with the onset of delayed contraction in the late-activated wall (typically the lateral free wall). This wall, coupled with already activated muscle and higher developed pressures, must contract at higher levels of regional wall stress. Yet this contraction also involves wasted effort, because part of it is converted to stretching the early activated wall that is now beginning to enter its relaxation phase. The result is generally mid- to late systolic septal motion toward the right ventricle, which has been traditionally termed *paradoxical* motion in the sense that it behaves as if the septum were ischemic without having this underlying pathophysiology. However, the motion is not paradoxical but really the consequence of a balance of forces. The septal myocardium is less capable of withstanding the systolic stresses being developed by the late-activating LV free wall and thus is pushed away from the central LV chamber toward the right heart.

Examples of regional stress strain loops, as they might be recorded in the early versus late-activated myocardium, are displayed in Figure 2–2*A*. The early activated territory shortens at low chamber stress (*a*) because most of the heart is yet to be stimulated. The inward motion of this territory is accompanied by prestretching (i.e., a higher preload) of the opposite region (*b*). As systole progresses, the late-activated region must develop higher load, relengthening the early activated muscle. The net result of this reciprocal *sloshing* of blood from early to late to early activated regions is a decline in ejection and depression of systolic chamber function. At the chamber level, the late systolic septal shift results in higher end-systolic volumes, effectively displacing the pressure-volume loops and end-systolic pressure-volume relation to the right (solid to dashed line, see Figure 2–2*B*). This phenomenon was first demonstrated in 1985 by Park et al.,[21] in a study of animals, and subsequently by Pak et al.[22] in a study of human subjects, both involving the use of single-site ventricular pacing to generate the discoordination. The pressure-volume loop itself narrows, indicating reduced stroke volume, often at similar if slightly reduced systolic pressures. As shown by the example, diastolic filling and filling pressures are minimally altered, at least acutely, by the imposition of contractile dyssynchrony due to an altered activation sequence.

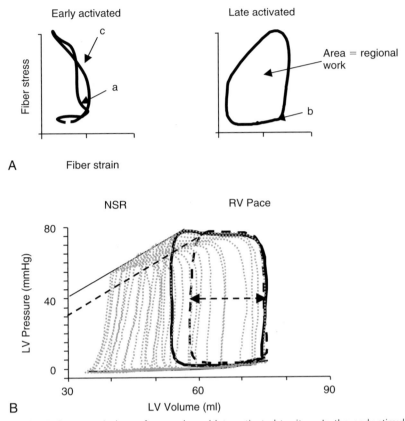

**FIGURE 2–2.** *A,* Stress-strain loops from early and late-activated territory. In the early stimulated region, there is initial shortening at little pressure load *(a),* as this motion is principally converted to prestretch of the still-inactive muscle. Stress then develops, but the region is pushed on by the later-activated myocardium and can stretch toward the right heart *(c).* The net loop is thin *(small area),* indicative of reduced regional work. The later-activated territory initiates stress development from a higher prestretch *(b, increased preload),* and the work loop is larger than normal. *B,* Pressure-volume (PV) loops and relations in synchronous and acutely dyssynchronous heart. With right ventricular (RV) pacing to induce delayed lateral contraction, there is a right shift of the PV loop, with reduced width (stroke volume) and area, and an increase in end-systolic pressure/volume point *(arrows).* The end-systolic PV relation shifts rightward. LV = left ventricular; NSR = normal sinus rhythm.

Table 2–1 summarizes the impact of infranodal conduction delay and loss of contractile coordination on the ventricle. Late-systolic septal stretch worsens function for several reasons. First, it effectively acts as an intracavitary sink for blood volume that would otherwise be ejected, reducing forward output. Second, the late stretch of the contracting muscle can break cross-bridges diminishing systolic force development and result in repolarization inhomogeneity and stretch-activated channel stimulation, triggering arrhythmias.[23-25] Inhomogeneous contraction is also a mechanism for delaying muscle relaxation and likely contributes to diastolic dysfunction.[26-29]

**TABLE 2–1. Mechanisms of Dysfunction Due to Contractile Discoordination**

- Reduced ejection volume
  - Internal *sloshing* from premature-activated region to late-activated region
  - Increased end-systolic volume (stress)
- Mechano-energetic Inefficiency
  - Reduced systolic function despite maintained or increased energetic cost
- Late systolic stretch
  - Cross-bride detachment, reduced force
  - Delayed relaxation
  - After-contractions/arrhythmia
- Mitral valve dysfunction
  - Papillary muscle discoordination

There are also important regional and global metabolic/energetic consequences that develop from dyssynchrony. The prematurely activated myocardium develops less overall work (e.g., the loop area in Figure 2–2A), consuming less energy.[16,30] The energy it does consume, however, is largely wasted with respect to ejection, because pressure remains low. The late-activated free wall, in contrast, operates under a higher load (larger loop area, see Figure 2–2A), with higher metabolic demand. It too wastes work in stretching the more compliant early activated territory rather than contributing to ejection, so the net effect is a reduction in chamber efficiency.[30-32]

Figure 2–3A shows data from a recent study of Prinzen et al.[16] These investigators employed magnetic resonance tagging methods to assess circumferential strain (normalized shortening in the circumferential direction), regional external work, and regional total work (combining both external and internal work, the latter reflecting metabolic demands, excitation-contraction coupling energy, heat, etc.) in normal canine hearts under sinus rhythm and RV apex versus LV basal pre-excitation. With RV apex pacing, regional work in the apex itself was reduced, whereas there was a reciprocal increase in the LV free wall. Similar results were obtained for total and external work, and the exact opposite pattern was observed with LV basal pacing. Now, if the geographic territory represented by each component were identical in size, the net result would be similar to a synchronous contraction. However, this is not the case. In particular, with an LBBB-type pattern (RV apex pacing), the territory represented by the LV zone is substantial in comparison with the smaller septum. Thus there can be a net increase in total work and thus energy consumption.

Figure 2–3B displays measures of regional wall mass in hearts rendered dyssynchronous by ventricular pacing, as noted in a study by Prinzen and colleagues.[33] Commensurate with a rise in wall stress of the late-activated myocardium, wall mass (i.e., hypertrophy) increased in the zones more distant from the pacing site. Regional dyssynchrony also acutely generated regional blood flow gradients, with higher flow in the late-activated myocardium (see Figure 2–3C). However, this was not sustained when pacing was chronically applied; rather, blood flow became more homogeneous.

Increased loading in the lateral wall is also accompanied by amplified molecular abnormalities. Using a canine model of heart failure with dyssynchronous contraction, we have found marked reductions in protein expression for gap junction proteins (connexin 43), excitation-contraction coupling proteins (SERCA2a and

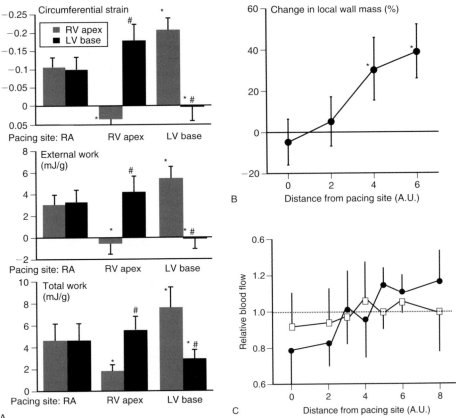

FIGURE 2–3. Regional disparities in myocardial work, hypertrophy, and blood flow associated with dyssynchronous contraction. *A,* Measured circumferential strains and estimated regional external (stroke) work and total work, based on magnetic resonance imaging (MRI) tagging analysis of canine hearts. Pacing is instituted from the right atrium (RA), right ventricular (RV) apex, or left ventricular (LV) base. Reciprocal increases and decreases in strain and work are observed, with reduced values in the early activated myocardium and higher values in the late-activated regions. *B,* Dyssynchronous contraction due to pacing generates myocardial hypertrophy in the territory remote to the pacing site (i.e., late-activated wall). This is consistent with predicted increases in wall stress in the same region. *C,* Relation of myocardial distance to pacing site and regional blood flow. Data show results following the acute institution of ventricular pacing (*lines with dots*) and after 6 months of chronic pacing (*lines with squares*). Acutely, there is a gradient of blood flow, with lower levels near the pacing site (reduced local work) and higher flow at the late-activated higher-stress region. Chronically, however, this is more homogeneous, with the development of hypertrophy and adaptive changes. AU = arbitrary unit. (*A, Reprinted from Prinzen FW, Hunter WC, Wyman BT, et al: Mapping of regional myocardial strain and work during ventricular pacing: experimental study using magnetic resonance imaging tagging. J Am Coll Cardiol 1999;33: 1735–1742, with permission from The American College of Cardiology Foundation. B, Used with permission from van Oosterhout MF, Arts T, Bassingthwaighte JB, et al: Relation between local myocardial growth and blood flow during chronic ventricular pacing. Cardiovasc Res 2002;53:831–840.*)

phospholamban), and increased stress kinase expression/activation in the late-activated (high-load) lateral endocardium. This is not observed in myocardium that is failing but contracts synchronously (Spragg et al., unpublished data).

## Hemodynamic Effects of Biventricular (or LV Free Wall) Pacing

Biventricular or univentricular pacing of the LV lateral free wall can recoordinate contraction, and both are associated with systolic improvement.[34-38] An example of resynchronization effects from biventricular stimulation is shown in Figure 2–4A (from Leclercq et al.[20]). These panels display magnetic resonance imaging (MRI)–tagged reconstructions of a failing heart with LBBB delay before (upper panel) and after (lower panel) biventricular stimulation. Early activation (coded in blue) occurs to the right and slowly spreads leftward, with evidence of reciprocal stretch (coded in yellow). With biventricular stimulation, shortening is initiated on both sides of the heart more simultaneously, and there is minimal reciprocal stretch with enhanced net ejection. Globally, the effect of resynchronization is immediate, as shown in Figure 2–4B. Hemodynamic parameters such as the maximal rate of pressure rise (dP/dt$_{max}$) or arterial pulse pressure are improved within one beat after initiation of pacing, the latter reflecting a rise in cardiac output.[37] From a pressure-volume loop perspective (see Figure 2–4C), the effect is the reverse of that shown in single-site (RV apex) pacing-induced dyssynchrony (see Figure 2–2B). CRT induced a leftward shift of the loop, lowering the end-systolic wall stress, increasing stroke work and stroke volume, and thus enhancing systolic performance. Although improvement of synchrony might be anticipated to enhance muscle relaxation, such diastolic properties appear to be minimally altered, at least in the short term.[37]

Recent advances in echo-Doppler imaging methods have provided direct evidence of wall motion resynchronization in humans receiving CRT.[39-41] Figure 2–4D displays the findings of enhanced contrast-echo imaging[41] in patients with DCM and LBBB undergoing long-term treatment with LV pacing. With pacing temporarily suspended (native LBBB delay), early inward septal motion is followed by stretch toward the RV. Pacing converts this to a more concordant inward motion, with LV-only and biventricular pacing producing similar responses. In the lateral wall, the intrinsic delay results in early stretch of the wall, followed by late lateral inward motion. With use of CRT, the major effect is shifting of the phase of lateral contraction earlier but not enhancement of its magnitude.

Long-term noninvasive studies have revealed systolic responses of similar magnitude.[39] For example, dP/dt$_{max}$ acutely increases from 600 to nearly 800 mm Hg/second. As shown in Figure 2–5B, similar results are observed after 1–12 weeks of chronic CRT. Although a short-term reduction in end-systolic volume is also observed (see Figure 2–4C), more chronic therapy is required to observe true reverse remodeling, with a decline in end-diastolic volume as well. As demonstrated by Yu et al.,[39] after 1 month or more of pacing, *both* end-systolic and end-diastolic chamber volumes decline (see Figure 2–5A). Particularly notable in that study was that when pacing was transiently suspended after 3 months of CRT, both volumes remained low, despite acute reversal of systolic augmentation (i.e., dP/dt$_{max}$ declined back toward baseline). This supports a true remodeling effect. When pacing was kept off for the ensuing month, chamber volumes gradually rose again, consistent with

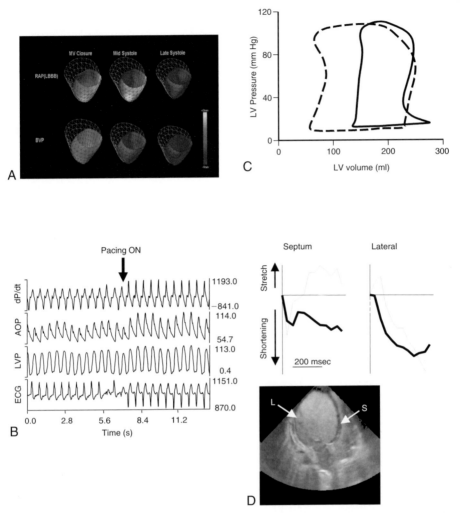

**FIGURE 2–4.** *A,* Magnetic resonance–tagged imaging shortening maps of left ventricle (LV) with underlying left bundle branch block (LBBB) and cardiac failure *(top images)* and the same heart paced with a biventricular stimulator (BVP; *lower images*). See text for details. *B,* Acute hemodynamic response in human ventricle with LBBB conduction delay before and after cardiac resynchronization therapy (CRT) pacing. There is an abrupt rise in pressure development and rate of development and increase in the arterial pulse pressure, indicative of enhanced cardiac output. *C,* Similar data displayed as pressure-volume loops. CRT induces a left shift of the loop, increasing the width and area and reducing end-systolic volumes. *D,* Regional wall motion improved by CRT. With pacing off, radial septal motion is initially inward but then shifts toward the RV as the lateral wall contracts (so-called *paradoxic motion*). CRT converts this to a more consistent inward motion. In the lateral wall, there is initial stretch followed by delayed contraction. CRT influences the phase but not the amplitude of motion, stimulating contraction earlier. MV = mitral valve; RAP = right atrial pacing.

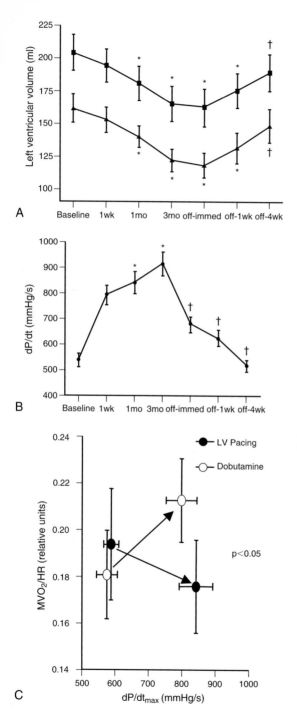

**FIGURE 2–5.** *A,* Reverse remodeling with chronic cardiac resynchronization therapy (CRT). See text for details. *B,* Unlike volume changes (which, once developed, do not acutely reverse when pacing is temporarily suspended), ventricular systolic function can be abruptly diminished by stopping pacing (*arrow*). *C,* Comparison of mechano-energetics of CRT versus dobutamine. Both stimuli increased cardiac systolic function, but with CRT, myocardial oxygen consumption (MVO$_2$/HR; dP/dt$_{max}$ = the maximal rate of pressure rise) declined, whereas it was increased by dobutamine. *$p < 0.05$ (B, Adapted with permission from Yu CM, Chau E, Sanderson JE, et al: Tissue Doppler echocardiographic evidence of reverse remodeling and improved synchronicity by simultaneously delaying regional contraction after biventricular pacing therapy in heart failure. Circulation 2002;105:438–445. C, From Nelson GS, Berger RD, Fetics BJ, et al: Left ventricular or biventricular pacing improves cardiac function at diminished energy cost in patients with dilated cardiomyopathy and left bundle-branch block. Circulation 2000;102:3053–3059.)*

re-initiation of chamber dilation/remodeling. Larger, long-term, blinded/controlled studies have also revealed significant reverse remodeling with long-term CRT.[10,12]

To date, the primary focus of therapy has been biventricular stimulation. However, many laboratories have shown similar short-term and now long-term benefits from single-site LV-free wall pacing alone.[36,37,42] Careful assessment of global function and regional wall motion has revealed remarkably similar benefits from both pacing modes, despite large disparities in electric activation pattern and time delay.[20] This suggests that electrical synchrony is not tantamount to mechanical synchrony and that the latter is more relevant to a hemodynamic benefit from CRT. This is addressed more fully in the subsequent discussion of how to identify responders.

## CRT Mechanoenergetics

During the 1980s and early 1990s, extensive efforts were made to develop novel cardiac failure therapies to enhance systolic function. The majority of these approaches targeted cAMP-dependent pathways, in particular by inhibiting phosphodiesterase III (e.g., with milrinone[43]). All of these agents, as well as dobutamine administered intermittently or in long-term therapy,[44,45] proved disappointing in that they worsened morbidity and mortality. One widely held hypothesis explaining these negative results was that these agents enhanced cardiac performance at an often substantial metabolic cost and that this ultimately worsened the underlying cardiac substrate.

With the demonstration that CRT could enhance systolic function acutely—literally within a single cardiac cycle—by as much as 25% to 40%, the same concerns over long-term energetic costs were raised. However, unlike inotropic interventions that target the contractility of the myocyte itself, CRT achieves its primary benefit from the improved temporal synchrony of muscle contraction, suggesting that it might enhance efficiency. This hypothesis was first tested by Nelson et al.[46] Patients underwent coronary catheterization with myocardial blood flow determined by Doppler and multiplied by the coronary sinus-arterial oxygen difference to determine myocardial oxygen consumption. Simultaneous ventricular mechanics were measured, and pacing data with both biventricular and LV-univentricular modes were tested in a group of patients with DCM and LBBB-type IVCD. Both stimulation modes enhanced ventricular systolic function substantially, yet cardiac oxygen consumption declined significantly at the same time. CRT was further contrasted with dobutamine, and the disparity in mechanoenergetics was made even more striking. As shown in Figure 2–5C, when dobutamine was titrated to enhance systolic function to the same extent as observed with CRT, there was a net increase in per-beat cardiac oxygen consumption, whereas this declined with CRT. Ukkonen et al.[47] recently employed positron-emission tomography (PET) scanning in a small group of patients to assess regional metabolism in septal and lateral walls. Whereas CRT enhanced function, global metabolism measured by [$C^{11}$]-acetate clearance was unchanged. However, regional metabolism was altered, with a net rise in the septum, increasing the septal/lateral wall ratio by 13%. This is consistent with greater regional work in the septum due to resynchronization. Because total metabolic activity was unchanged, there was presumably a decline elsewhere in the myocardium, and the data suggested this occurred in the lateral wall, although these data did not achieve statistical significance.

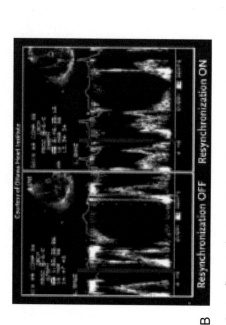

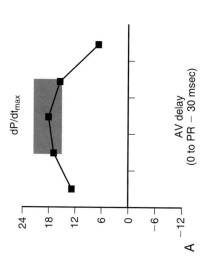

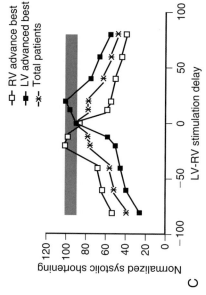

**FIGURE 2-6.** A, Influence of atrioventricular (AV) interval optimization on systolic response to cardiac resynchronization therapy (CRT). There is diminished efficacy at very short or long AV delays but also a fairly flat maximal response over a broad range of delays in the middle. This suggests that AV delay is not a critical parameter if a reasonable delay (typically in the physiologic range of 110–140 msec) is used. B, Example of mitral inflow Doppler filling in patient with CRT off (left) and on (right). At baseline there is only an early filling wave with fast E-wave deceleration. With CRT, this is converted to an E and A wave (still frame from echo video). C, Influence of right ventricular–left ventricular (RV-LV) timing delay on systolic function. In a group of patients with left bundle branch block (LBBB), some display enhanced response with RV slightly pre-excited over LV, whereas about half show the opposite effect. Even with subselection on this basis, the difference between maximal response and response with simultaneous activation is small. Furthermore, the combined analysis shows a maximal response at simultaneous RV and LV, with only modest decline when RV or LV is advanced by 20 msec. dP/dt$_{max}$ = the maximal rate of pressure rise. (Adapted from Sogaard P, Egeblad H, Pedersen AK, et al: Sequential versus simultaneous biventricular resynchronization for severe heart failure: evaluation by tissue Doppler imaging. Circulation 2002;106:2078–2084.)

## Effects of AV and RV-LV Timing

The magnitude of systolic benefit depends in part on the AV timing delay selected.[36,37] Clearly, when atrial and ventricular activation are synchronous, there is a detrimental effect on chamber filling and increased atrial pressures. Increasing the delay enhances AV mass transfer while still maintaining pre-excitation of the portion of the myocardium with delayed activation. Too long a delay, however, reduces the efficacy of pacing because pre-excitation is lost. The net magnitude of this effect, however, is not very large. This is shown by data from a study by Auricchio et al.,[36] in which AV delay was varied broadly and in a highly controlled manner (Figure 2–6$A$). Although the relation between percentage of improvement in dP/dt$_{max}$ and AV delay displays an optimal decrease at either extreme, there is a broad mid-region (shaded) where the precise delay makes little difference. Instead, mechanical responses to CRT are frequently similar over a fairly broad range of physiologic AV intervals (typically ranging from 40-100 msec). However, for some individuals with a very long basal AV delay, shortening this delay can improve the dynamics of LV filling. An example of this is shown in the Doppler tracings in Figure 2–6$B$. With CRT inactive (left), there is a single filling wave (E-wave) as atrial contraction occurs during early rapid filling, whereas with CRT activated and shortening of the AV delay, there is a more clear early (E) and late (A) wave, the normal filling pattern. This may be used to set the AV delay; however, in most patients, setting the delay at 100-140 msec appears to be similarly effective without such detailed analysis.

Another timing factor that can be manipulated by biventricular pacing is between ventricular stimulation of right and left ventricles (RV-LV delay). Virtually all published studies involving biventricular stimulation have employed simultaneous stimulation, but normal activation involves slight LV (versus RV) pre-excitation by about 25 msec. Thus it has been proposed that optimization of the RV-LV interval might further augment the therapeutic response. In this regard, Sogaard and colleagues[48] examined the influence of varying the RV-LV delay in 20 patients with cardiac failure, LBBB, and sinus rhythm. In 11 patients, the peak systolic response occurred with the RV slightly advanced (12-20 msec), whereas the remaining patients did better with the LV advanced by a similar amount.

Several features of this study deserve comment. The response to simultaneous stimulation in each subgroup fell to within 10% of the peak response, suggesting that the effect of RV-LV delay is modest at best. Furthermore, this separation was performed post hoc, whereas combining all subjects yielded a relation with its peak occurring at simultaneous stimulation and only a 10% decline at a ±20-msec delay (see Figure 2–6$C$). This suggests that optimization of this interval appears to be a minor factor in most patients, although it may play a role in a select subset that has particularly delayed conduction from the pacing electrode. In addition, it is interesting that more pronounced pre-excitation of the LV versus RV led to a decline in response in this study. As already noted, LV-only pacing, which maximally preactivates the left ventricle, produced similar if not greater acute mechanical responses in several studies. The cause of this discrepancy remains unresolved.

## Mitral Regurgitation

MR is very common in patients with dilated cardiomyopathy. As noted previously, adjustment of the AV delay can modify the extent of pre-ejection MR, particularly in patients with very long basal delays. In addition, the rate of LV pressure rise itself is an important factor for determining how much MR may accrue. Dyssynchronous hearts develop pressure slowly (i.e., have a reduced $dP/dt_{max}$), so the effective mitral valve orifice area is larger and regurgitation is greater. Because CRT often can increase $dP/dt_{max}$ by 25%, this might itself limit MR. This mechanism was examined by Briethardt et al.,[49] who demonstrated an acute 50% decline in effective regurgitant orifice area, which was strongly and inversely correlated with improvement in $dP/dt_{max}$ ($r = -0.83$; $P < 0.0001$). Papillary muscle discoordination can also worsen MR, and resynchronization of contraction timing of these muscles can enhance normal leaflet coaptation. Because this particular effect is difficult to assess, there is no direct evidence to date. Last, chronic CRT can result in reverse remodeling, and this could alter cardiac preload and afterload to further limit MR. Neither short-term nor long-term studies have shown that MR is required for CRT to be beneficial, but there is little doubt that reducing MR is a further benefit of CRT in many patients.

## Criteria for Identifying Responders

Table 2–2 summarizes the factors that are believed to influence the responsiveness of patients to CRT and used to identify candidates. The most widely used marker to identify patients with cardiac dyssynchrony has been a widened QRS complex on the surface electrocardiogram. To date, all clinical trials have enrolled subjects on the basis of systolic dysfunction with dilated cardiomyopathy and a widened QRS duration. The precise amount of widening used as an enrollment criterion has varied from >120 msec to 150 msec. The notion that QRS duration should index dyssynchrony at first seemed logical in that substantial LV conduction delay should result in widening, in concordance with experimental data.[18] Indeed, many studies have shown that the wider the basal QRS duration, the greater the systolic improvement with biventricular or LV pacing. Figure 2–7A shows an example of this relation with data combined from two studies.[36,38] Although it is statistically significant, this relation displays considerable scatter, even for the acute mechanical response; only 25% of the systolic response is predicted by basal QRS duration. Clearly, some responsive patients have narrow complexes and, by contrast, some less-responsive ones have wide QRS complexes.

Figure 2–7B provides further evidence of the correlative and indirect nature of basal QRS width versus cardiac functional response to resynchronization. Despite substantial systolic improvement with LV or biventricular pacing, QRS duration does not consistently narrow: many subjects have no change or even widening of the duration.[38] This may reflect the reliance on intramyocardial conduction and that

TABLE 2–2. **Factors Related to CRT Response**

- Wide QRS complex
- Interventricular
- Intraventricular dyssynchrony*
- Successful lead placement*
- Adequate preload
- Physiologic AV

*Most important.

abnormal wall geometry (dilation) as well as gap-junction and other ion channel abnormalities may slow this process further. These data highlight the notion that QRS duration is at best an indirect correlate but not a direct reflection of mechanical synchrony; the latter is the real substrate that causes a decline in chamber function.

Recently investigators have begun examining the utility of QRS duration in predicting the chronic response to CRT. The data have generally confirmed the short-term findings, showing a general correlation between basal QRS duration and efficacy,[50] but usually with a poor predictive value for identifying responders versus nonresponders.[51,52] For example, baseline New York Heart Association (NYHA) functional class, age, sex, QRS duration, and ejection fraction were no different between responders and nonresponders in a recent study of 45 subjects.[53] In a larger cohort of 102 consecutive patients, both responders and nonresponders had similar basal QRS duration, and both displayed near-identical shortening of complex duration,[54] a finding mirrored in other recent reports.[55] Clinical outcome showed no correlation with basal QRS in the larger Multicenter InSync Randomized Clinical Evaluation (MIRACLE) trial.[10] Patients with reduced baseline $dP/dt_{max}$ who have greater than 22% short-term improvement have been reported to be consistent responders to long-term treatment (with very few false negatives),[50] concordant with an earlier reported observation in an acute hemodynamic study.[38]

## Basal Mechanical Dyssynchrony as a Predictor of CRT Response

The use of QRS duration was generally recognized as a surrogate for mechanical discoordination, but one whose value resided in its clinical simplicity. However, because electrical markers have proved to be disappointing, recent studies have begun to quantify mechanical dyssynchrony directly and to test this as a prognostic index. Dyssynchrony was first comprehensively examined by means of tagged MRI.[38,56] This approach provided full three-dimensional strain measurements throughout the left ventricle and allowed calculation of a variety of synchrony indexes from these maps. Investigators employing this approach in recent animal studies have further shown that dissociation can exist between electrical delay times and mechanical dyssynchrony.[20] The latter appears increasingly to be the primary target for identifying responders and a good candidate parameter to monitor efficacy.

MRI analysis is complex and has limited clinical use; thus simpler echo-based methods have been developed. The simplest is M-mode imaging, used to assess timing. Both interventricular (RV versus LV) and intraventricular (within the LV) delays can be assessed. The former has been illustrated by plotting instantaneous RV and LV pressure tracings. When synchronous, this plot appears as a straight line, whereas a phase delay results in an open contour whose area is mathematically related to the delay. Whereas analysis of pressures requires invasively obtained data, interventricular delay (IVD) can also be determined by the difference between two time intervals, $T_2$ and $T_1$, with $T_1$ denoting the time from QRS to the onset of pulmonary artery flow and $T_2$ denoting the time from QRS to aortic flow. On the basis of 95% confidence intervals of normal hearts, an IVD of greater than 30 msec has been considered significant, although this remains somewhat arbitrary and might be changed in prospective analysis. One problem with the echo-derived IVD is that it incorporates several components that may not relate to phase delay, for example, underlying contractile function of each ventricle (which determines the isovolumic

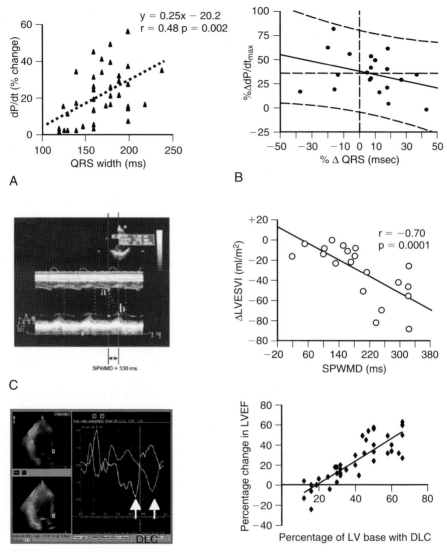

**FIGURE 2–7.** Predicting responders to cardiac resynchronization therapy (CRT). *A,* QRS duration correlates with the acute mechanical response, although there is considerable scatter in these data, raising questions as to its predictive value. dP/dt$_{max}$ = the maximal rate of pressure rise. *B,* Correlation between QRS duration change from biventricular only or left ventricular (LV) only pacing and mechanical response. Although mechanical changes are substantial, there is no correlation between them and QRS duration change. *C,* M-mode echo assessment of intraventricular dyssynchrony. The time of initial inward septal motion is identified, and the delay between this time and inferolateral motion is assessed. This delay (SPWMD) is then plotted against the chronic change in ventricular end-systolic volume (*right upper panel*). There is a significant negative correlation, suggesting the predictive value of SPWMD in identifying chronic response. *D,* Analysis of intraventricular dyssynchrony with strain-rate tissue Doppler. Left panel shows color-coded long-axis view of the left ventricle, with two regions of interest selected (lateral wall = green; septum = yellow).

*Continued*

contraction time) and impedance loading on each ventricle. Furthermore, recent studies have raised questions about the predictive utility of such an IVD for defining responders and support analysis of intraventricular delay.[51,52]

Intraventricular delay reflects the mechanical dispersion of motion between septal and lateral walls. This can be assessed in various ways. Echo-contrast imaging indexes regional inward wall motion, from which one can calculate a dyssynchrony index.[41] M-mode echo imaging has been used to determine the delay between initial septal inward motion and inferolateral motion.[51] An example of the latter is shown in Figure 2–7C. This delay time appears to be correlated with chronic improvement in LV end-systolic volume (reverse remodeling) in patients receiving CRT. In contrast, there is little or no significant correlation with QRS duration. Other investigators have applied tissue Doppler imaging to assess absolute or relative wall velocities (the latter is termed *strain rate imaging*), thereby determine timing delays between opposing portions of the left ventricle. This imaging is commonly applied in long-axis views and thus quantifies longitudinal motion. An example of such analysis is shown in Figure 2–7D, from Sogaard et al.[57] As with other measures of dyssynchrony, the delay in lateral contraction (DLC, in Figure 2–7D) has been shown to correlate with long-term improvement in ejection fraction as well as with reduced cardiac volumes. These and other investigators are prospectively evaluating the utility of dyssynchrony measures for predicting responders to CRT. All data from long-term controlled trials have been derived solely from QRS duration on the basis of the enrollment criterion and yet they have demonstrated substantial improvements. However, the previously cited and ongoing trials support mechanical synchrony assessment, and it is likely that such an approach will be strongly recommended in the near future to better stratify patients and identify the most likely responders.

Last, a few other factors should be noted that may play an important role in response to CRT. One is whether or not the lead in the LV has been optimally positioned. The closer the lead is to the already (early) activated septum/anterior wall, the less the mechanical effect on resynchronization and hemodynamic benefit. Pacing the anterior wall can actually make function worse in some patients, as demonstrated by Butter and colleagues,[58] and overall yielded less than 50% of the systolic benefit of lateral free wall placement. Another factor is the AV delay: if it is too long it will not provide sufficient pre-excitation of the lateral wall, and if it is too short, it will compromise function by adverse AV timing. Tissue viability is also a factor because the paced region must be excitable and cannot be diffusely infiltrated by scar tissue. These latter factors should be considered particularly when a candidate is unresponsive to CRT despite evidence of dyssynchrony and QRS widening.

---

Relative tissue velocity in the orientation of the transducer (i.e., longitudinal motion) in each region is determined and plotted versus time. The dominant negative deflection identifies time at maximal systolic motion, and the delay between septal and lateral deflections (delayed lateral contraction, or DLC) can be measured. The right panel shows the correlation between the extent of discoordination (percentage of regions with DLC) at baseline versus chronic improvement in ejection fraction (EF). There is a good overall positive correlation between the measures. (C, Reprinted from Pitzalis MV, Iacoviello M, Romito R, et al: Cardiac resynchronization therapy tailored by echocardiographic evaluation of ventricular asynchrony. J Am Coll Cardiol 2002;40:1615–1622, with permission from The American College of Cardiology Foundation. D, From Sogaard P, Egeblad H, Kim WY, et al: Tissue Doppler imaging predicts improved systolic performance and reversed left ventricular remodeling during long-term cardiac resynchronization therapy. J Am Coll Cardiol 2002;40:723–730.)

## Summary

CRT based on biventricular or LV pre-excitation or both to resynchronize the discoordinate heart has been established recently as a novel method to enhance systolic function in a subset of patients with dilated cardiomyopathy. Optimal identification of candidates remains a high priority. Although investigators initially focused on electrical markers, recent data have highlighted the value of more direct assessment of mechanical discoordination by means of tissue Doppler, echo-Doppler, or MRI. Ongoing efforts to prospectively test the utility of these measures to predict responders will likely provide a major advance in targeting this therapy to those most likely to benefit.

## REFERENCES

1. Xiao HB, Roy C, Fujimoto S, et al: Natural history of abnormal conduction and its relation to prognosis in patients with dilated cardiomyopathy. *Int J Cardiol* 1996;53:163–170.
2. Murkofsky RL, Dangas G, Diamond JA, et al: A prolonged QRS duration on surface electrocardiogram is a specific indicator of left ventricular dysfunction [see comment]. *J Am Coll Cardiol* 1998;32:476–482.
3. Hamby RI, Weissman RH, Prakash MN, et al: Left bundle branch block: a predictor of poor left ventricular function in coronary artery disease. *Am Heart J* 1983;106:471–477.
4. Iuliano S, Fisher SG, Karasik PE, et al: QRS duration and mortality in patients with congestive heart failure. *Am Heart J* 2002;143:1085–1091.
5. Baldasseroni S, Opasich C, Gorini M, et al: Left bundle–branch block is associated with increased 1-year sudden and total mortality rate in 5517 outpatients with congestive heart failure: a report from the Italian network on congestive heart failure. *Am Heart J* 2002;143:398–405.
6. Leclercq C, Kass DA: Retiming the failing heart: principles and current clinical status of cardiac resynchronization. *J Am Coll Cardiol* 2002;39:194–201.
7. Trautmann SI, Kloss M, Auricchio A: Cardiac resynchronization therapy. *Curr Cardiol Rep* 2002;4:371–378.
8. Abraham WT. Cardiac resynchronization therapy for heart failure: biventricular pacing and beyond. *Curr Opin Cardiol* 2002;17:346–352.
9. Cazeau S, Leclercq C, Lavergne T, et al: Effects of multi-site biventricular pacing in patients with heart failure and intraventricular conduction delay. *N Engl J Med* 2001;344:873–880.
10. Abraham WT, Fisher WG, Smith AL, et al: Cardiac resynchronization in chronic heart failure. *N Engl J Med* 2002;346:1845–1853.
11. Auricchio A, Stellbrink C, Sack S, et al: Long-term clinical effect of hemodynamically optimized cardiac resynchronization therapy in patients with heart failure and ventricular conduction delay. *J Am Coll Cardiol* 2002;39:2026–2033.
12. Stellbrink C, Breithardt OA, Franke A, et al: Impact of cardiac resynchronization therapy using hemodynamically optimized pacing on left ventricular remodeling in patients with congestive heart failure and ventricular conduction disturbances. *J Am Coll Cardiol* 2001;38:1957–1965.
13. Meisner JS, McQueen DM, Ishida Y, et al: Effects of timing of atrial systole on LV filling and mitral valve closure: computer and dog studies. *Am J Physiol* 1985;249:H604–H619.
14. Yellin EL, Nikolic S, Frater RWM: Left ventricular filling dynamics and diastolic function. *Prog Cardiovasc Dis* 1990;32:247–271.
15. Brecker SJ, Xiao HB, Sparrow J, et al: Effects of dual-chamber pacing with short atrioventricular delay in dilated cardiomyopathy. *Lancet* 1992;340:1308–1312.
16. Prinzen FW, Hunter WC, Wyman BT, et al: Mapping of regional myocardial strain and work during ventricular pacing: experimental study using magnetic resonance imaging tagging. *J Am Coll Cardiol* 1999;33:1735–1742.
17. Wyman BT, Hunter WC, Prinzen FW, et al: Mapping propagation of mechanical activation in the paced heart with MRI tagging. *Am J Physiol* 1999;276:H881–H891.
18. Burkhoff D, Oikawa RY, Sagawa K: Influence of pacing site on canine left ventricular contraction. *Am J Physiol* 1986;251:H428–H435.
19. Park RC, Little WC, O'Rourke RA: Effect of alteration of the left ventricular activation sequence on the left ventricular end-systolic pressure-volume relation in closed-chest dogs. *Circ Res* 1985; 57:706–717.

20. Leclercq C, Faris O, Tunin R, et al: Systolic improvement and mechanical resynchronization does not require electrical synchrony in the dilated failing heart with left bundle-branch block. *Circulation* 2002;106:1760–1763.
21. Park RC, Little WC, O'Rourke RA. Effect of alteration of left ventricular activation sequence on the left ventricular end-systolic pressure-volume relation in closed-chest dogs. *Circ Res* 1985;57:706–717.
22. Pak PH, Maughan WL, Baughman KL, et al: Mechanism of acute mechanical benefit from VDD pacing in hypertrophied heart: Similarity of responses in hypertrophic cardiomyopathy and hypertensive heart disease. *Circulation* 1998;98:242–248.
23. Eckardt L, Kirchhof P, Breithardt G, et al: Load-induced changes in repolarization: evidence from experimental and clinical data. *Basic Res Cardiol* 2001;96:369–380.
24. Taggart P, Sutton PM: Cardiac mechano-electric feedback in man: clinical relevance. *Prog Biophys Mol Biol* 1999;71:139–154.
25. Franz MR, Cima R, Wang D, et al: Electrophysiological effects of myocardial stretch and mechanical determinants of stretch-activated arrhythmias. *Circulation* 1992;86:968–978.
26. Crozatier B: Stretch-induced modifications of myocardial performance: from ventricular function to cellular and molecular mechanisms. *Cardiovasc Res* 1996;32:25–37.
27. Su JB, Hittinger L, Laplace M, et al: Loading determinants of isovolumic pressure fall in closed chest dogs. *Am J Physiol* 1991;260:H690–H697.
28. Gillebert TC, Brutsaert DL: Regulation of left ventricular pressure fall. *Eur Heart J* 1990;11 (Suppl I):124–132.
29. Gillebert TC, Sys SU, Brutsaert DL: Influence of loading patterns on peak length-tension relation and on relaxation in cardiac muscle. *J Am Coll Cardiol* 1989;13:483–490.
30. Prinzen FW, Augustijn CH, Arts T, et al: Redistribution of myocardial fiber strain and blood flow by asynchronous activation. *Am J Physiol* 1990;259:H300–H308.
31. Baller D, Wolpers HG, Zipfel J, et al: Comparison of the effects of right atrial, right ventricular apex and atrioventricular sequential pacing on myocardial oxygen consumption and cardiac efficiency: a laboratory investigation. *Pacing Clin Electrophysiol* 1988;11:394–403.
32. Owen CH, Esposito DJ, Davis JW, et al: The effects of ventricular pacing on left ventricular geometry, function, myocardial oxygen consumption, and efficiency of contraction in conscious dogs. *Pacing Clin Electrophysiol* 1998;21:1417–1429.
33. van Oosterhout MF, Arts T, Bassingthwaighte JB, et al: Relation between local myocardial growth and blood flow during chronic ventricular pacing. *Cardiovasc Res* 2002;53:831–840.
34. Blanc JJ, Etienne Y, Gilard M, et al: Evaluation of different ventricular pacing sites in patients with severe heart failure: results of an acute hemodynamic study. *Circulation* 1997;96:3273–3277.
35. Leclercq C, Cazeau S, Le Breton H, et al: Acute hemodynamic effects of biventricular DDD pacing in patients with end-stage heart failure. *J Am Coll Cardiol* 1998;32:1825–1831.
36. Auricchio A, Stellbrink C, Block M, et al: Effect of pacing chamber and atrioventricular delay on acute systolic function of paced patients with congestive heart failure. The Pacing Therapies for Congestive Heart Failure Study Group. The Guidant Congestive Heart Failure Research Group. *Circulation* 1999;99:2993–3001.
37. Kass DA, Chen CH, Curry C, et al: Improved left ventricular mechanics from acute VDD pacing in patients with dilated cardiomyopathy and ventricular conduction delay. *Circulation* 1999;99:1567–1573.
38. Nelson GS, Curry CW, Wyman BT, et al: Predictors of systolic augmentation from left ventricular preexcitation in patients with dilated cardiomyopathy and intraventricular conduction delay. *Circulation* 2000;101:2703–2709.
39. Yu CM, Chau E, Sanderson JE, et al: Tissue Doppler echocardiographic evidence of reverse remodeling and improved synchronicity by simultaneously delaying regional contraction after biventricular pacing therapy in heart failure. *Circulation* 2002;105:438–445.
40. Sogaard P, Egeblad H, Kim WY, et al: Tissue Doppler imaging predicts improved systolic performance and reversed left ventricular remodeling during long-term cardiac resynchronization therapy. *J Am Coll Cardiol* 2002;40:723–730.
41. Kawaguchi M, Murabayashi T, Fetics BJ, et al: Quantitation of basal dyssynchrony and acute resynchronization from left or biventricular pacing by novel echo-contrast variability imaging. *J Am Coll Cardiol* 2002;39:2052–2058.
42. Touiza A, Etienne Y, Gilard M, et al: Long-term left ventricular pacing: assessment and comparison with biventricular pacing in patients with severe congestive heart failure. *J Am Coll Cardiol* 2001;38:1966–1970.
43. Packer M, Carver JR, Rodeheffer RJ, et al: Effect of oral milrinone on mortality in severe chronic heart failure. The PROMISE Study Research Group. *N Engl J Med* 1991;325:1468–1475.

44. O'Connor CM, Gattis WA, Uretsky BF, et al: Continuous intravenous dobutamine is associated with an increased risk of death in patients with advanced heart failure: insights from the Flolan International Randomized Survival Trial (FIRST). *Am Heart J* 1999;138:78–86.

45. Capomolla S, Febo O, Opasich C, et al: Chronic infusion of dobutamine and nitroprusside in patients with end-stage heart failure awaiting heart transplantation: safety and clinical outcome. *Eur J Heart Fail* 2001;3:601–610.

46. Nelson GS, Berger RD, Fetics BJ, et al: Left ventricular or biventricular pacing improves cardiac function at diminished energy cost in patients with dilated cardiomyopathy and left bundle-branch block. *Circulation* 2000;102:3053–3059.

47. Ukkonen H, Beanlands RS, Burwash IG, et al: Effect of cardiac resynchronization on myocardial efficiency and regional oxidative metabolism. *Circulation* 2003;107:28–31.

48. Sogaard P, Egeblad H, Pedersen AK, et al: Sequential versus simultaneous biventricular resynchronization for severe heart failure: evaluation by tissue Doppler imaging. *Circulation* 2002;106:2078–2084.

49. Breithardt OA, Sinha AM, Schwammenthal E, et al: Acute effects of cardiac resynchronization therapy on functional mitral regurgitation in advanced systolic heart failure. *J Am Coll Cardiol* 2003;41:765–770.

50. Oguz E, Dagdeviren B, Bilsel T, et al: Echocardiographic prediction of long-term response to biventricular pacemaker in severe heart failure. *Eur J Heart Fail* 2002;4:83–90.

51. Pitzalis MV, Iacoviello M, Romito R, et al: Cardiac resynchronization therapy tailored by echocardiographic evaluation of ventricular asynchrony. *J Am Coll Cardiol* 2002;40:1615–1622.

52. Fauchier L, Marie O, Casset-Senon D, et al: Interventricular and intraventricular dyssynchrony in idiopathic dilated cardiomyopathy. A prognostic study with fourier phase analysis of radionuclide angioscintigraphy. *J Am Coll Cardiol* 2002;40:2022–2030.

53. Krahn AD, Snell L, Yee R, et al: Biventricular pacing improves quality of life and exercise tolerance in patients with heart failure and intraventricular conduction delay. *Can J Cardiol* 2002;18:380–387.

54. Reuter S, Garrigue S, Barold SS, et al: Comparison of characteristics in responders versus nonresponders with biventricular pacing for drug-resistant congestive heart failure. *Am J Cardiol* 2002;89:346–350.

55. Lunati M, Paolucci M, Oliva F, et al: Patient selection for biventricular pacing. *J Cardiovasc Electrophysiol* 2002;13:S63–S67.

56. Curry CC, Nelson GS, Wyman BT, et al: Mechanical dyssynchrony in dilated cardiomyopathy with intraventricular conduction delay as depicted by 3–D tagged magnetic resonance imaging. *Circulation* 2000;101:2.

57. Sogaard P, Kim WY, Jensen HK, et al: Impact of acute biventricular pacing on left ventricular performance and volumes in patients with severe heart failure. A tissue doppler and three–dimensional echocardiographic study. *Cardiology* 2001;95:173–182.

58. Butter C, Auricchio A, Stellbrink C, et al: Effect of resynchronization therapy stimulation site on the systolic function of heart failure patients. *Circulation* 2001;104:3026–3029.

# 3

# Clinical Trials of Resynchronization Therapy

### Kenneth A. Ellenbogen • Leslie A. Saxon

In this chapter we review the status of clinical trials with cardiac resynchronization therapy (CRT). The concept of this therapy has evolved through three distinct stages. In the first stage, from 1990 to 1997, a number of acute and a few intermediate-term observational studies of CRT were conducted. In the second stage, several pivotal studies were performed and completed between 1997 and 2000 that measured the effect of CRT on exercise capacity, functional status, and quality of life. The third stage of the evolution of CRT, from 2000 to the present, is characterized by the continuation and/or completion of several large-scale randomized trials of CRT and its effects on endpoints of mortality and hospitalizations, including nonelective hospitalization for heart failure. The status of each of the major clinical trials is summarized in Table 3–1.

A brief mention of several of the early observational studies of biventricular pacing is timely. A number of these studies have been presented in abstract form only and are not discussed in detail. An early report in 1994 from Cazeau and colleagues in France described acute and 6-week follow-up of a single patient with New York Heart Association (NYHA) functional class IV heart failure who experienced significant clinical improvement after undergoing four-chamber pacing, with a left ventricular (LV) epicardial lead to provide LV pacing.[1] Several other groups, including Bakker et al., studied the acute and short-term effects of biventricular pacing.[2-4] These reports include the description by Daubert et al. of a small group of patients with end-stage heart failure followed for a mean of 7.5 months who underwent biventricular pacing with a transvenous LV lead.[5] A large prospective multicenter feasibility registry was undertaken in the mid-1990s. The InSync registry was initiated at European and Canadian sites investigating the safety and efficacy of biventricular pacing.[6,7] Between August 1997 and November 1998, 117 patients were enrolled. Inclusion criteria for the patients studied included NYHA functional classes III and IV during medical therapy, QRS duration >150 msec, left ventricular ejection fraction (LVEF) <35%, LVend-diastolic dimension >60 mm, and stable medical therapy for 1 month or more.

TABLE 3–1. **Overview of Status and Enrollment of Major Clinical Trials in CRT Therapy**

|            | NYHA   | QRS    | Sinus  | ICD? | Status    |
|------------|--------|--------|--------|------|-----------|
| MIRACLE    | III, IV | ≥130   | Normal | No   | Published |
| MUSTIC SR  | III    | >150   | Normal | No   | Published |
| MUSTIC AF  | III    | >200*  | AF     | No   | Published |
| PATH CHF   | III, IV | ≥120   | Normal | No   | Published |
| CONTAK CD  | II–IV  | ≥120   | Normal | Yes  | Published |
| MIRACLE ICD | II–IV | ≥130   | Normal | Yes  | Published |
| PATH-CHF II | III, IV | ≥120  | Normal | No   | Published |
| CARE HF    | III, IV | ≥120†  | Normal | No   | Complete  |
| COMPANION  | III, IV | ≥120   | Normal | No   | Presented |
| InSync III | III, IV | ≥130   | Normal | No   | Presented |

*If QRS is paced.
†Plus a measure of dyssynchrony.

Patients underwent baseline and follow-up evaluations, with quality of life measured by means of the Minnesota Living with Heart Failure questionnaire and on the basis of distance covered during a 6-minute walk test. Echocardiographic measurements were determined for a subset of 46 patients. Transvenous implantation of an LV lead was successful in 103 of 117 patients (88%). The atrioventricular (AV) pacing interval was individually adjusted to optimize hemodynamic function on the basis of Doppler echocardiographic measurements. Clinical outcome measures were obtained at 1, 3, 6, and 12 months after implantation and included NYHA functional class, QRS duration, 6-minute walking distance, and quality of life. Over a period of 1 year, 21 patients died, resulting in an actual survival rate of 78% (confidence interval [CI]: 70% to 87%). Significant improvements in mean NYHA functional class, 6-minute walking distance, and quality of life were observed.

For the 46 patients for whom echocardiographic data were available, LVEF increased from $21.7 \pm 6.4\%$ (mean ± standard deviation) at baseline to $26.1 \pm 9.0\%$ at last follow-up ($P = 0.006$), LV end-diastolic dimension decreased from $72.7 \pm 9.2$ to $71.6 \pm 9.1$ mm ($P = 0.233$), interventricular mechanical delay decreased from $27.5 \pm 32.1$ to $20.3 \pm 25.5$ msec ($P = 0.243$), mitral regurgitation (MR) area decreased from $7.66 \pm 5.5$ to $6.69 \pm 5.9$ cm$^2$ ($P = 0.197$), and LV filling time increased from $363 \pm 127$ to $408 \pm 111$ msec ($P = 0.002$). It is noteworthy that 25 patients were too sick to perform a 6-minute walk test at baseline because of the severity of heart failure, and on follow-up 19 of these 25 patients were able to perform the 6-minute walk test, scoring an average of $395 \pm 130$ meters (range: 100–700 meters). Additional registry information comes from the Italian InSync Registry.[8] They enrolled 190 patients from 39 centers who were followed prospectively after implantation of a biventricular pacemaker. The results from the Italian InSync registry were similar to the results reported from the main registry.

The second stage of experience with CRT is marked by reports of several prospective randomized studies of larger numbers of patients. This phase of CRT is marked by a movement away from observational studies toward prospective, randomized trials. The hallmark of these trials is a period with no pacing, by programming the CRT device to either OVO or backup VVI pacing at 30–40 bpm (e.g., in the "placebo" arm). These trials were instrumental in providing the scientific data that convinced the regulatory bodies in the United States and Europe to grant approval for these devices.

Several additional remarks should be made about these trials. Patients studied were required to be stable without pressors for at least 1 month. Patients were also required to be receiving optimal medical therapy for congestive heart failure (CHF), which included administration of diuretics, angiotensin-converting enzyme (ACE) inhibitors or angiotensin receptor blockers, digitalis preparations, beta-adrenergic blockers, and aldosterone receptor blockers. Finally, in all studies except for the Multisite Stimulation in Cardiomyopathy (MUSTIC) trial, patients with CHF who received devices did not meet any of the conventional indications for device implantation, such as symptomatic bradycardia.

The Pacing Therapies in Congestive Heart Failure (PATH-CHF I) trial was begun in 1995 and completed in 1998.[9-11] It was performed in Europe and included patients with NYHA class III–IV CHF, sinus rate >55 bpm, and QRS duration greater than 120 msec. Forty-two patients were studied, and the LV lead was placed surgically (e.g., epicardially). This trial was unique in its design (Figure 3–1). It was a single-blind study. Patients underwent surgical implantation of the LV lead and at the time of device implantation underwent hemodynamic study. Acute hemodynamic data, consisting of aortic pulse pressure +dP/dt, were measured at different AV intervals and then analyzed later to determine the optimal univentricular pacing site and the optimal AV interval for the best univentricular and biventricular stimulation. Patients also received two separate DDD pacemakers: one connected to a right atrial and right ventricular (RV) lead and the other connected to another right atrial lead and an epicardial LV pacing lead. This study design allowed for a change in pacing site from RV to LV and then to biventricular pacing during long-term follow-up. Biventricular pacing was achieved by programming one device in the VDD mode and the second device in the VVT mode. Patients were then randomized to 1 month of optimized univentricular or biventricular pacing, followed by 1 month of no pacing.

During the third month of the protocol, the patients crossed over to the other pacing mode. After 3 months all patients were paced in the mode that provided the optimal acute response during intra-operative testing. Pacing was continued for the ensuing year. The follow-up was at 1, 2, 3, and 12 months. All patients studied were in sinus rhythm. The functional capacity of the patients was assessed by a physician blinded to the pacing mode. Echocardiographic findings at 6 months were also compared to baseline findings. The primary endpoints were improvement in functional capacity, as measured by peak oxygen consumption and 6-minute walking distance. The secondary endpoints were quality of life, as measured by the Minnesota Living with Heart Failure score, need for recurrent hospitalization, and NYHA functional class.

This trial demonstrated a 25% improvement in 6-minute walking time with the optimized pacing mode ($357 \pm 20$ m to $446 \pm 15$ m, $P < 0.001$), a 59% improvement in quality of life ($48.6 \pm 4.3$ to $20 \pm 4.1$; $P < 0.001$), a 24% improvement in peak oxygen consumption ($12.57 \pm 0.63$ to $15.63 \pm 0.86$ ml/kg/min, $P < 0.001$). Exercise performance improved significantly only during the two periods of active pacing. Continuous CRT was associated with sustained hemodynamic improvement at 12 months that was not different from the changes measured at 3 months. Twenty-one of 29 patients followed to 12 months improved from NYHA functional class III/IV to class I/II. LV volumes and dimensions decreased during the 6-month

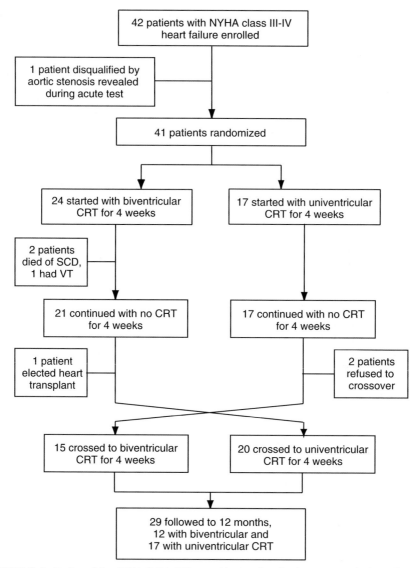

**FIGURE 3–1.** Design of the PATH-CHF I. SCD = sudden cardiac death; VT = ventricular tachycardia. *(Reproduced from Auricchio A, Stellbrink C, Sack S, et al: The Pacing Therapies for Congestive Heart Failure (PATH-CLIF) Study: Rationale, design, and endpoints of a prospective randomized multicenter study.* Am J Cardiol *1999;83:130–135D, with permission from* The American College of Cardiology Foundation.)

follow-up, and ejection fraction increased with hemodynamically optimized pacing. There was no difference in fractional shortening, LV mass, sphericity index, or heart rate change with pacing in comparison with baseline. Hospitalization for heart failure was reduced from the year prior to implantation (76%) to 31% during the year following implantation. Limitations of this trial include the fact that the majority of patients had heart failure due to nonischemic cardiomyopathy, and only 60% of patients received beta-blockers. This was the first study to show that clinical effects of LV stimulation alone were similar to those provided by biventricular stimulation. In fact, there were no demonstrable differences between hemodynamically optimized biventricular and LV pacing.

The results of the PATH-CHF II trial were recently published. In this trial, 86 patients with NYHA class II–IV CHF, LV ejection fraction less than 30%, and peak oxygen consumption less than 18 ml/kg per minute on maximum exercise testing who were also in sinus rhythm were eligible for enrollment (Figure 3–2). Half of the patients had a QRS duration between 120 and 150 msec (short) and the other half had a QRS duration greater than 150 msec (long). Patients were stratified into long and short QRS groups on the basis of QRS duration. Patients underwent an invasive procedure to evaluate their acute hemodynamic response to pacing and to select the best site for permanent ventricular pacing. The device was implanted in a second procedure. All patients received either a pacemaker or an implantable cardioverter-defibrillator (ICD), depending on clinical indications. Early in the trial patients received an epicardial lead, and later they received the Guidant EASYTRAK endocardial lead. At baseline and after each crossover period, patients underwent a maximum bicycle exercise test to measure peak oxygen consumption and oxygen consumption at anaerobic threshold, submaximal exercise test with a 6-minute walk, quality-of-life assessment by the Minnesota Living with Heart Failure questionnaire, and evaluation of NYHA functional class.

Patients from nine centers were enrolled in the trial between September 1998 and January 2001.[12] The study design was a 6-month randomized crossover comparing 3 months of active pacing (univentricular) with 3 months of inactive pacing at a lower rate of 40 bpm, with the two pacing modes in random order for each patient. Three patients who received RV pacing for right bundle branch block (RBBB) were excluded from analysis. Optimal medical therapy consisted

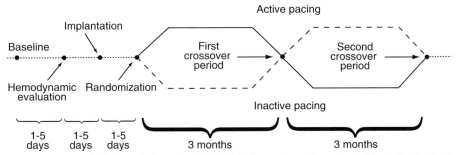

**FIGURE 3–2.** Study design of the PATH-CHF II trial. *(Reproduced from Auricchio A, Stellbrink C, Butter C, et al: Clinical efficacy of cardiac resynchronization therapy using left ventricular pacing in heart failure patients stratified by severity of ventricular conduction delay. J Am Coll Cardiol 2003 [in press], with permission from The American College of Cardiology Foundation.)*

of administration of ACE inhibitors or angiotensin II receptor blockers to 99% of patients and beta-blockers to 73%. The best univentricular pacing mode was LV pacing for all 85 patients with left bundle branch block (LBBB) or nonspecific intraventricular conduction defect (IVCD) and for one patient with RBBB. The best LV pacing site was in a lateral or posterior vein.

Seventeen patients did not complete the two crossover periods, and three patients were withdrawn following randomization (one had misplaced leads, another received an LV assist device, and the third received an ICD and a pacemaker). Five patients dropped out during an active pacing period: two had sudden cardiac death, two were unwilling to comply with the study protocol, and one had a left-sided pleural effusion related to epicardial lead placement. Nine patients dropped out during an inactive pacing period: two died (sudden cardiac death), one developed ventricular tachycardia, one developed atrial arrhythmias, one developed bronchitis requiring frequent hospitalization, three developed acute heart failure (two were switched to active pacing and one received an LV assist device), and one died (nonsudden cardiac death).

For the 69 patients who completed the crossover period, the results showed an improvement in NYHA class with active pacing of 0.25 points ($P = 0.001$, CI: 0.11–0.38), improvement in quality of life score with active pacing of 4.7 points ($P = 0.015$, CI: 0.9–8.5 points), improvement of 26 m during the 6-minute walk test ($P = 0.021$, 95% CI: 5–48 m), increase in peak oxygen uptake of 1.37 ml/kg per minute ($P < 0.001$, CI: 0.76–1.99 ml/kg per minute) and oxygen uptake at anaerobic threshold of 0.87 ml/kg per minute ($P < 0.001$, CI: 0.40–1.35 ml/kg per minute). The clinical effects of active pacing were most marked in the long QRS group (Figure 3–3). For example, 71% of the patients in the long QRS group and 38% of the patients in the short QRS group had an increase in peak oxygen uptake of more than 1 ml/kg per minute with active pacing. The short QRS group did not have an improvement in peak oxygen uptake or any other endpoint measure.

The Vigor in Congestive Heart Failure (VIGOR-CHF) trial was a prospective randomized sequential trial involving patients with heart failure designed to evaluate the effects of CRT[13,14] (Figure 3–4). Patients underwent epicardial placement of an LV lead. The study consisted of two short-term therapy phases of 6 weeks each and an additional pacing therapy mode for 6 weeks, until the week-18 visit, at which time the physician could decide which pacing mode to employ for long-term therapy. Randomization occurred about 2 weeks after implantation, at the time of a postoperative visit; some patients were randomized to VDD pacing during the first and second 6-week pacing phases, and another patient group was assigned to no pacing (ODO) in the first period and the VDD pacing mode during the second period. Randomization was blocked by each center with a 2:1 ratio (ODO:VDD mode). The primary study endpoint was peak oxygen uptake during maximal exercise, and the secondary endpoints included 6-minute walking distance, quality of life assessment, and hemodynamic status, as assessed by echocardiography. The trial was terminated prior to completion because of declining enrollment, when a transvenous lead became available in competing clinical trials.

Saxon and colleagues published data from this trial on the effects of biventricular stimulation for resynchronization on echocardiographic measures of remodeling. Echocardiographic data from 53 patients taken at the time of randomization, at 6 weeks, and after 12 weeks of CRT were analyzed. There was no change in heart rate or QRS duration after 12 weeks. Serum norepinephrine levels

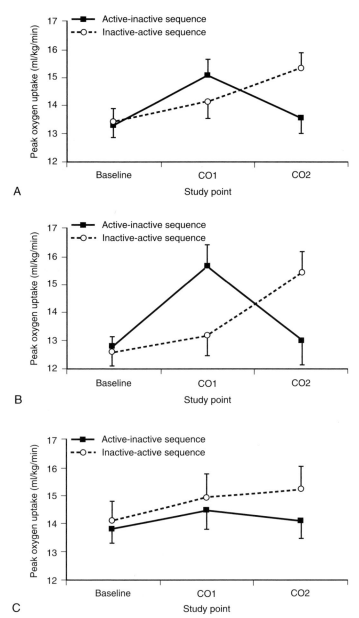

**FIGURE 3–3.** Peak oxygen uptake at each evaluation point during the study. CO1 is the first crossover period and CO2 is the second crossover period. *A*, Mean peak oxygen uptake (*bars* = standard error of the mean) for patients in the active first and inactive first pacing sequences. *B*, Same as panel *A* for the subset of patients in the long QRS group (QRS > 150 msec). *C*, Same as in panel *A* for the subset of patients in the short QRS group (120 < QRS < 150 msec). *(Reproduced with permission from Auricchio A, Stellbrink C, Butter C, et al: Clinical efficacy of cardiac resynchronization therapy using left ventricular pacing in heart failure patients stratified by severity of ventricular conduction delay. J Am Coll Cardiol 2003 [in press].)*

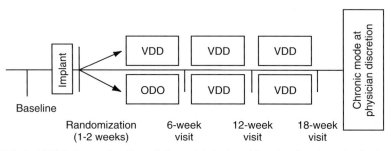

**FIGURE 3–4.** VIGOR Congestive Heart Failure trial design. After the first 6 weeks, both patient groups receive active pacing therapy.

did not change with CRT. LV and left atrial volumes decreased, whereas the LV sphericity index was unchanged (Figure 3–5). Measurements of LV systolic function, including LV outflow tract and aortic velocity time integral, and myocardial performance index improved. The severity or grade of mitral regurgitation improved as well as mitral deceleration, a measure of diastolic LV function.

The MUSTIC trial was the first multicenter randomized, controlled trial in which all patients received transvenous LV pacing with a biventricular pacing system.[15-18] The trial design was a randomized crossover type (Figure 3–6). Two groups of patients were studied: one included 67 patients with sinus rhythm and the second included 43 patients with atrial fibrillation (AF). The study design for both groups was identical. Patients underwent implantation of a CRT pacemaker. Two weeks later they were randomized to resynchronization therapy "on" and "off" groups. Three months later they crossed over to the other therapy. Following completion of the trial, patients were left in the pacing mode they preferred and then followed up for 1 year. The primary endpoint was the 6-minute walk test result. Secondary endpoints were quality of life (measured by the Minnesota heart failure score), oxygen consumption, hospitalization for heart failure, mortality, and patient preference for a particular pacing mode.

Patients enrolled in the sinus rhythm portion of this clinical trial had NYHA class III CHF with a QRS duration of greater than 150 msec. Successful implantation of a transvenous lead at a target site was achieved in 80% of patients, with access to the LV veins achieved in 88%. Patients with biventricular pacing demonstrated a 23% improvement in 6-minute walk distance (Figure 3–7), 32% improvement in quality of life (Figure 3–8), 8% improvement in peak oxygen uptake, and 7.5% improvement in mortality at 7.5 months. At the end of the crossover phase, patients (blinded to their treatment) were asked to choose which period they preferred. Eighty-five percent of patients preferred the 3-month period in which they were programmed to active pacing (VDD), 4% preferred the period of no pacing (ODO), and 10% had no preference. Ten patients did not complete the two crossover periods: two lost LV capture, four patients had severe decompensation during the ODO period, one patient died suddenly, one patient withdrew consent, one patient died of an acute myocardial infarction, and one patient withdrew after the diagnosis of lung cancer. This was the first published report of a clinical trial involving patients with severe heart failure and CRT that showed an improvement in exercise tolerance and quality of life.

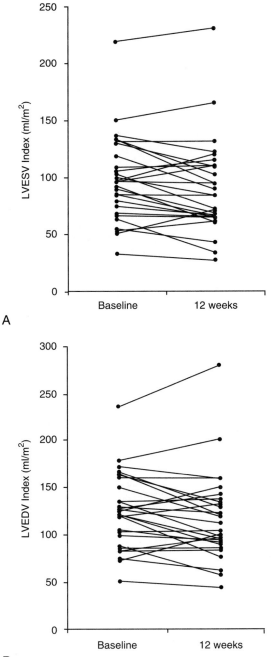

**FIGURE 3–5.**  Individual changes in *A,* LV end-systolic (ES) volume (V) index; *B,* LV end-diastolic (ED) volume index;                                                                    *Continued*

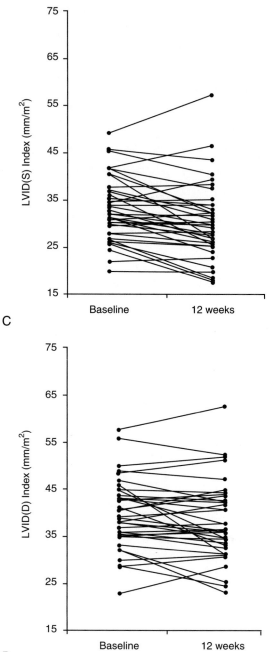

C

D

FIGURE 3–5, Cont'd. *C, D* dimension (D) indexrom the VIGOR trial. ID(S) = LV internal dimension (diastole); ID(D) = LV internal dimension (systole). *(Reproduced with permission from Saxon LA, Marco TD, Schafer J,et al: Effects of long-term biventricular stimulation for resynchronization on echocardiographic measures of remodeling.* Circulation *2002;105:1304–1310.)*

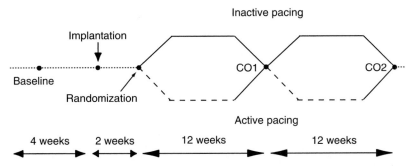

**FIGURE 3–6.** MUSTIC study design. Patients were randomly assigned to 3 months each of inactive pacing (ventricular, inhibited at a basic rate of 40 bpm) and active pacing (atriobiventricular). CO1 denotes the end of crossover period 1 and CO2 the end of crossover period 2. *(Reprinted from Cazeau S, Leclercq C, Lavergne T, et al: Effects of multisite biventricular pacing in patients with heart failure and intraventricular conduction delay. N Engl J Med 2001;344:873–880, with permission from Massachusetts Medical Society.)*

MUSTIC-AF was a substudy of the MUSTIC trial that involved patients with chronic AF, a slow ventricular rate, and NYHA class III CHF and patients with an implanted pacemaker with a wide QRS duration during RV pacing greater than 200 msec.[17] The trial was designed as a single-blinded, randomized, controlled crossover study comparing two 3-month treatment periods of conventional RV apical pacing versus transvenous biventricular pacing. The primary endpoint was the 6-minute walk test result, and secondary endpoints were peak oxygen uptake, quality of life, hospitalizations, patients' preferred study period, and mortality. There was a

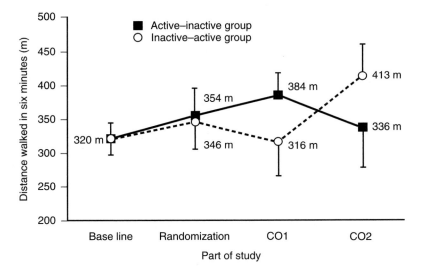

**FIGURE 3–7.** Distance walked in 6 minutes at specified times during the study. The mean (±SD) values are given for each part of the study. *(Used with permission from Cazeau S, Leclercq C, Lavergne T, et al: Effects of multisite biventricular pacing in patients with heart failure and intraventricular conduction delay. N Engl J Med 2001;344:873–880.)*

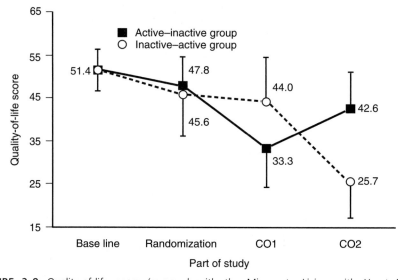

**FIGURE 3–8.** Quality-of-life score (assessed with the Minnesota Living with Heart Failure questionnaire) at specified times during the study. The mean (±SD) values are given for each phase of the study. *(Used with permission from Cazeau S, Leclercq C, Lavergne T, et al: Effects of multisite biventricular pacing in patients with heart failure and intraventricular conduction delay.* N Engl J Med *2001;344:873–880.)*

higher-than-expected dropout rate during this study, of 42%: only 37 of 59 patients completed the protocol. Of the 22 dropouts, 5 left prior to pacemaker implantation, 6 left because of the inability to adequately position an LV lead, 2 died of CHF, 1 died suddenly, 4 met exclusion criteria with respect to QRS duration, and several others dropped out for a variety of other reasons. On the basis of an intention to treat analysis, there was no statistically significant difference in primary or secondary endpoints. In the patients with "effective" therapy, the mean distance walked improved by 9.3% with CRT ($P = 0.05$), and peak oxygen uptake increased by 13% ($P = 0.04$). The hospitalization rate was very low. When the entire 6-month crossover phase is considered, 10 of 44 patients were hospitalized for heart failure decompensation during RV pacing, and only 3 patients were hospitalized for heart failure during the CRT period. Eighty-five percent of the patients preferred the CRT period ($P < 0.001$). There was a trend toward a better quality of life among patients with CRT, but it did not reach statistical significance (11% improvement, $P = 0.09$). QRS duration decreased by a mean of 18% in patients with CRT.

The MUSTIC trial also reported long-term follow-up of CRT.[18] Follow-up of 42 of 67 patients in sinus rhythm and 33 of 64 in atrial fibrillation took place over a 12-month period, and assessments included 6-minute walking distance, peak oxygen uptake, quality-of-life score, NYHA functional class, and LV ejection fraction by radionuclide measurement and echocardiography (Figure 3–9). At 12 months all patients in sinus rhythm and 88% of the patients with atrial fibrillation remained and were programmed to biventricular pacing. The clinical improvements in the 6-minute walking distance (20% increase over baseline in sinus rhythm [$P = 0.0001$]

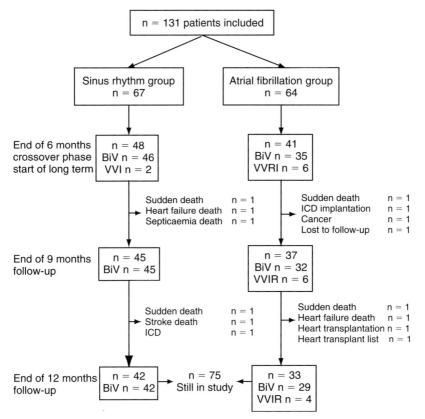

**FIGURE 3–9.** Study profile: number of patients active in the study at each follow-up between inclusion and the 12 months in the sinus rhythm (*A*) and atrial fibrillation (*B*) groups. BiV = biventricular; ICD = implantable cardioverter-defibrillator; VVI = ventricular inhibited pacing; VVIR = rate-adaptive ventricular inhibited pacing. *(Reprinted from Linde C, Leclercq C, Rex S, et al: Long-term benefits of biventricular pacing in congestive heart failure: Results from the Multisite Stimulation in Cardiomyopathy (MUSTIC) study. J Am Coll Card 2002;40:111–118, with permission from The American College of Cardiology Foundation.)*

and 17% increase in atrial fibrillation [$P = 0.004$]), peak oxygen consumption (increased over baseline by 11% in sinus rhythm and by 9% in atrial fibrillation), quality of life (36% improvement in sinus rhythm [$P = 0.0001$] and 32% improvement in atrial fibrillation [$P = 0.002$]), and NYHA functional class (25% improvement in sinus rhythm [$P = 0.0001$] and 27% improvement in atrial fibrillation [$P = 0.00001$]) were maintained at 12 months (Table 3–2). Improvements in the degree of mitral regurgitation (45% decrease in mitral regurgitation during sinus rhythm and 50% decrease during atrial fibrillation) and in ejection fraction (5% increase in sinus rhythm and 4% in atrial fibrillation) were maintained at 12 months also (Table 3–3).

The next large multicenter trial of CRT was the Multicenter InSync Randomized Clinical Evaluation (MIRACLE trial).[19] This trial was a randomized parallel design (Figure 3–10). Four hundred fifty-three patients with NYHA class III–IV CHF were enrolled. Patients were required to have a QRS duration of

TABLE 3–2. **Long-Term Results from MUSTIC**

| | Randomization | M6 | Sinus Rhythm Group M9 | M12 |
|---|---|---|---|---|
| 6-min walked distance (m) | 354 ± 92 (n = 43) | 396 ± 104 (n = 43) | | |
| | 346 ± 96 (n = 38) | | 411 ± 113 (n = 38) | |
| | 348 ± 98 (n = 38) | | | 418 ± 112 (n = 38) p = 0.0001 |
| Peak VO$_2$ (ml/kg/min) | 14.2 ± 4.6 (n = 41) | 15.5 ± 4.6 (n = 41) | NA | |
| | 14.9 ± 4.7 (n = 32) | | | 16.6 ± 3.6 (n = 32) p = NS |
| QoL score (0–105) | 47 ± 22 (n = 46) | 31 ± 22 (n = 46) | | |
| | 45 ± 21 (n = 41) | | 30 ± 20 (n = 41) | |
| | 47 ± 23 (n = 41) | | | 30 ± 22 (n = 41) p = 0.0001 |
| NYHA (I–IV) | 2.8 ± 0.4 (n = 46) | 2.1 ± 0.5 (n = 46) | | |
| | 2.8 ± 0.4 (n = 40) | | 2.1 ± 0.4 (n = 40) | |
| | 2.8 ± 0.4 (n = 41) | | | 2.1 ± 0.5 (n = 41) p = 0.0001 |

| | Randomization | M6 | Atrial Fibrillation Group M9 | M12 |
|---|---|---|---|---|
| 6-min walked distance (m) | 338 ± 87 (n = 37) | 363 ± 101 (n = 37) | | |
| | 320 ± 82 (n = 27) | | 368 ± 97 (n = 27) | |
| | 315 ± 80 (n = 27) | | | 370 ± 87 (n = 27) p = 0.004 |
| Peak VO$_2$ (ml/kg/min) | 12.8 ± 4.7 (n = 37) | 14.3 ± 4.1 (n = 37) | NA | |
| | 12.8 ± 3.6 (n = 24) | | | 13.9 ± 3.5 (n = 24) p = NS |
| QoL score (0–105) | 44 ± 22 (n = 40) | 34 ± 20 (n = 40) | | |
| | 45 ± 22 (n = 31) | | 34 ± 22 (n = 31) | |
| | 45 ± 23 (n = 28) | | | 31 ± 17 (n = 28) p = 0.002 |
| NYHA (I–IV) | 3.0 ± 0 (n = 38) | 2.3 ± 0.5 (n = 38) | | |
| | 3.0 ± 0 (n = 29) | | 2.1 ± 0.4 (n = 29) | 2.2 ± 0 5 (n = 28) p = 0.0001 |
| | 3.0 ± 0 (n = 28) | | | |

M6 = 6 months; M9 = 9 months; M12 = 12 months; NA = not applicable; NS = nonsignificant (p > 0.0125 Bonferroni adjustment); NYHA = New York Heart Association; QoL = quality of life.
Reproduced from Linde C, Leclercq C, Rex S, et al: Long-term benefits of biventricular pacing in congestive heart failure: Results from the Multisite Stimulation in Cardiomyopathy (MUSTIC) study. *J Am Coll Card* 2002;40:111–118, with permission from *The American College of Cardiology Foundation.*

130 msec or greater, an LV ejection fraction of less than 35%, and a 6-minute walking distance of less than 450 m and to be receiving appropriate CHF therapy. The primary endpoints were the NYHA functional class, quality-of-life score, and 6-minute walking distance. Secondary endpoints included peak oxygen uptake, treadmill time, LV ejection fraction, LV end-diastolic dimension, severity of MR, QRS duration, clinical composite response (one of three response groups: improved, worsened, or unchanged), death or worsening heart failure, and number of days spent in the hospital. Results at the 6-month follow-up were reported in the literature.

Patients who underwent CRT had a 13% improvement in 6-minute walking distance (*P* = 0.005), 13% improvement in quality of life (*P* = 0.001), and improvement in functional class (*P* < 0.001; Figures 3–11 and 3–12). Differences in favor of CRT were apparent as early as after 1 month of treatment. The degree of improvement was maintained without attenuation during the entire 6-month study period. The magnitude of primary endpoints was not influenced by the use of beta-blockers, etiology of CHF (ischemic versus nonischemic), QRS configuration (LBBB versus RBBB), or baseline QRS duration. Secondary endpoints were also improved with CRT. An improvement in peak oxygen consumption of about 1 ml/kg per minute ($P = 0.009$), increase in total exercise time of approximately 60 seconds ($P = 0.001$), and improvement in clinical composite score ($P < 0.001$) were noted. The LV ejection fraction increased and the end-diastolic dimension and area of the MR jet decreased in patients undergoing CRT. There was a trend toward fewer hospitalizations for patients with CRT (Table 3–4). Plasma neurohormonal levels are shown in Table 3–5.

Unlike previous studies that analyzed only those patients completing the 6-month randomization period, the composite response accounts for the status of all patients randomized. Sixty-seven percent of the CRT patients showed improvement in their composite response at 6 months, in comparison with 39% of the control group, but the composite response of 16% of the CRT patients (versus 27% of control patients) was considered to have worsened ($P < 0.001$). A patient's condition was considered improved if the functional class changed by one or more levels (as determined by the [blinded to pacing mode] heart failure physician) or if there was moderate or marked improvement in the global assessment score. A patient's condition was considered worsened on the basis of any of the following occurrences: death, hospitalization for worsening CHF since implantation, crossover from the assigned group because of worsening heart failure, withdrawal of consent, worsening of NYHA functional class, or moderately/markedly worse ranking in the global assessment.

Echocardiographic results were recently reported by the MIRACLE Study Group.[20] Echocardiographic studies performed after 3 and 6 months of therapy were performed for 172 patients randomized to CRT and 151 patients randomized to CRT "off." At 6 months, CRT was associated with a reduction in LV end-diastolic and end-systolic volumes (both $P < 0.001$), reduced LV mass ($-12.0$ g versus 10.6 g, $P < 0.01$), and increased ejection fraction (3.6% versus 0.6%, $P < 0.001$; Figures 3–13 and 3–14). MR was reduced ($-2.5$ cm$^2$ versus 0.5 cm$^2$ jet area, $P < 0.001$), and improvement in the myocardial performance index was noted in comparison with controls ($P < 0.001$). Beta-blocker treatment status did not influence the outcome or effect of CRT, but patients with nonischemic cardiomyopathy had twofold greater improvement in LV end-diastolic volume (LVEDV) and ejection fraction from baseline to 6 months than did patients with ischemic cardiomyopathy (Figure 3–15). Significant but weak correlations were observed between changes in clinical outcomes and changes in echocardiographic parameters.

Clinical trials of patients receiving biventricular pacing and ICD (CRT-D) therapy have been reported only in abstract form. The InSync ICD and CONTAK Cardiac Defibrillator (CD) trials were completed in 2001. These trials included patients of NYHA class II–IV receiving optimal drug therapy for CHF in sinus rhythm and met conventional (pre–MADIT II) criteria for implantation of an ICD. Trial design was similar for both studies (Figure 3–16). The majority of patients enrolled in both trials had heart failure of ischemic etiology. The U.S. Food and Drug Administration (FDA) approved CRT-D on the basis of an analysis of trial data for patients of NYHA functional class III–IV only. At the time of this writing, these devices have not been approved for NYHA class II patients.

TABLE 3–3. Echocardiographic Data and Ejection Fraction for the Sinus Rhythm Group and the Atrial Fibrillation Group at M6, M9, and M12

| | Randomization | Sinus Rhythm Group M6 | M9 | M12 |
|---|---|---|---|---|
| LVEDD (mm) | 74 ± 9 (n = 46)<br>73 ± 9 (n = 42)<br>74 ± 10 (n = 40) | 69 ± 11 (n = 46) | 68 ± 10 (n = 42) | 67 ± 12 (n = 40) |
| LVESD (mm) | 64 ± 10 (n = 46)<br>64 ± 10 (n = 42)<br>63 ± 10 (n = 40) | 58 ± 12 (n = 46) | 57 ± 11 (n = 42) | 58 ± 12 (n = 40) |
| MR area (cm²) | 7.4 ± 6.8 (n = 44)<br>8.0 ± 7.8 (n = 39)<br>7.8 ± 7.8 (n = 39) | 5.6 ± 8.3 (n = 44) | 4.9 ± 4.6 (n = 39) | 4.3 ± 4.0 (n = 39) |
| DFT (ms) | 376 ± 134 (n = 44)<br>372 ± 132 (n = 42)<br>375 ± 136 (n = 40) | 430 ± 137 (n = 44) | 471 ± 154 (n = 42) | 425 ± 129 (n = 40) |
| LVEF (%) radionuclides | 24.5 ± 7.8 (n = 26) | NA | NA | 30.0 ± 12.1 (n = 26) |
| CT ratio | 0.60 ± 0.07 (n = 41)<br>0.59 ± 0.07 (n = 34)<br>0.60 ± 0.07 (n = 36) | 0.60 ± 0.07 (n = 41) | 0.56 ± 0.06 (n = 34) | 0.56 ± 0.06 (n = 36) |

|  | Randomization | Atrial Fibrillation Group | | |
|  |  | M6 | M9 | M12 |
| --- | --- | --- | --- | --- |
| LVEDD (mm) | 69 ± 8 (n = 28) <br> 70 ± 9 (n = 28) | NA | 68 ± 10 (n = 28) | 68 ± 8 (n = 28) |
| LVESD (mm) | 59 ± 9 (n = 28) <br> 60 ± 10 (n = 28) | NA | 56 ± 11 (n = 28) | 58 ± 9 (n = 28) |
| MR area (cm$^2$) | 10.2 ± 13.7 (n = 27) <br> 10.8 ± 13.7 (n = 26) | NA | 6.4 ± 6.2 (n = 27) | 5.4 ± 3.9 (n = 26) |
| DFT (msec) | 349 ± 95 (n = 27) <br> 346 ± 99 (n = 24) | NA | 357 ± 133 (n = 27) | 405 ± 143 (n = 24) |
| LVEF (%) radionuclides | 26.7 ± 6.9 (n = 19) | NA | NA | 30.4 ± 7.8 (n = 19) |
| CT ratio | 0.61 ± 0.07 (n = 36) <br> 0.61 ± 0.07 (n = 26) <br> 0.61 ± 0.07 (n = 27) | 0.60 ± 0.07 (n = 36) | 0.60 ± 0.06 (n = 26) | 0.60 ± 0.07 (n = 27) |

M6 = 6 months; M9 = 9 months; M12 = 12 months; NA = not applicable

Reproduced from Linde C, Leclercq C, Rex S, et al: Long-term benefits of biventricular pacing in congestive heart failure: Results from the Multisite Stimulation in Cardiomyopathy (MUSTIC) study. *J Am Coll Card* 2002;40:111–118, with permission from *The American College of Cardiology Foundation.*

MIRACLE Program: Study Design

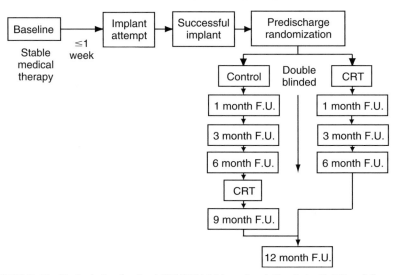

FIGURE 3–10. Study design for the MIRACLE trial (see description in text). F.U. = follow-up.

The CONTAK CD study was originally called the VENTAK CHF biventricular pacing study and enrolled patients with epicardial LV leads. Later, the study protocol was modified to add the CONTAK CD/EASYTRAK lead system and the study name was changed to the VENTAK CHF/CONTAK CD biventricular pacing study. The study is now commonly referred to as the CONTAK CD study for shorthand, because that was the device for which approval was sought. Only 53 patients received a nontransvenous system. The original study (phase I) was of a crossover design with two 3-month observation periods and endpoints of peak oxygen consumption, 6-minute walking distance, and quality of life. The study design was later modified (phase II) at the request of the FDA because of regulatory concerns about the length of follow-up in the randomized mode. No changes were made to the study's eligibility criteria. Study design was changed from a crossover to a parallel design. The primary endpoint was changed from peak oxygen consumption to a composite endpoint consisting of events associated with worsening heart failure. A total of 581 patients were enrolled at 47 investigational centers in the United States between February 1998 and December 2000. Fourteen patients withdrew informed consent or did not meet eligibility criteria, 66 patients did not receive an investigational system because the coronary venous lead could not be placed and instead received a conventional ICD system. Thus 501 patients were implanted with the investigational system.

Phase I included 222 patients (51 with epicardial leads), and 279 were enrolled in phase II (two patients received epicardial leads).[21,22] Ten patients died and one withdrew within the 30-day postimplantation recovery period before randomized therapy could be programmed. Four-hundred ninety patients were available for analysis. All patients were required to have a heart failure physician as a co-investigator and to be receiving a stable dose of heart failure medication. Angiotensin-converting

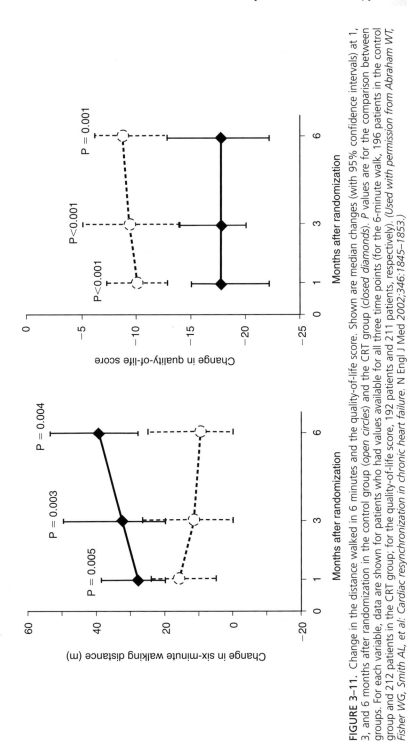

**FIGURE 3–11.** Change in the distance walked in 6 minutes and the quality-of-life score. Shown are median changes (with 95% confidence intervals) at 1, 3, and 6 months after randomization in the control group (*open circles*) and the CRT group (*closed diamonds*). *P* values are for the comparison between groups. For each variable, data are shown for patients who had values available for all three time points (for the 6-minute walk, 196 patients in the control group and 212 patients in the CRT group; for the quality-of-life score, 192 patients and 211 patients, respectively). (*Used with permission from Abraham WT, Fisher WG, Smith AL, et al: Cardiac resynchronization in chronic heart failure. N Engl J Med 2002;346:1845–1853.*)

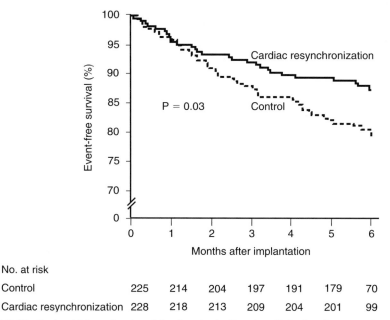

**FIGURE 3–12.** Kaplan-Meier estimates of the time to death or hospitalization for worsening heart failure in the control and resynchronization groups. The risk of an event was 40% lower in the resynchronization group (95% confidence interval, 4% to 63%; P = 0.03). *(Used with permission from Abraham WT, Fisher WG, Smith AL, et al: Cardiac resynchronization in chronic heart failure.* N Engl J Med *2002;346:1845–1853.)*

enzyme (ACE) inhibitor therapy and beta-blocker therapy was given to the majority of patients. Patients enrolled had an LVEF less than 35%, QRS duration greater than 120 msec, NYHA functional class II–IV, heart failure symptoms, and a conventional indication for an ICD. The primary endpoint was an adjusted composite endpoint consisting of a heart failure morbidity index: mortality due to any cause, hospitalization due to heart failure, worsening heart failure requiring intervention, and ventricular tachycardia/ventricular fibrillation (VT/VF) events requiring treatment.

There was an overall 15% relative reduction in the composite endpoint for patients during CRT, but it did not reach statistical significance (P = 0.35; Figure 3–17). No statistically significant reductions were found when patients were stratified into NYHA class I/II (12% reduction) and NYHA class III/IV groups (22% reduction). The reductions with CRT were seen in all components of the composite endpoint, including a 23% decrease in death, 13% decrease in heart failure–related hospitalization, 26% decrease in worsening heart failure, and 9% decrease in VT/VF. Secondary endpoints evaluated demonstrated significant improvement in functional measures of heart failure status in the patients assigned to CRT, in comparison with controls. These included improvements in NYHA functional class (P = 0.10), 6-minute walking distance (P = 0.043), quality of life (Minnesota score; P = 0.39), and peak oxygen consumption (P = 0.030). Peak oxygen uptake improved by 1.8 ml/kg per minute in the group receiving CRT. Patients of NYHA class III/IV demonstrated improvement in peak oxygen consumption (P = 0.003), 6-minute walking distance (P = 0.029),

TABLE 3–4.  Clinical Events During the Double-Blind Treatment Period

| Event | Control Group (N = 225) | Cardiac Resynchronization Group (N = 223) | Hazard Ratio (95% CI) | P Value |
|---|---|---|---|---|
| | no. of patients | | | |
| Death from any cause | 16 | 12 | 0.73 (0.34–1.54) | 0.40 |
| Death or worsening heart failure requiring hospitalization | 44 | 28 | 0.60 (0.37–0.96) | 0.03 |
| Death or worsening heart failure requiring hospitalization or intravenous treatment | 55 | 36 | 0.61 (0.40–0.93) | 0.02 |
| Hospitalization for worsening heart failure | 34 | 18 | 0.50 (0.28–0.88) | 0.02 |
| Worsening heart failure leading to the use of intravenous diuretic agents | 24 | 13 | 0.51 (0.26–1.00) | 0.05 |
| Worsening heart failure leading to the use of intravenous vasodilators or positive inotropic agents | 14 | 6 | 0.41 (0.16–1.08) | 0.06 |
| Worsening heart failure leading to the use of intravenous medication for heart failure | 35 | 16 | 0.43 (0.24–0.77) | 0.004 |

*Events are not mutually exclusive. Hazard ratios are based on Cox proportional-hazards regression models applied to an analysis of the time to the first event. CI denotes confidence interval.
Reproduced from Linde C, Leclercq C, Rex S, et al: Long-term benefits of biventricular pacing in congestive heart failure: Results from the Multisite Stimulation in Cardiomyopathy (MUSTIC) study. *J Am Coll Card* 2002;40:111–118, with permission from *The American College of Cardiology Foundation.*

**TABLE 3–5. Plasma Neurohormonal Levels from the MIRACLE Trial\***

|  | Control | Treatment | P Value |
|---|---|---|---|
| Plasma BNP (pg/ml) | 279.5 ± 1071.5<br>n = 170 | 184.0 ± 1221.3<br>n = 181 | 0.46 |
| Aldosterone (ng/dl) | 8.4 ± 17.0<br>n = 155 | 9.7 ± 11.4<br>n = 153 | 0.6 |
| Renin (ng/ml/min) | 10.2 ± 16.7<br>n = 149 | 11.0 ± 9.7 | 0.775 |
| Dopamine (pg/ml) | 9.0 ± 39.9<br>n = 150 | 9.0 ± 326.5<br>n = 170 | 0.656 |
| Norepinephrine (pg/ml) | 441.5 ± 281.3<br>n = 160 | 362.0 ± 369.9<br>n = 170 p = 0.144 | 0.144 |
| Epinephrine (pg/ml) | 18.0 ± 21.4<br>n = 159 | 14.5 ± 21.7<br>n = 170 | 0.192 |

\*No Significant changes were seen in the levels of any of the substances measured during CRT pacing compared with no pacing at 6 months.

NYHA class ($P = 0.006$), and quality of life ($P = 0.017$), whereas patients with NYHA class I/II did not show significant improvement in any of these parameters (Figures 3–18 to 3–21). LV size also decreased after 6 months of resynchronization therapy, but in control patients there was no decrease in LV size (Figures 3–22 and 3–23). Implant success rate for the coronary sinus over the wire lead used to achieve LV stimulation was 87% and markedly improved with increased implant experience.

The results from the two InSync ICD trials have been reported. One was a prospective multicenter trial evaluating the safety and efficacy of a CRT-D device.[23] This study was performed at 20 different centers in Europe. A total of 84 patients with standard ICD indications and fulfilling the following criteria were enrolled: NYHA class II–IV, CHF symptoms, LVEF less than 35%, LV end-diastolic diameter greater than 55 mm, and QRS duration greater than 130 msec. Patients significantly improved in the 6-minute walking distance, quality of life, and NYHA heart failure class. The results of this trial are similar to those of the InSync pacemaker trial. Patients significantly improved in the 6-minute hall-walking distance, from a baseline of 304 ± 131 m to 397 ± 142 m at 3 months ($P < 0.001$); quality of life improved from a baseline score of 38.9 ± 21.2 to 26.5 ± 21.2 ($P < 0.001$), and the NYHA classification improved from a baseline class of 2.8 ± 0.6 to 2.2 ± 0.5 at 3 months. LV end-diastolic size decreased from 79.6 ± 13.0 mm to 73.6 ± 12.9 mm ($P = 0.002$), end-systolic diameter decreased from 68.3 ± 13.5 mm to 63.9 ± 12.9 mm ($P < 0.001$), and fractional shortening increased from 16 ± 6% to 18 ± 6% ($P = 0.018$). Biventricular pacing was more effective at terminating ventricular tachycardia than RV pacing ($P < 0.001$).

The InSync ICD (MIRACLE-ICD) study performed in North America enrolled a larger number of patients with NYHA class II–IV CHF and a QRS duration of 130 msec or greater.[24,25] Patients were undergoing therapy with a stable medical regimen for heart failure and had an LV ejection fraction ≤35%, sinus rhythm, and conventional ICD indications. The study design was similar to that of the MIRACLE trial (multicenter, randomized, parallel). The primary endpoints were quality of life (measured with the Minnesota Living with Heart Failure questionnaire), NYHA functional class, and 6-minute hall-walking distance.

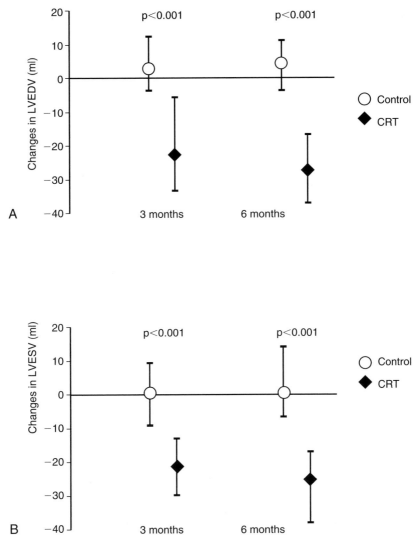

**FIGURE 3–13.** Median change (with 95% confidence intervals) in left ventricular (LV) end-diastolic volumes (LVEDV, *A*) and end-systolic volumes (LVESV, *B*) at 3 and 6 months after randomization in the control group (*circles*) and the cardiac resynchronization group (*diamonds*). *(Used with permission from St. John Sutton MG, Plappert T, Abraham WT, et al: Effect of cardiac resynchronization therapy on left ventricular size and function in chronic heart failure.* Circulation *2003;107:1985–1990.)*

Secondary endpoints were analyzed in the core laboratory and included cardiopulmonary exercise stress time, echocardiographic measurements of LV size and MR, and neurohormonal measurements. Patients with NYHA class II heart failure were analyzed separately from the patients with NYHA class III/IV heart failure. Four hundred twenty-one patients of NYHA class III/IV were enrolled,

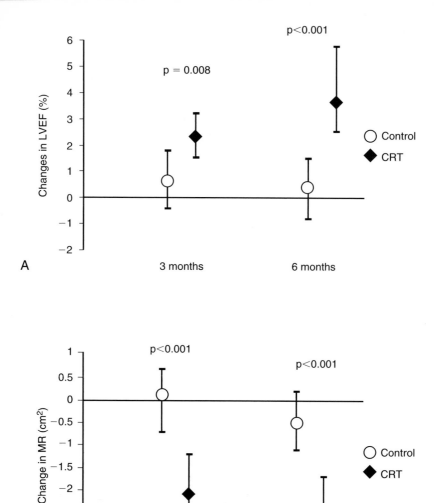

A          3 months          6 months

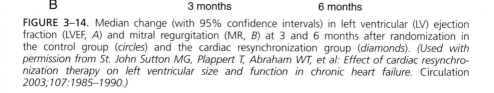

B          3 months          6 months

**FIGURE 3–14.** Median change (with 95% confidence intervals) in left ventricular (LV) ejection fraction (LVEF, *A*) and mitral regurgitation (MR, *B*) at 3 and 6 months after randomization in the control group (*circles*) and the cardiac resynchronization group (*diamonds*). *(Used with permission from St. John Sutton MG, Plappert T, Abraham WT, et al: Effect of cardiac resynchronization therapy on left ventricular size and function in chronic heart failure.* Circulation *2003;107:1985–1990.)*

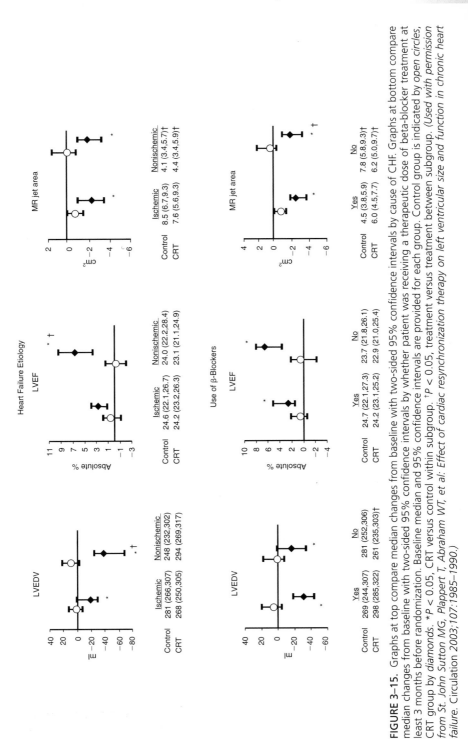

**FIGURE 3-15.** Graphs at top compare median changes from baseline with two-sided 95% confidence intervals by cause of CHF. Graphs at bottom compare median changes from baseline with two-sided 95% confidence intervals by whether patient was receiving a therapeutic dose of beta-blocker treatment at least 3 months before randomization. Baseline median and 95% confidence intervals are provided for each group. Control group is indicated by open circles, CRT group by diamonds. *P < 0.05, CRT versus control within subgroup. †P < 0.05, treatment versus control between subgroup. (Used with permission from St. John Sutton MG, Plappert T, Abraham WT, et al: Effect of cardiac resynchronization therapy on left ventricular size and function in chronic heart failure. Circulation 2003;107:1985–1990.)

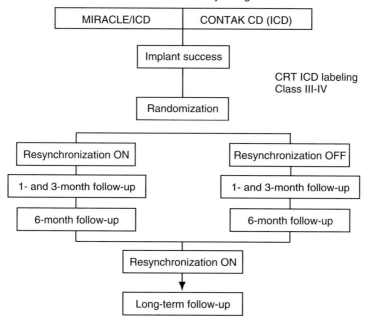

**FIGURE 3–16.** Designs of the controlled clinical trials MIRACLE ICD and CONTAK CD.

and 364 were randomized (177 were randomized to control therapy and 187 to CRT-D). Of the 215 patients with NYHA class II CHF, 191 were randomized (106 to control or no pacing and 85 to resynchronization therapy). With an intention-to-treat approach for patients with paired data, quality of life improved in patients with CRT ($P = 0.02$), and only the patients with biventricular pacing experienced a sustained improvement in quality of life during the double-blind 6-month study period. There was a significant improvement in NYHA functional class: 65% of the treatment patients improved by at least one functional class, versus 50% of the control patients ($P = 0.01$). In other words, 90% of the patients were in NYHA class III at baseline, and at 6 months 63% of the patients receiving resynchronization therapy were at NYHA class I or II, whereas only 48% of the control patients were at NYHA class I or II. There was no significant improvement in the 6-minute hall-walking distance at 6 months. The composite score improvement was similar to that observed in the MIRACLE study (Figure 3–24). There was a trend toward decreased hospitalization and decreased CHF-related hospitalizations in patients receiving CRT-D (Figure 3–25). The overall results for CRT (from MIRACLE) and CRT-D for the endpoints of death or worsening heart failure requiring hospitalization or intravenous medications are shown in Figure 3–26.

Secondary endpoints showed a statistically significant improvement in peak oxygen consumption, with the treatment group improving 1.1 ml/kg per minute and no change in the control group ($P = 0.03$). The exercise duration data showed a significant improvement of a mean of 56 seconds in total exercise time for patients

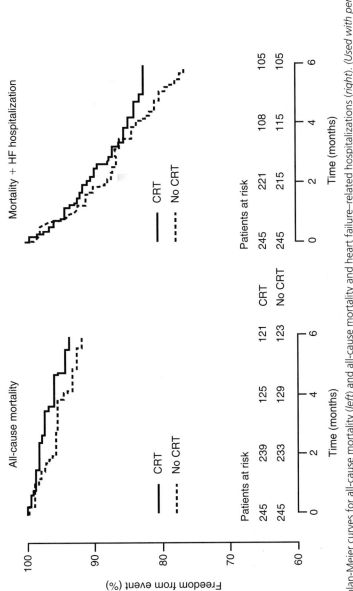

FIGURE 3–17. Kaplan-Meier curves for all-cause mortality (*left*) and all-cause mortality and heart failure–related hospitalizations (*right*). (*Used with permission from Higgins SL, Hummel JD, Niazi IK, et al: Cardiac resynchronization therapy for the treatment of heart failure in patients with intraventricular conduction delay and malignant ventricular tachyarrhythmias. J Am Coll Cardiol 2003 [in press].*)

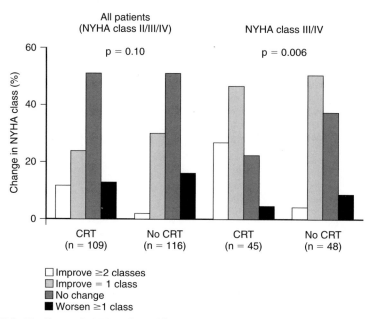

**FIGURE 3–18.** Change in NYHA class with CRT and without CRT in CONTAK CD study. Patients are stratified by NYHA class.

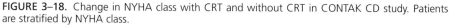

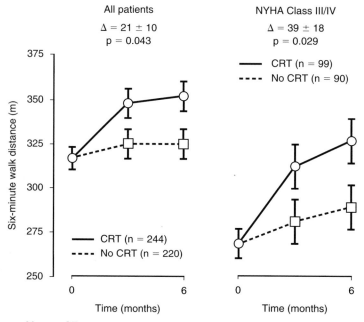

Mean ± SE

**FIGURE 3–19.** Six-minute walking distance with CRT and no CRT for all patients (*left panel*) and class III/IV CHF patients (*right panel*). P <0.05. *Left*, P = 0.04; *Right*, P = 0.03.

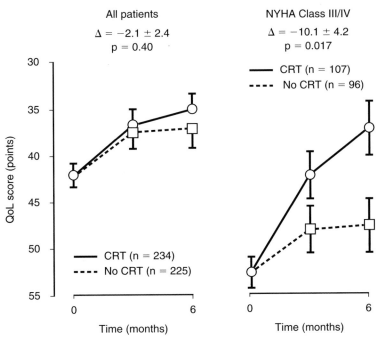

**FIGURE 3–20.** Quality-of-life (QL) data with CRT and no CRT for all patients (*left panel*) and class III/IV CHF patients (*right panel*). $P <0.05$. B, $P = 0.002$.

receiving CRT, in comparison with a decrease in exercise time of 9 seconds in the control group.

The overall success rate of terminating spontaneous episodes of VT and VF was 99.1%. All episodes of VT were eventually terminated. There was no difference in the number of VT/VF episodes between the control and CRT groups. Over time, however, there was a trend toward reduction in the number of VT/VF episodes with CRT during follow-up, but this did not reach statistical significance. Antitachycardia pacing (ATP) with combined RV + LV pacing was more effective than RV pacing alone (95% termination versus 88% termination, $P = 0.0009$). These findings are similar to those observed in the CONTAK CD trial.

An overview of the effect of CRT and CRT-D on NYHA functional class, quality of life, peak oxygen consumption, and 6-minute walking distance from clinical trial data is provided in Figures 3–27 to 3–30 and Tables 3–6 to 3–8. A recently published meta-analysis of randomized controlled trials of CRT reviewed 5681 reports, and 11 reports were selected from four studies including 1634 patients.[26] The pooled data from these trials were used to estimate CIs for treatment effects. These studies include the CONTAK CD, MIRACLE, MUSTIC, and InSync ICD trials. The reduction in death associated with CRT was 51% in comparison with controls (odds ratio [OR], 0.49; 95% CI: 0.25–0.93). Progressive heart failure–associated mortality was 1.7% for CRT patients and 3.5% for controls. Cardiac resynchronization therapy also reduced hospitalizations due to heart failure by 29%

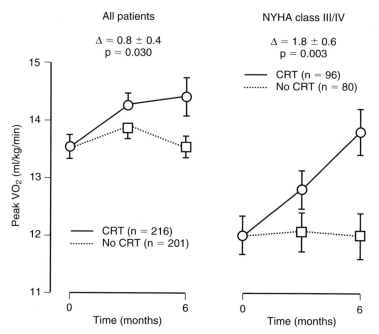

**FIGURE 3–21.** Peak oxygen consumption (VO₂) data with CRT and no CRT for all patients (*A*) and class III/IV CHF patients (*B*). *P* <0.05. *A, P* = 0.003; *B, P* = 0.003.

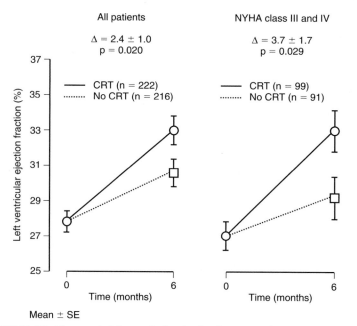

Mean ± SE

**FIGURE 3–22.** Changes in left ventricular ejection fraction in the CONTAK CD trial.

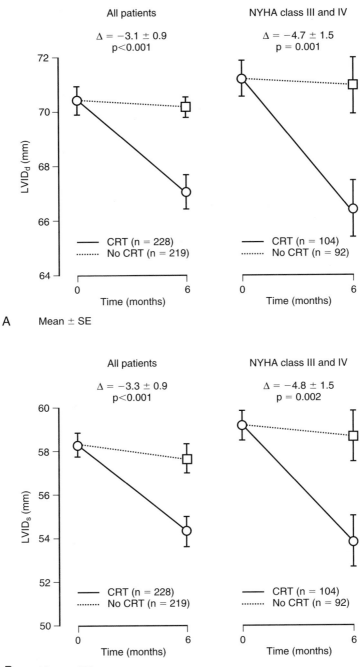

**FIGURE 3–23.** Changes in left ventricular internal diastolic dimension during systole (LVID$_s$, A) and diastole (LVID$_d$, B) in the CONTAK CD trial.

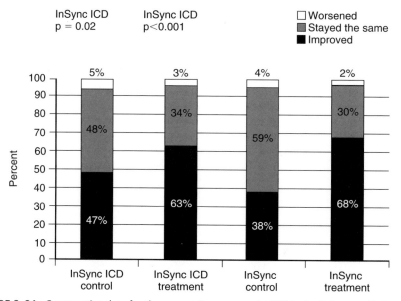

FIGURE 3–24. Comparative data for the composite response to CRT in the InSync and InSync ICD trials, with regard to overall change in clinical status at baseline to 6 months.

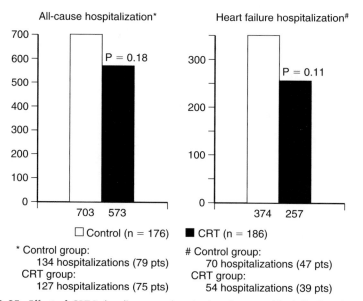

FIGURE 3–25. Effect of CRT-D (cardiac resynchronization therapy with defibrillator) on all-cause hospitalization and heart failure–associated hospitalization in the InSync ICD study. pts = patients.

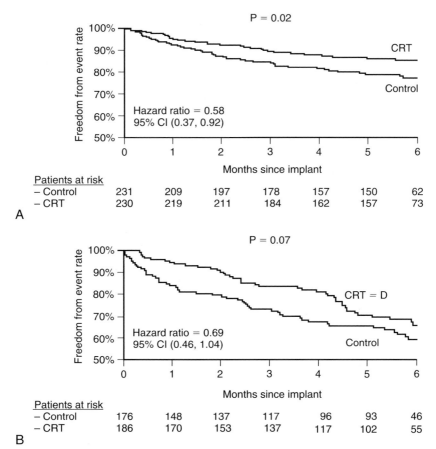

**FIGURE 3–26.** Results of the InSync (CRT; *A*) and InSync ICD (CRT-D; *B*) trials, with comparison of secondary endpoints (death or worsening heart failure requiring hospitalization or requiring intravenous medications).

(OR, 0.71; 95% CI: 0.53–0.96) and showed a trend toward reducing all-cause mortality (OR, 0.77; 95% CI: 0.51–1.18). CRT was not associated with a statistically significant effect on non–heart failure mortality (OR, 1.15; 95% CI: 0.65–2.02). Among patients with an ICD, CRT had no clear impact on VT or VF (OR, 0.92; 95% CI: 0.67–1.27).

## Future and Ongoing Studies

The goals of any therapy for patients with symptomatic CHF are to improve symptoms, slow disease progression, and prolong survival. The results of the trials reviewed in the previous section demonstrate that CRT and CRT-D significantly improve symptoms and slow disease progression when echocardiographic measures of ventricular size are analyzed. The COMPANION and CARE-HF trials are designed to determine whether CRT improves the outcomes of all-cause hospitalization and mortality rates. In the CARE-HF trial, a European study, patients are randomized to

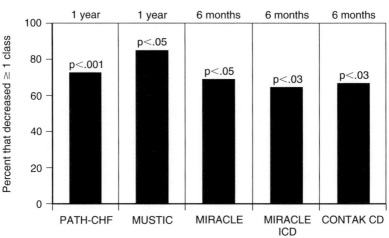

FIGURE 3–27. Change in NYHA functional class at 6 months or 1 year in the PATH-CHF, MUSTIC, MIRACLE, MIRACLE ICD, and CONTAK CD trials.

a resynchronization device or optimal drug therapy (Figure 3–31).[27] This trial was completed in March 2003, with enrollment of 800 patients at 82 clinical centers. The minimum follow-up is 1.5 years. Entry criteria include a QRS duration greater than 150 msec or 120–150 msec and dyssynchrony demonstrated by echocardiography. The primary study endpoint is the rate of all-mortality death or unplanned

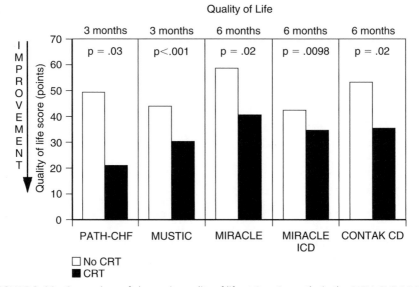

FIGURE 3–28. Comparison of change in quality of life at 3 or 6 months in the PATH-CHF, MUSTIC, MIRACLE, MIRACLE ICD, and CONTAK CD trials.

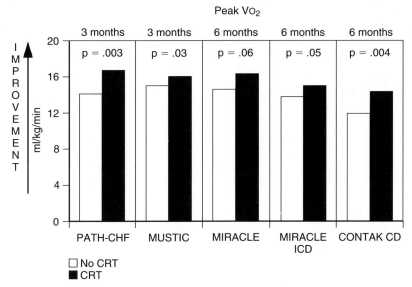

**FIGURE 3–29.** Comparison of change in peak oxygen consumption ($VO_2$) at 3 months or 6 months in the PATH-CHF, MUSTIC, MIRACLE, MIRACLE ICD, and CONTAK CD trials.

cardiovascular hospitalization. Cardiovascular hospitalization is defined as hospitalization for or with worsening heart failure, angina, myocardial infarction, stroke, syncope, arrhythmia, transient ischemic attack, pulmonary embolism, or other cardiovascular event. Secondary endpoints include all-cause mortality, the composite of all-cause mortality or rates of unplanned hospitalization for or with worsening heart failure, days alive and not in hospital for unplanned cardiovascular cause during the minimum period of follow-up, days alive and not in hospital for any

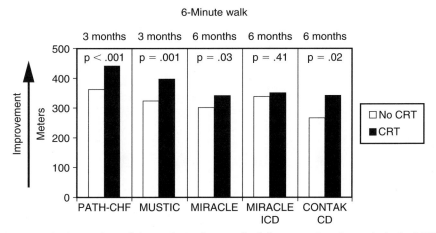

**FIGURE 3–30.** Comparison of change in 6-minute walked distance at 3 or 6 months in the PATH-CHF, MUSTIC, MIRACLE, MIRACLE ICD, and CONTAK CD trials.

TABLE 3–6. **Overview of Biventricular Clinical Trials: Functional Status**

|  | QoL Score (p <0.05) | NYHA Class (p <0.05) |
|---|:---:|:---:|
| MIRACLE (n = 453) | ↓ | ↓ |
| MIRACLE ICD (n = 247) | ↓ | ↓ |
| MUSTIC (n = 67) | ↓ | NA |
| PATH-CHF (n = 41) | ↓ | ↓ |
| CONTAK CD (n = 203) | ↓ | ↓ |
| French Pilot (n = 50) | NA | ↓ |
| InSync (Europe) (n = 103) | ↓ | ↓ |
| InSync ICD (Europe) (n = 84) | ↓ | ↓ |
| InSync III | ↓ | ↓ |

NA = not available; NYHA = New York Heart Association; QoL = quality of life.

reason during the minimum period of follow-up, NYHA classification at 90 days, quality of life at 90 days, and patient status at the end of the study.

The COMPANION trial was performed in the United States and randomized NYHA functional class III–IV patients with QRS duration of ≥120 msec, with no standard ICD indication, and who had had a heart failure–related hospitalization within the previous year. Patients were randomized with a 1:2:2 sequence to optimal medical therapy (OPT) versus OPT + CRT versus OPT + CRT-D (Figure 3–32).[28,29] The study was powered to enroll 2200 patients. Roughly half of all patients enrolled had heart failure of a nonischemic etiology. The Data and Safety Monitoring Board recommended stopping the trial after an interim review of the data in November 2002 after 1520 patients were enrolled. The trial was terminated in December of that year because of a significant benefit in the combined endpoint of all-cause hospitalization and mortality for patients randomized to CRT. The primary endpoint was time to death or hospitalization (including treatment of decompensated CHF with vasoactive drugs for a period of greater than 4 hours in an urgent care setting). Secondary endpoints included all-cause mortality, cardiac morbidity, and maximal exercise, and the tertiary endpoints included submaximal exercise tolerance and quality of life.

A preliminary analysis presented at the March 2003 American College of Cardiology meeting included data from the November 2002 Data and Safety Monitoring Boards and all patients or events censored at the date of withdrawal.

TABLE 3–7. **Overview of Biventricular Clinical Trials: Exercise**

|  | 6-Min Walk | Peak VO$_2$ | Exercise Time |
|---|:---:|:---:|:---:|
| MIRACLE (n = 453) | ↑ | ↑ | ↑ |
| MIRACLE ICD (n = 247) | ↔ | ↑ | ↑ |
| MUSTIC (n = 67) | ↑ | ↑ | NA |
| PATH-CHF (n = 41) | ↑ | ↑ | NA |
| CONTAK CD (n = 203) | ↑ | ↑ | NA |
| French Pilot (n = 50) | NA | ↑ | NA |
| InSync (Europe) (n = 103) | ↑ | NA | NA |
| InSync ICD (Europe) (n = 84) | ↑ | NA | NA |
| InSync III | ↑ | NA | NA |

NA = not available.

TABLE 3–8. **Overview of Biventricular Clinical Trials: LV Function**

| | LVEF | MR | LVEDV/ LVESV | LV Filling Time |
|---|---|---|---|---|
| Queen Mary Hospital | ↑ | ↓ | ↓ | ↑ |
| MIRACLE | ↑ | ↓ | ↓ | ↑ |
| PATH-CHF | ↑ | NA | ↓ | ↑ |
| MUSTIC | NA | ↓ | NA | ↑ |
| MIRACLE ICD | ↔ | ↔ | ↓ | ↑ |

NA = not available.

The overall implant success rate was 88% to 92%, and mean total implantation time was 200 minutes for the CRT pacemaker and 213 minutes for the CRT-D. The reduction in the combined endpoints of death and hospitalizations due to cardiovascular or heart failure was due to CRT because CRT and CRT-D resulted in similar effect sizes. Both reduced the 12-month event rate by approximately 19% (Figure 3–33). The secondary endpoint of all-cause mortality was reduced by 24% with CRT and by 43% with CRT-D (Figures 3–34 and 3–35). There was no obvious difference in mortality benefit of CRT-D between patients with ischemic versus nonischemic cardiomyopathy. Similar benefits were seen in other subgroups, including age, gender, NYHA class III or IV, LVEF, and LV end-diastolic dimension. Moderate or severe device-related adverse events were seen in 7% to 9% of patients. The 30-day crude mortality was 1% in the medical therapy group, 0.9% in the CRT-D group, and 1.8% in the CRT group. Further analysis of the data will answer many more questions about this therapy.

One of the critical questions that has important implications for patient care and for reimbursement issues is related to the selection CRT pacemaker versus CRT ICD for patients who are identified to be candidates for resynchronization therapy.

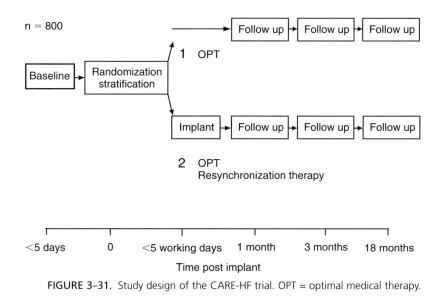

FIGURE 3–31. Study design of the CARE-HF trial. OPT = optimal medical therapy.

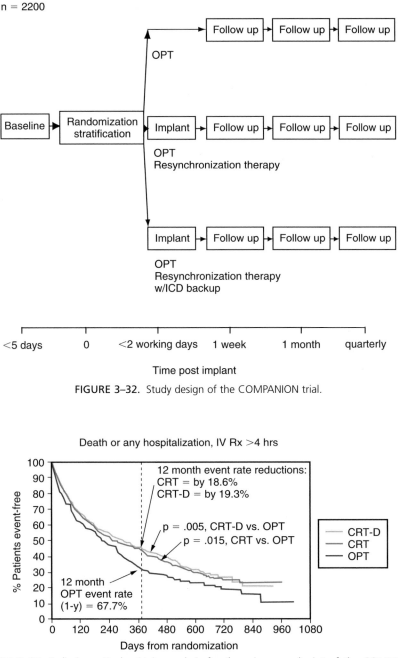

FIGURE 3–32. Study design of the COMPANION trial.

FIGURE 3–33. Preliminary Kaplan-Meier analysis for the primary endpoint of the COMPANION trial: preliminary results reported at the ACC March 2003 Late-Breaking Clinical Trials Session (www.uchsc.edu/cvi/clb.pdf). IV Rx = intravenous medication.

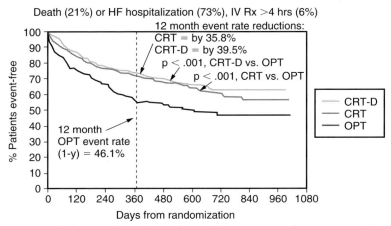

**FIGURE 3–34.** Preliminary Kaplan-Meier analysis of death or heart failure–associated hospitalization in the COMPANION trial. Preliminary results from the ACC March 2003 Late Breaking Clinical Trials Session (www.uchsc.edu/cvi/clb.pdf). IV Rx = Intravenous medication.

With the results of MADIT II, there will be a strong inclination to implant CRT-Ds in patients with ischemic cardiomyopathy, and now with the results of the COMPANION trial there will also be an impetus to implant more CRT-D devices in patients with nonischemic cardiomyopathy.[30]

A second key issue is whether patients with CHF due to systolic dysfunction who present with heart block and will be paced all or most of the time should have a device with CRT. This question remains largely unanswered, although nonrandomized data from the Emory group suggest that these patients may also benefit from CRT. They studied 20 patients with NYHA class III/IV CHF, ejection fraction less than 35%, and chronic AF with prior AV junction ablation and RV pacing

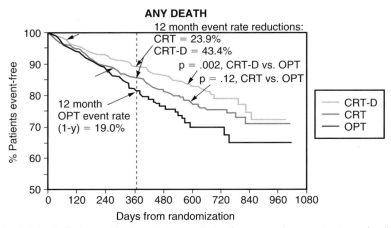

**FIGURE 3–35.** Preliminary Kaplan-Meier analysis for secondary endpoint of all-cause mortality: results reported at the ACC March 2003 Late-Breaking Clinical Trials Session (www.uchsc.edu/cvi/clb.pdf).

who underwent upgrades to biventricular systems. The number of hospitalizations of these patients decreased by 81% ($P < 0.001$), the quality of life according to questionnaire/survey improved by 31% ($P < 0.01$), and the NYHA functional class improved 29% ($P < 0.001$).[31] Unfortunately, these data are limited by the nonblinded nature of the study, the small sample size, and the fact that all patients had AF. Results of the recently completed DAVID trial also support the observation that chronic RV pacing–induced LBBB may have adverse effects on survival.[32] A recently proposed trial, Pacing Efficiently by Resynchronization for Efficiency in CHF (PERFECT), will answer this question definitively.[33] This European trial will enroll 1000 patients and randomize them to groups that will continue with standard RV pacing alone or undergo upgrade to a CRT device. Study design is parallel with minimum follow-up (planned to last 1.5 years). Enrolled patients will be of NYHA class I–IV with an LVEF of less than 40% or diastolic heart failure. The primary endpoint proposed is all-cause mortality or unplanned cardiovascular hospitalization rate.

PAVE (LV-based cardiac stimulation Post-AV-node ablation Evaluation) is a double-blinded randomized trial designed to evaluate the effect of RV pacing versus biventricular pacing in patients with heart failure requiring AV nodal ablation because of chronic AF. The primary study endpoint is to compare exercise capacity and safety of the implanted system. Exercise capacity is measured during the 6-minute walking test. The secondary endpoints are quality-of-life scores and functional capacity as measured by peak oxygen consumption. Additional data to be collected include LV diameter, left atrial diameter, ejection fraction, 24-hour Holter monitoring findings, and MR. Enrollment criteria include AV junction ablation for chronic AF that results in complete AV block. A minimum enrollment of 261 patients is anticipated, and the minimum enrollment criterion was met in January 2003. Selected ongoing clinical trials are summarized in Table 3–9.

The next era of clinical trials in CRT pacing will focus on further refinements in therapy, including testing of new device features and better selection of patients. Studies evaluating the use of nonsimultaneous LV and RV stimulation, AV interval programming, and LV stimulation alone to achieve CRT are now in progress. CRT devices with more advanced diagnostic and therapeutic features are being evaluated.

Several additional issues are touched upon in other chapters. For example, the clinical trials presented demonstrate that up to one third of patients may not benefit from CRT. The lack of an agreed-upon methodology other than QRS duration to assess dyssynchrony and the failure of QRS width or any other clinical parameter to predict improvement with CRT present other important goals for future research. The utility of CRT for patients with no or only mild CHF will also need to undergo study in the future. Use of simple echo-cardiographic indices of mechanical dyssynchrony to identify potential candidates, to assess the effects of therapy, and to fine tune therapy is contemplated for future trials.

Another type of pacemaker is currently undergoing active clinical evaluation for patients with CHF due to systolic dysfunction. Patients who may benefit from this therapy do not have to have underlying interventricular conduction disturbances. The implanted device delivers nonexcitatory stimuli during the absolute refractory period. These nonexcitatory stimuli cause an increase in intracellular calcium levels via pacing-stimuli modification of calcium channel gating. The pacemaker stimulus

TABLE 3–9. **Ongoing Clinical Trials in Biventricular Pacing**

| Trial | Patients | Design | Primary Endpoint |
|---|---|---|---|
| CARE-HF | NYHA Class III, IV | Randomized BiV + OPT $R_x$ | Death/ CHF admission |
| | LVEF < 35% | vs. | $VO_2$ Max |
| | QRS > 150 ms or QRS > 120 ms + Echo-based dyssynchrony | OPT $R_x$ | 6-min walk |
| BELIEVE | NYHA Class II–IV | LV + ICD | Echocardiography |
| | LBBB | vs. | endpoints |
| | QRS > 130 ms | BiV + ICD | |
| | LVEF > 55 ms | | |
| | ICD indicated | | |
| PAVE | Post AV junction | RV | 6-min walk |
| | Ablation | vs. | and |
| | Stable medical $R_x$ at 3 mo | LV vs. | QoL |
| | NYHA Class II–III | BiV | |
| VECTOR | NYHA Class II–IV | OPT $R_x$ | Mortality |
| | LVEF < 35% | vs. | 6-min walk |
| | QRS > 140 ms | BiV Pacing | Echo measurements |
| | LVEDD > 54 mm | | |
| RELEVENT | NYHA Class II–IV | OPT $R_x$ | Safety |
| | LVEF < 35% | vs. | 6-min walk |
| | QRS > 140 ms | OPT $R_x$ + | |
| | LVEDD > 55 mm | BiV or LV | |
| PACMAN | NYHA Class II | OPT $R_x$ | 6-min walk |
| | LVEF < 35% | vs. | |
| | QRS > 150 ms | BiV ± ICD | |
| LV 3P | NYHA Class II–IV | LV | 6-min walk |
| | Require PM | vs. | $VO_2$ Max |
| | | RV | |

BiV = biventricular; OPT = optimal.

modulates cardiac contractility by allowing for enhanced calcium release from the sarcolemma and increased sarcoplasmic reticulum loading. In one study of 18 patients with dilated cardiomyopathy, involving acute assessment of the benefit of cardiac contractility modulation (CCM) with use of signals applied in the left ventricle via an epicardial vein ($n = 12$) or to the RV aspect of the septum ($n = 6$), both LV and RV CCM stimulation increased $dP/dt_{max}$ to a similar degree (by 7% to 9%), with associated increases in aortic pulse pressure of 10% (Figures 3–36 and 3–37). Regional systolic wall motion was markedly enhanced as well near the CCM electrode, and the area of contractility involved approximately 3–5 segments (Figure 3–38). There was no relationship between QRS duration and increased dP/dt response. In one animal model, CCM with nonexcitatory stimuli improved LV function (as measured by LV dP/dt, LV ejection fraction, and LV pulse pressure) more than biventricular pacing. In a preliminary clinical study, there was a significant improvement in 6-minute walking distance (by greater than 20%), increased oxygen consumption, improved anaerobic threshold, and improved rate pressure product in a small number of patients in whom this device was implanted. Quality of life improved significantly over a 2-month study period. Ongoing trials in Europe and soon in the United States

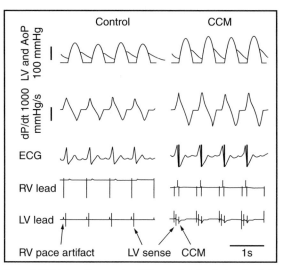

**FIGURE 3–36.** Timing of CCM (cardiac contractility modulation) signal relative to hemodynamic and electrical events. From *top* to *bottom*: simultaneous recordings of LV and aortic (AoP) pressures, dP/dt, surface electrocardiography (*ECG*), and endocardial electrography with LV and RV leads. After detecting right atrial and RV activation, the CCM generator waits for detection of local activation of the left ventricle ("local sense") and delivers the signal after a preset delay for a specified duration and amplitude. *(Reprinted from Pappone C, Rosanio S, Burkhoff D, et al: Cardiac contractility modulation by electric currents applied during the refractory period in patients with heart failure secondary to ischemic or idiopathic dilated cardiomyopathy. Am J Cardiol 2002;90:1307–1313, with permission from Excerpta Medica Inc.)*

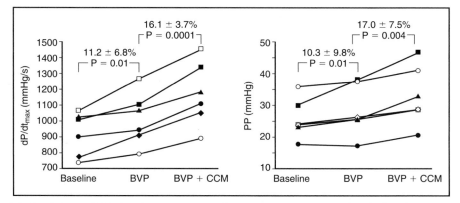

**FIGURE 3–37.** Individual patient responses and average percent changes (±SD) of dP/dt$_{max}$ (maximal pressure change) and aortic pulse pressure (*PP*) during simultaneous biventricular pacing (*BVP*) and CCM. *(Used with permission from Pappone C, Rosanio S, Burkhoff D, et al: Cardiac contractility modulation by electric currents applied during the refractory period in patients with heart failure secondary to ischemic or idiopathic dilated cardiomyopathy. Am J Cardiol 2002;90:1307–1313.)*

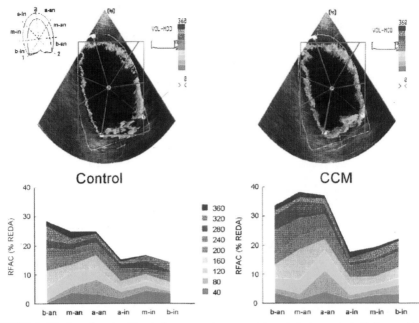

**FIGURE 3–38.** Systolic color kinesis images and segmental analysis in controls (*left panels*) and during CCM delivery from the anterior vein (*right panels*). A-an = apical anterior; a-in = apical inferior; b-in = basal inferior; m-an = mid-anterior; m-in = mid-inferior; REDA = regional end-diastolic area; RFAC = regional incremental fractional area change. *(Reprinted from Pappone C, Rosanio S, Burkhoff D, et al: Cardiac contractility modulation by electric currents applied during the refractory period in patients with heart failure secondary to ischemic or idiopathic dilated cardiomyopathy.* Am J Cardiol *2002;90:1307–1313, with permission from* Excerpta Medica Inc.*)*

will answer more questions about this device's role in treatment of patients with CHF and without conduction system disease.

The device as it is currently designed has three pacing leads (one in the right atrium) and two active fixation leads in the right ventricle (one in the RV septum). Lead positions for the CCM lead are confirmed by an improvement in hemodynamics as measured by a Millar catheter during stimulation.

CRT has changed much in a little less than 10 years, and it is likely that the next 10 years will see an even greater understanding of this new therapy.

## REFERENCES

1. Cazeau S, Ritter P, Bakdach S, et al: Four-chamber pacing in dilated cardiomyopathy. *Pacing Clin Electrophysiol* 1994;17:1974–1979.
2. Bakker PA, Meijburg H, De Jouge N, et al: Beneficial effects of bi-ventricular pacing in congestive heart failure (abstract). *Pacing Clin Electrophysiol* 1994;17:820.
3. Blanc JJ, Etienne Y, Gilard M, et al: Evaluation of different ventricular pacing sites in patients with severe heart failure: Results of an acute hemodynamic study. *Circulation* 1997;96:3273–3277.
4. Foster AH, Gold MR, McClaughlan JS: Acute hemodynamic effects of atrio-biventricular pacing in humans. *Ann Thorac Surg* 1995;59:294–300.
5. Daubert JC, Ritter P, Le Breton H, et al: Permanent left ventricular pacing with transvenous leads inserted into the coronary veins. *Pacing Clin Electrophysiol* 1998;21:239–245.

6. Gras D, Mabo P, Tang T, et al: Multisite pacing as a supplemental treatment of congestive heart failure: Preliminary results of the Medtronic Inc. InSync study. *PACE* 1998;21:2249–2255.

7. Gras D, Leclercq C, Tang ASL, et al: Cardiac resynchronization therapy in advanced heart failure the multicenter InSync clinical study. *Eur J Heart Fail* 2002;4:311–320.

8. Ricci R, Ansalone G, Toscano S, et al: Cardiac resynchronization: materials, technique and results. The InSync Italian Registry. *Eur Heart J Suppl* 2000;2:J6–J15.

9. Auricchio A, Stellbrink C, Sack S, et al: The Pacing Therapies for Congestive Heart Failure (PATH-CHF) Study: Rationale, design, and endpoints of a prospective randomized multicenter study. *Am J Cardiol* 1999;83:130–135D.

10. Auricchio A, Stellbrink C, Sack S, et al: Long-term clinical effect of hemodynamically optimized cardiac resynchronization therapy in patients with heart failure and ventricular conduction delay. *J Am Coll Card* 2002;39:2026–33.

11. Breithardt O-A, Stellbrink C, Franke A, et al: Acute effects of cardiac resynchronization therapy in left ventricular Doppler indices in patients with congestive heart failure. *Am Heart J* 2002;143:34–44.

12. Auricchio A, Stellbrink C, Butter C, et al: Clinical efficacy of cardiac resynchronization therapy using left ventricular pacing in heart failure patients stratified by severity of ventricular conduction delay. *J Am Coll Cardiol* 2003 (in press).

13. Saxon LA, Boehmer JP, Hummel J, et al: Bi-ventricular Pacing in patients with congestive heart failure: Two prospective randomized trials. *Am J Cardiol* 1999;83:120D–130D.

14. Saxon LA, Marco TD, Schafer J, et al: Effects of long-term biventricular stimulation for resynchronization on echocardiographic measures of remodeling. *Circulation* 2002;105:1304–1310.

15. Cazeau S, Leclercq C, Lavergne T, et al: Effects of multisite biventricular pacing in patients with heart failure and intraventricular conduction delay. *N Engl J Med* 2001;344:873–880.

16. Varma C, Sharma S, Firoozi S, et al: Atriobiventricular pacing improves exercise capacity in patients with heart failure and intraventricular conduction delay. *J Am Coll Cardiol* 2003;41:582–588.

17. Leclercq C, Walker S, Linde C, et al: Comparative effects of permanent biventricular and right-univentricular pacing in heart failure patients with chronic atrial fibrillation. *Eur Heart J* 2002;23:1780–1787.

18. Linde C, Leclercq C, Rex S, et al: Long-term benefits of biventricular pacing in congestive heart failure: Results from the Multisite Stimulation in Cardiomyopathy (MUSTIC) study. *J Am Coll Card* 2002;40:111–118.

19. Abraham WT, Fisher WG, Smith AL, et al: Cardiac resynchronization in chronic heart failure. *N Engl J Med* 2002;346:1845–1853.

20. St. John Sutton MG, Plappert T, Abraham WT, et al: Effect of cardiac resynchronization therapy on left ventricular size and function in chronic heart failure. *Circulation* 2003;107:1985–1990.

21. Higgins SL, Hummel JD, Niazi IK, et al: Cardiac resynchronization therapy for the treatment of heart failure in patients with intraventricular conduction delay and malignant ventricular tachyarrhythmias. *J Am Coll Cardiol* 2003 (in press).

22. Guidant Corporation. *P010012. CONTAK CD and Easy Track Lead System.* <*http://www.fda.gov/ohrms/dochets/ac/cdrh01.html*> Circulatory System.

23. Kühlkamp V, InSync 7272 ICD Worldwide Investigators: Initial experience with an implantable cardioverter defibrillator incorporating cardiac resynchronization therapy. *J Am Coll Card* 2002;39:790–7.

24. *Medtronic InSync ICD Cardiac Resynchronization System.* <*www.fda.gov/ohrms/dockets/ac/02/bnefing/3843b2.html*>.

25. *Summary of Safety and Effectiveness: Medtronic InSync ICD Model 7272.* <*www.fda.gov/ohrms/dockets/ac/02/briefing/3843b2.html*>.

26. Bradley DJ, Bradley EA, Baughman KL, et al: Cardiac resynchronization and death from progressive heart failure: A meta-analysis of randomized controlled trials. *JAMA* 2003;289:730–740.

27. Cleland JGF, Daubert JC, Erdmann E, et al: The CARE-HF study (Cardiac Resynchronization in Heart Failure study): rationale, design, and end-points. *Eur J Heart Fail* 2001;3:481–9.

28. Bristow MR, Feldman AM, Saxon LA: Heart failure management using implantable devices for ventricular resynchronization: Comparison of medical therapy, pacing, and defibrillation in chronic heart failure (COMPANION) trial. *J Card Fail* 2000;6:276–85.

29. *Late Breaking Clinical Trials.* American College of Cardiology, March 2003.

30. Moss AJ, Zareba W, Hall WJ, et al: Prophylactic implantation of a defibrillator in patients with myocardial infarction and reduced ejection fraction. *N Engl J Med* 2002;346:877–883.

31. Leon AR, Greenberg JM, Kanuru N, et al: Cardiac resynchronization patients with congestive heart failure and chronic right ventricular pacing. *J Am Coll Cardiol* 2002;39:1258–1263.

32. The DAVID trial investigations: Dual chamber pacing as ventricular backup pacing in patients with an implantable defibrillation: The Dual chamber and VVI Implantable Defibrillator (DAVID) Trial. *JAMA* 2002;288:3115–3123.

33. Cleland JGF, Ghosh J, Khan NK, et al: Multi-chamber pacing: a perfect solution for cardiac mechanical dyssynchrony. *Eur Heart J* 2003;24:384–390.

34. Pappone C, Rosanio S, Burkhoff D, et al: Cardiac contractility modulation by electric currents applied during the refractory period in patients with heart failure secondary to ischemic or idiopathic dilated cardiomyopathy. *Am J Cardiol* 2002;90:1307–1313.

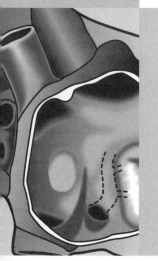

# 4

# Clinical Pacemakers Trials in Systolic Cardiac Dysfunction: Nonresynchronization

Michael R. Gold • J. Marcus Wharton

With advances of medical and surgical therapy for patients with left ventricular dysfunction (e.g., the use of beta-blockers, angiotensin-converting enzyme [ACE] inhibitors, off-pump coronary artery bypass surgery, and mitral valve repair), survival of this cohort has improved significantly. There are currently more than 2 million people with heart failure due to left ventricular (LV) systolic dysfunction in the United States.[1] The number is growing by approximately 400,000 new cases each year and will undoubtedly increase further with a population that is gradually aging. Despite the optimizing of medical therapy to reduce morbidity and mortality, the potential cost of treatment and hospitalization of this population is staggering. In addition, the rate of sudden death in the setting of LV dysfunction and heart failure has remained disappointingly high, with most of these deaths being presumed arrhythmic. In the present chapter we review right-sided pacing therapies that are available or are being developed for patients with LV systolic dysfunction, and we explore the possible mechanisms underlying their beneficial and detrimental effects.

## Pacing in Heart Failure Patients for Standard Bradycardic Indications

Before discussion of pacing to improve hemodynamic function, it should be noted that patients with severe myocardial dysfunction often have involvement of the specialized conduction system and that symptomatic bradyarrhythmias are relatively common, often requiring permanent pacing. There is now some evidence that bradycardia may be a relatively important mechanism of sudden cardiac death in advanced heart failure,[2] providing further impetus for permanent pacemaker implantation, especially in symptomatic individuals. In addition, medications such as amiodarone, beta-blockers, and digitalis, which are used frequently in this population, may produce chronotropic incompetence and/or conduction disturbances, requiring permanent pacing.

More recently, dual-chamber pacing defibrillators have become readily available. Because subjects undergoing implantable cardiac defibrillator (ICD) placement typically have LV dysfunction, there is an increasing use of dual-chamber pacing in this population. Many of these subjects receive dual-chamber pacing defibrillators for less stringent bradycardic indications than those subjects who receive "stand alone" pacemakers.[3] Thus permanent pacemakers are used relatively often in patients with LV systolic dysfunction.

# Pacing in Heart Failure Patients for Hemodynamic Indications

## Heart Rate

Within the normal physiologic range, an increase in heart rate may have several beneficial hemodynamic effects. Cardiac output is determined by the heart rate and stroke volume; thus increasing heart rate will result in an increase of cardiac output. Cardiac output may be enhanced further by the accompanying increase in venous return as well as by an increase in contractility (the Treppe phenomenon).[4] In addition, cardiac output may be enhanced by neurohumoral activation. Conversely, increases in heart rate may be associated with other changes, which may adversely affect cardiac output and myocardial performance. For instance, the reduction of diastolic ventricular filling time that accompanies an increased heart rate may compromise cardiac output, especially if venous return does not increase proportionately. Among patients with coronary artery disease, it is likely that an increase in rate might induce myocardial ischemia, with resulting worsening LV dysfunction.

Although the effect of heart rate on cardiac hemodynamic function is not well understood, this issue is even less clear with regard to patients with heart failure. Whereas it seems obvious that very slow and very rapid rates are poorly tolerated by heart failure patients, the most appropriate heart rate within the physiologic range (the lower and upper rate settings used in pacemaker-dependent patients) has yet to be determined. It is likely that the optimal heart rate will vary considerably between individuals, based upon etiology of heart disease, the degree of LV systolic and diastolic dysfunction and multiple other factors, and even, at different times, in the same individual, depending upon the state of hydration, autonomic tone, and the use of vasoactive medications.

Patients with congestive heart failure and permanent pacemakers are often paced at higher rates than those patients with preserved systolic function. The rationale for this strategy is to use the pacemaker to increase cardiac output. However, the effect of paced heart rate on functional status in this population has not been evaluated. There is clear evidence that beta-blockers improve survival among patients with left ventricular systolic dysfunction and heart failure,[5–7] but it is uncertain whether this beneficial effect is related to their negative chronotropic effect or to some other anti-adrenergic property. However, the greatest benefit of beta blocker therapy is observed in those patients with the highest resting heart rate.[8] These data call into question the strategy of rapid pacing for patients with heart failure.

## Atrioventricular Synchrony

In individuals with normal systolic function, it has been estimated that the atrial contribution adds approximately 15% to 30% to the total cardiac output.[9]

Atrial contraction assists in diastolic filling of the ventricle, and the increased ventricular volume may augment contractility by the Frank-Starling mechanism.[10] Conversely, the absence of proper atrioventricular (AV) synchrony may produce systolic mitral and tricuspid valve insufficiency, diastolic insufficiency due to delayed valve closure, pulmonary and systemic venous congestion due to atrial contraction against closed AV valves, and an inappropriate decrease in peripheral resistance caused by autonomic activation associated with atrial distention. All of these factors have the potential to decrease cardiac output and cause symptomatic hypotension. The term *pacemaker syndrome* was originally applied to individuals with pacemakers in the VVI mode who became symptomatic from the loss of a properly timed atrial contraction.[11] Although syncope and severe symptomatic hypotension are relatively uncommon, it has become clear that many patients experience some adverse effects with chronic pacing in the VVI mode. There is also evidence from experimental studies to suggest that long-term ventricular pacing may be associated with adverse structural and functional alterations in the ventricular muscle.[12,13] In contrast, improved cardiac performance with dual-chamber pacing has now been well documented clinically.[14]

The loss of the atrial contribution can be especially deleterious in individuals who have abnormal ventricular diastolic filling due to a stiff, noncompliant ventricle (e.g., LV hypertrophy or restrictive cardiomyopathies), outflow obstruction (e.g., mitral stenosis or aortic stenosis), or both (hypertrophic cardiomyopathy). The importance of the atrial contraction in patients with congestive heart failure (who may have continuously elevated filling pressures) is more controversial. Despite some reports to the contrary,[15] the preponderance of evidence indicates that individuals with heart failure (CHF) tolerate loss of the atrial "kick" poorly.[16] In one study, the acute effect of pacing mode on hemodynamic function was measured in 21 subjects with CHF and conduction system disease.[17] Comparisons were made between pacing in AAI, VVI, and DDD (150-msec AV delay) modes at the same paced rates. Hemodynamic function worsened with VVI pacing, with no difference between the atrial-based pacing modes. Other larger series of subjects with CHF and left bundle branch block (LBBB) have demonstrated the lack of benefit of right ventricular (RV) pacing (VDD mode) in comparison with intrinsic conduction.[18,19]

### Atrioventricular Delay

Hemodynamic parameters during dual-chamber pacing can be markedly affected by the AV conduction time. This relationship is complex, however, and may be influenced by multiple variables such as interatrial conduction time, level of hydration (preload), peripheral vascular resistance (afterload), degree of diastolic dysfunction, and presence of interventricular conduction defects. Several studies have correlated the programmed AV delay with hemodynamic parameters, and the data suggest that cardiac performance, both in patients with a reduced left ventricular ejection fraction (LVEF) and in those with normal LV function, is impaired at long AV delays, especially when associated with diastolic mitral regurgitation (MR).[20,21] This issue is especially important in the heart failure population, where small improvements in cardiac performance may markedly improve functional status.

### Clinical Studies of Right Ventricular Pacing

One of the first investigations of chronic pacing, as a primary therapy for the treatment of congestive heart failure, was performed by Hochleitner and associates.[22] In an uncontrolled study of 16 patients with severe idiopathic dilated cardiomyopathy, they reported dramatic functional improvement with dual-chamber pacing using a short AV delay of 100 msec. In a subsequent long-term follow-up study, they found that the beneficial effects persisted for up to 5 years.[23] Although the 100-msec AV delay was apparently chosen empirically, subsequent case studies using short AV delay pacing in heart failure patients yielded similar findings.[24,25] Several additional investigators have reported that optimizing AV delay may produce acute hemodynamic improvement in patients with heart failure, although there is some suggestion that the major benefit is confined to individuals with prolonged PR intervals and diastolic MR.[26,27]

More recent studies using instantaneous or beat-by-beat hemodynamic measures have failed to confirm the benefit of RV pacing on measures of contractility or cardiac output.[19,28] Another problem with the evaluation of different AV delays is identifying which hemodynamic parameter should be optimized. Traditionally, the optimal AV delay is defined as that associated with the maximal cardiac output. However, it is possible that minimizing filling pressures or reducing the amount of MR may be more appropriate endpoints for predicting long-term functional improvement.

The preliminary studies of pacing in subjects with LV dysfunction provided the stimulus for controlled clinical trials, which unfortunately have failed to confirm the benefits of short AV delay RV pacing in this population. There are many possible reasons for this discrepancy; among them are the use of subjective endpoints (in the uncontrolled and unblinded studies), spontaneous variability in the clinical course of the disease, and the possibility that changes in the medical regimens (e.g., addition of ACE inhibitors or beta-blockers) rather than pacing may have been primarily responsible for the observed symptomatic improvement. Accordingly, it is not surprising that, in a controlled randomized study using a crossover design, Gold and coworkers failed to demonstrate a hemodynamic benefit with VDD pacing with a 100-msec AV delay (compared with VVI pacing at 40 bpm) in 12 patients with class III or IV congestive heart failure refractory to medical management.[29] Similar findings were reported by Innes et al.,[30] who, in a randomized crossover study of patients with symptomatic CHF, used VDD pacing and a short AV delay. Linde and associates also failed to demonstrate any benefit of AV synchronous pacing and "optimum" AV delay over a 3-month follow-up period for 10 patients with severe symptomatic heart failure.[31]

More recently, the DAVID trial was completed, which is the largest trial to date evaluating the role of RV pacing in patients with LV systolic dysfunction and no traditional pacing indication.[32] In this study, patients were required to have an ejection fraction less than 40% and have a standard indication for ICD implantation but no class I pacemaker indication. All subjects received a dual-chamber ICD and were then randomized to pacing in DDDR mode at a lower rate of 70 bpm or back-up pacing in VVI mode at 40 bpm. The primary composite endpoint of this trial was time to death or first hospitalization for CHF. One-year event-free survival was significantly better in the group programmed to VVI pacing (hazard ratio, 1.61; $P < 0.03$; Figure 4–1). The most likely explanation for this finding was that the mean proportion of ventricular pacing was 61% in the DDDR group but only 2.9% in the VVI group ($P < 0.001$). These results imply that frequent RV pacing is deleterious in patients with LV dysfunction.

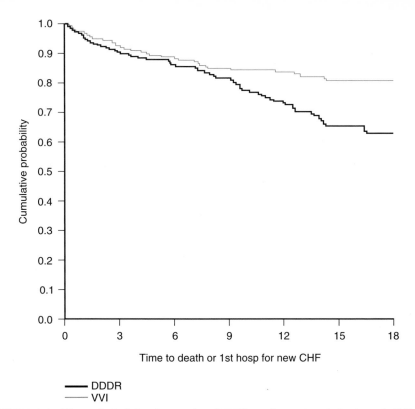

FIGURE 4–1. Effect of dual-chamber pacing (DDDR) mode on hospitalization of CHF and death. Results from the DAVID trial. *(From The DAVID Trial Investigators: Dual-chamber pacing or ventricular backup pacing in patients with an implantable defibrillator: the Dual Chamber and VVI Implantable Defibrillator [DAVID] Trial. JAMA 2002;288:3115–3123.)*

These findings are consistent with results from the MOST pacemaker trial. In a subanalysis of patients with normal QRS duration, it was observed that the risk of hospitalization for heart failure was directly proportional to the amount of ventricular pacing in patients programmed to DDDR and VVIR modes.[33] The risk of atrial fibrillation was also increased as a function of the percentage of ventricular pacing.

Thus, despite the promising results described initially, controlled studies have not verified that the application of short AV delay pacing in the VDD or DDD modes to an unselected population of symptomatic patients with CHF and LV systolic dysfunction provides any sustained hemodynamic benefit. In fact, recent studies indicate that there is a long-term deleterious effect of frequent RV pacing, a finding suggesting that, rather than being optimized, AV delays should be prolonged or the AAI mode should be utilized to minimize such pacing.

## Right Ventricular Stimulation Site

When ventricular pacing techniques were initially developed, the RV apex was selected preferentially because it was readily accessible and provided good pacing and sensing characteristics, with an acceptable incidence of lead dislodgment. However, there are a number of potential reasons why RV pacing in general and RV apical pacing in particular might be suboptimal (Table 4–1). RV pacing has been shown to produce paradoxical septal motion and to interfere with the normal functioning of the mitral apparatus, potentially causing mitral insufficiency. In addition, there is evidence that RV pacing affects diastolic function[34] and that diastolic filling time may be diminished. There are also important metabolic effects of RV pacing, including changes in regional myocardial blood flow and perfusion.[35,36] Pacing from the apex increases serum catecholamine levels, which could have deleterious long-term effects on functional status and survival.[37] Finally, it has also been demonstrated that atrial (AAI) pacing in patients with intact AV conduction produces a higher cardiac output than dual-chamber pacing, suggesting that the ventricular activation pattern may influence cardiac performance.[38]

Initial data from animal studies and from uncontrolled clinical investigations suggested that the site of RV pacing and the accompanying difference in contraction pattern did, in fact, affect hemodynamic parameters, with RV septal or outflow tract pacing being superior to apical pacing.[39–41] These observations were supported by a prospective study of Mera and colleagues. They performed a randomized crossover trial of 12 patients in chronic AF following His-bundle ablation and showed that QRS duration was shorter with septal pacing than with apical pacing. LV fractional shortening and ejection fraction were better with septal pacing, although exercise times did not differ significantly. The improvements of ejection fraction correlated with the change in QRS duration.[42] However, in a randomized double-blind study, Gold et al. found that VDD pacing from the outflow tract offered no hemodynamic advantage to no pacing among patients with heart failure and intact AV conduction, over a wide range of AV delays.[43] Furthermore, in a subsequent prospective randomized study, it was shown that RV apical pacing was comparable hemodynamically to pacing from the RV outflow tract.[17] Pacing mode (VVI versus DDD) was more important than pacing site (right ventricular apex versus outflow tract) hemodynamically (Figure 4–2). Kass and colleagues also found no acute hemodynamic effects of RV pacing (septal or apical) in subjects with LBBB, but they did report an increase of pulse pressure with RV pacing in the few patients with RBBB.[19]

One possible explanation for the discrepant findings noted previously as to the benefit of right ventricular outflow tract pacing is the variability of pacing site.

TABLE 4–1. **Potential Adverse Effects of Right Ventricular Pacing**

1. Dyssynchronous left ventricular contraction
2. Decreased left ventricular ejection fraction
3. Myocardial perfusion defects
4. Mitral and tricuspid valvular insufficiency
5. Altered diastolic function
6. Diminution of diastolic filling time
7. Increase in serum catecholamine concentration

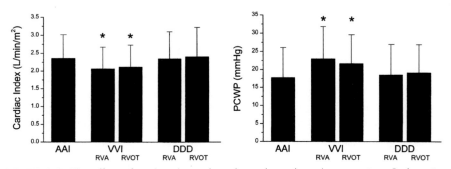

FIGURE 4–2. The effect of pacing site and mode on hemodynamic parameters. Pacing at a fixed rate were compared in AAI, VVI, and DDD modes from the RV apex (*RVA*) or outflow tract (*RVOT*). *Top panel,* Cardiac index. *Bottom panel,* Pulmonary capillary wedge pressure (*PCWP*). *(From Gold MR, Brockman R, Peters RW, et al. Acute hemodynamic effects of right ventricular pacing site and pacing mode in patients with congestive heart failure. Am J Cardiol 2000;85:1106–1109.)*

In this regard, Schwaab and co-workers investigated subjects with sinus rhythm and complete AV block to determine whether pacing from the RV apex or outflow tract produced QRS narrowing and if this was accompanied by improved ventricular performance.[44] In each patient, the AV delay was optimized to produce the maximum cardiac output. They observed that pacing-induced QRS narrowing did improve the LV contraction pattern, but that they could not predict whether the improvement would occur with pacing from the outflow tract or from the apex. However, using a different approach to synchronize activation, Buckingham et al. evaluated the acute hemodynamic effects of simultaneous dual-site RV pacing (apex and outflow tract) and found no significant improvement with dual-site pacing, despite a narrowing of QRS duration.[45]

Several studies have evaluated the chronic effects of RV outflow tract pacing. Victor and colleagues compared the long-term hemodynamic and functional effects of RV apical and outflow tract pacing in 16 patients with chronic AF and complete AV block.[46] All patients underwent implantation of a dual-chamber pacemaker with one lead in the apex and the other in the outflow tract. In this way, ventricular pacing from both sites could be evaluated in the same subject. They found that neither pacing site offered a distinct advantage in those with either normal or reduced LV function. The Right Ventricular Outflow Versus Apical Pacing (ROVA) trial involved 103 patients with chronic AF, LVEF less than 40%, and a fully paced ventricular rhythm due to either AV junctional ablation or intrinsic AV node disease.[47] A dual-chamber pacemaker was implanted (with both leads in the right ventricle), and the effects of outflow tract and apical pacing were compared with a randomized double-blind crossover design, followed by an open-label period of dual-site right ventricular pacing. The primary endpoint of this study was quality of life; however, functional class, exercise capacity, and LVEF were also assessed. Again, no benefit of outflow tract pacing or of dual-site pacing was noted in comparison with pacing from the RV apex. Recently, Tse and colleagues reported a study of 24 patients with complete heart block who were randomized to RV apical or outflow tract pacing.[48] They observed significantly more perfusion defects and a greater decline in ejection fraction in those patients paced from the apex, but these effects were not noted until

18 months of pacing. This is a longer clinical follow-up than evaluated previously. Thus it is possible that a functional difference between RV pacing sites may take years rather than weeks to manifest.

In summary, despite early promising results from uncontrolled studies, the location of the pacing site in the right ventricle does not appear to be an important determinant of cardiac performance. Accordingly, at this time the routine use of RV septal or outflow tract pacing cannot be recommended as a means of improving cardiac function in patients with CHF.[48] Further studies will be necessary to assess the more chronic effects of pacing site on function status to determine whether there is a long-term benefit of outflow tract pacing or if there are specific patient subgroups that might benefit, such as those with significant MR, those with concomitant diastolic dysfunction, or those with specific conduction defects (such as RBBB).

A more novel approach to pacing in the right ventricle without causing asynchronous ventricular activation is to stimulate the His bundle directly. This results in a narrow QRS complex that is similar to that observed with normally conducted beats. Deshmukh and colleagues demonstrated the feasibility of permanent pacing of the His bundle in a series of patients with chronic AF, LV systolic dysfunction, and a narrow conducted QRS complex.[50] Although there are a number of technical challenges with this approach, such as high thresholds, failure to pace the His bundle in some patients, and probable parahisian pacing with QRS widening chronically in other subjects, this is a promising approach to avoid the deleterious effects of chronic RV pacing. However, this will not be a useful means of resynchronization among patients with bundle branch block, because the conduction disturbance is distal to the site of His bundle pacing. Controlled studies of this technique, after the development of improved tools and leads to achieve reliable His bundle pacing, will be needed to evaluate this approach more fully.

## Pacing for Patients with Atrial Fibrillation and Heart Failure

AF is the most common sustained arrhythmia and is encountered frequently in a population with LV dysfunction and CHF. Indeed, it is likely that there is a vicious cycle involving these disorders with the atrial distention, sympathetic stimulation, and hypoxia produced by heart failure predisposing to AF and the loss of atrial contraction exerting deleterious effects upon cardiac function. Although permanent pacing has been traditionally utilized for symptomatic AF with a slow ventricular response, the availability of AV nodal ablation/modification has helped introduce the concept of pacing in AF to improve hemodynamic function. In addition to preventing tachycardia-induced LV dysfunction, there is considerable clinical evidence that regularization of the ventricular rate alone in patients with AF may be helpful hemodynamically.[51,52] However, RV pacing may promote atrial fibrillation. In a small crossover study, VVI pacing increased dispersion of refractoriness, sinus node dysfunction, and left atrial size in comparison with dual-chamber pacing.[53,54] It cannot be determined from these studies if the adverse effect of pacing is due to the loss of AV synchrony or to RV pacing. Several recent studies have examined the effects of AV node ablation with permanent pacemaker implantation among patients with a reduced LVEF.

Brignole and colleagues reported a randomized controlled multicenter study of radiofrequency catheter AV junction ablation with VVIR permanent pacemaker implantation versus best pharmacologic therapy in 66 patients with heart failure and chronic (longer than 6 months' duration) AF with a rapid ventricular response.[55] Patients in the ablation/pacing group experienced greater symptomatic improvement, but there was no demonstrable difference in cardiac performance as assessed by serial echocardiographic and exercise studies. Twidale and colleagues analyzed predictors of outcome after radiofrequency catheter ablation of the AV node in 44 consecutive patients with heart failure and AF with a poorly controlled ventricular response.[56] They found that significant mitral regurgitation, severe LV dysfunction (ejection fraction less than 30%), and failure to exhibit any improvement in cardiac performance within 1 month of ablation predicted a poor outcome and high mortality. They also reported that AV node ablation was more effective than AV nodal modification in improving cardiac performance in this cohort.[57] Vanderheyden and colleagues found that LV systolic and diastolic dilation were more predictive of worsening heart failure than fractional shortening among patients with heart failure undergoing AV junctional ablation.[58] Marshall and associates reported the results of a prospective, randomized study of ablation and permanent pacing in 56 patients with paroxysmal AF.[59] Although heart failure was present in only a minority of the population, they found that ablation and DDDR pacing with mode-switching produced greater symptomatic relief than either medical therapy or ablation with VVIR pacing. It is noteworthy, however, that patients receiving antiarrhythmic drugs were less likely to have recurrence of AF.

The Ablate and Pace Trial was a prospective multicenter study of 153 subjects undergoing AV junction ablation and permanent pacemaker implantation as treatment of drug-refractory AF. There were significant improvements in quality of life, functional class, and LVEF following ablation, but no effects were observed on exercise parameters. Subjects with LV dysfunction showed the greatest increase in ejection fraction following ablation.[60] A meta-analysis of clinical trials of ablation and pacing for atrial fibrillation was performed by Wood et al.[61] They summarized the results of 21 studies with a total of 1181 patients. Significant improvements of quality of life, ejection fraction, exercise duration, and healthcare use were improved with this procedure (Table 4–2).

In summary, heart block and symptomatic bradycardia are frequently observed in the cohort with LV dysfunction, so pacemaker therapy is common in this group. Despite early promise, there are little controlled data to suggest that RV pacing,

**TABLE 4–2. Meta-Analysis of AV Junctional Ablation and Pacing for Atrial Fibrillation**

| Measure | Effect Size | 95% Confidence Intervals | P Value |
|---|---|---|---|
| Treadmill | 107 ± 8 sec | 94 – 120 sec | <0.001 |
| LVEF | 4.4 ± 0.1% | 2.9 – 5.8% | <0.001 |
| General QoL | 0.25 ± 0.02 | 0.21 – 0.28 | <0.001 |
| Activity scale | −0.46 ± 0.18 | −0.17 – −0.76 | 0.005 |
| Improved patients | 87 ± 5% | 78 – 95% | <0.001 |
| NYHA class | −0.83 ± 0.07 | −0.72 – −0.95 | <0.001 |
| Hospital admissions | −2.3 ± 0.4 | −1.7 – −3.0 | <0.001 |
| Outpatient visits | −3.1 ± 0.4 | −2.6 – −3.6 | <0.001 |

in the absence of symptomatic bradycardia, has any long-term hemodynamic or functional benefit. In fact, recent studies suggest that there is a cumulative deleterious effect of chronic RV pacing that has led to the emerging strategy of minimizing ventricular pacing with implanted systems.

## REFERENCES

1. Konstam M, Dracup K, Baker D, et al: *Heart failure: Evaluation and care of patients with left ventricular systolic dysfunction.* Rockville, MD: Agency for Health Care Policy and Research, 1994 [Clinical Practice Guideline No. 11: AHCPR Publication No. 94-0612].
2. Luu M, Stevenson WG, Stevenson LW, et al: Ventricular tachycardia is not the predominant cause of monitored sudden death in heart failure. *Circulation* 1989;80:1675.
3. Higgins SL, Williams SK, Pak JP, et al: Indications for implantation of a dual-chamber pacemaker combined with an implantable cardioverter-defibrillator. *Am J Cardiol* 1998;81:1360.
4. Koch-Wesser J, Blinks JR: The influence of the interval between beats on myocardial contractility. *Pharmacol Rev* 1963;15:601.
5. Heidenreich PA, Lee TT, Massie BM: Effect of beta-blockade on mortality in patients with heart failure: A meta-analysis of randomized clinical trials. *J Am Coll Cardiol* 1997;30:27.
6. Packer M, Bristow MR, Cohn JN, et al: The effect of carvedilol on morbidity and mortality in patients in chronic heart failure. *N Engl J Med* 1996;334:1349.
7. Fisher ML, Gottlieb SS, Plotnick GD, et al: Beneficial effects of metoprolol in heart failure associated with coronary artery disease: a randomized trial. *J Am Coll Cardiol* 1994;23:943.
8. De Lenarda A, Gregori D, Sinagra G, et al: Metoprolol in dilated cardiomyopathy: is it possible to identify factors predictive of improvement? *J Card Failure* 1996;2:87.
9. Barold SS, Zipes DP: Cardiac pacemakers and antiarrhythmic devices. In: Braunwald E, ed: *Heart Disease: A Textbook of Cardiovascular Medicine.* 5th ed. Philadelphia: WB Saunders, 1997:705–741.
10. Linden RJ, Mitchell JH: Relation between left ventricular diastolic pressure and myocardial segment length and observations on the contribution of atrial systole. *Circ Res* 1960;8:1092.
11. Reynolds DW: Hemodynamics of cardiac pacing. In: Ellenbogen KA, ed: *Cardiac Pacing.* 2nd ed. Cambridge: Blackwell Science, 1996:124–167.
12. Lee MA, Dae MW, Langberg JJ, et al: Effects of long-term right ventricular apical pacing on left ventricular perfusion, innervation, function and histology. *J Am Coll Cardiol* 1994;24:225.
13. Tse H-F, Lau CP: Long-term effect of right ventricular pacing on myocardial perfusion and function. *J Am Coll Cardiol* 1997;29:744.
14. Nielsen JC, Andersen HR, Thomsen PEB, et al: Heart failure and echocardiographic changes during long-term follow-up of patients with sick sinus syndrome randomized to single-chamber atrial or ventricular pacing. *Circulation* 1998;97:987.
15. Greenberg B, Chatterjee K, Parmley W, et al: The influence of left ventricular filling pressure on atrial contribution to cardiac output. *Am Heart J* 1979;98:742.
16. Matsuda Y, Toma Y, Ogawa H, et al: Importance of left atrial function in patients with myocardial infarction. *Circulation* 1983;67:566.
17. Gold MR, Brockman R, Peters RW, et al: Acute hemodynamic effects of right ventricular pacing site and pacing mode in patients with congestive heart failure. *Am J Cardiol* 2000;85:1106–1109.
18. Blanc J-J, Etienne Y, Mansourati J, et al: Evaluation of different ventricular pacing sites in patients with severe heart failure: results of an acute hemodynamic study. *Circulation* 1997;96:3273.
19. Kass DA, Chen C-H, Curry C, et al: Improved left ventricular mechanics from acute VDD pacing in patients with dilated cardiomyopathy and ventricular conduction delay. *Circulation* 1999;99:1567.
20. Jutsy RV, Feenstra L, Pai R, et al: Comparison of intrinsic versus pace ventricular function. *PACE* 1992;15:1919.
21. Ishikawa T, Sumita S, Kimura K, et al: Critical PQ interval for the appearance of diastolic mitral regurgitation and optimal PQ interval in patients implanted with DDD pacemakers. *PACE* 1994;17:1989.
22. Hochleitner M, Hortnagl H, Ng C-K, et al: Usefulness of physiologic dual-chamber pacing in drug-resistant idiopathic cardiomyopathy. *Am J Cardiol* 1990;66:198.
23. Hochleitner M, Hortnagl H, Hortnagl H, et al: Long-term efficacy of physiologic dual-chamber pacing in the treatment of end-stage idiopathic dilated cardiomyopathy. *Am J Cardiol* 1992;70:1320.
24. Kataoka H: Hemodynamic effect of physiological dual chamber pacing in a patient with end-stage dilated cardiomyopathy: a case report. *PACE* 1991;14:1330.

25. Auricchio A, Sommariva S, Salo RW, et al: Improvement of cardiac function in patients with severe congestive heart failure and coronary artery disease by dual chamber pacing with shortened AV delay. *PACE* 1993;16:2034.

26. Brecker SJD, Xiao HB, Sparrow J, et al: Effects of dual-chamber pacing with short atrioventricular delay in dilated cardiomyopathy. *Lancet* 1992;340:1308.

27. Nishimura RA, Hayes DL, Holmes DR, et al: Mechanism of hemodynamic improvement by dual-chamber pacing for severe left ventricular dysfunction: an acute Doppler and catheterization hemodynamic study. *J Am Coll Cardiol* 1995;25:281.

28. Auricchio A, Stellbrink C, Block M, et al: Effect of pacing chamber and atrio-ventricular delay on acute systolic function of paced patients with congestive heart failure. *Circulation* 1999;99:2993–3001.

29. Gold MR, Feliciano Z, Gottlieb SS, et al: Dual-chamber pacing with a short atrioventricular delay in congestive heart failure: a randomized study. *J Am Coll Cardiol* 1995;26:967.

30. Innes D, Leitch JW, Fletcher PJ, et al: VDD pacing at short atrioventricular intervals does not improve cardiac output in patients with dilated heart failure. *PACE* 1994;17:959.

31. Linde C, Gadler F, Edner M: Results of atrioventricular synchronous pacing with severe congestive heart failure. *Am J Cardiol* 1995;75:919.

32. The DAVID Trial Investigators: Dual-chamber pacing or ventricular backup pacing in patients with an implantable defibrillator: the Dual Chamber and VVI Implantable Defibrillator (DAVID) Trial. *JAMA* 2002;288:3115–3123.

33. Sweeney MO, Hellkamp AS, Ellenbogen K, et al: Adverse Effect of Ventricular Pacing on heart failure and atrial fibrillation among patients with normal baseline QRS duration in a clinical trial of pacemaker therapy for sinus node dysfunction. *Circulation,* 2003;107:2932.

34. Betocchi S, Piscione F, Billiari B, et al: Effects of induced asynchrony on left ventricular diastolic function in patients with coronary artery disease. *J Am Coll Cardiol* 1993;21:1124.

35. Nielsen JC, Bottcher M, Nielsen TT, et al: Regional myocardial blood flow in patients with sick sinus syndrome randomized to long-term single chamber atrial or dual chamber pacing—effect of pacing mode and rate. *J Am Coll Cardiol* 2000;35:1453–1461.

36. Skalidia EI, Kochiadakis GE, Koukouraki SI, et al: Myocardial perfusion in patients with permanent ventricular pacing and normal coronary arteries. *J Am Coll Cardiol* 2001;37:124–129.

37. Saxon LA, DeMarco T, Chatterjee K, et al: Chronic biventricular pacing decreases serum norepinephrine in dilated heart failure patients with the greatest sympathetic activation at baseline [abstract]. *PACE* 1999;22:830.

38. Rosenqvist M, Isaaz K, Botvinick EH, et al: Relative importance of activation sequence compared to atrioventricular synchrony in left ventricular function. *Am J Cardiol* 1991;67:148.

39. Karpawich PP, Vincent JA: Ventricular pacing site does make a difference: improved left ventricular function with septal pacing. *PACE* 1994;17:820.

40. Giudici MC, Thornburg GA, Buck DL, et al: Comparison of right ventricular outflow tract and apical lead permanent pacing on cardiac output. *Am J Cardiol* 1997;79:209.

41. Cowell R, Morris-Thurgood J, Ilsley C, et al: Septal short atrioventricular delay pacing: additional hemodynamic improvements in heart failure. *PACE* 1994;17:1980.

42. Mera F, DeLurgio DB, Patterson RE, et al: A comparison of ventricular function during high right ventricular septal and apical pacing after his-bundle ablation for refractory atrial fibrillation. *PACE* 1999;22:1234–1239.

43. Gold MR, Shorofsky SR, Metcalf MD, et al: The acute hemodynamic effects of right ventricular septal pacing in patients with congestive heart failure secondary to ischemic or idiopathic dilated cardiomyopathy. *Am J Cardiol* 1997;79:679.

44. Schwaab B, Frohlig G, Alexander C, et al: Influence of right ventricular stimulation site on left ventricular function in atrial synchronous ventricular pacing. *J Am Coll Cardiol* 1999;33:317.

45. Buckingham TA, Candinas R, Schlapfer J, et al: Acute hemodynamic effects of atrioventricular pacing at differing sites in the right ventricle individually and simultaneously. *PACE* 1997;20:909.

46. Victor F, Leclerq C, Mabo P, et al: Optimal right ventricular pacing site in chronically implanted patients: a prospective randomized cross-over comparison of apical and outflow tract pacing. *J Am Coll Cardiol* 1999;33:311.

47. Stambler BS, Ellenbogen KA, Zhang X, et al: Right ventricular outflow versus apical pacing in pacemaker patients with congestive heart failure and atrial fibrillation. *J Cardiovasc Electrophysiol* (in press), 2003.

48. Tse H-F, Yu C, Wond K-K, Tsang V, et al: Functional abnormalities in patients with permanent right ventricular pacing: The effect of sites of electrical stimulation. *J Am Coll Cardiol* 2002;40:1451–8.

49. Gold MR: Optimization of ventricular pacing: where should we implant the leads? *J Am Coll Cardiol* 1999;33:324.

50. Deshmukh P, Casavant DA, Romanyshyn M, Anderson K. Permanent, direct his-bundle pacing: A novel approach to cardiac pacing in patients with normal his-purkinje activation. *Circulation* 2000;101:869–877.
51. Daoud E, Weiss R, Bahu M, et al: Effect of irregular ventricular rhythm on cardiac output. *Am J Cardiol* 1996;78:1433.
52. Clark D, Plumb V, Epstein A, et al: Hemodynamic effects of irregular sequence of ventricular cycle lengths during atrial fibrillation. *J Am Coll Cardiol* 1997;30:1039.
53. Sparks PB, Mond HG, Vohra JK, et al: Mechanical remodeling of the left atrium after loss of atrioventricular synchrony: A long-term study in humans. *Circulation* 1999;100:1714–1721.
54. Sparks PB, Mond HG, Vohra JK, et al: Electrical remodeling of the atria following loss of atrioventricular synchrony: A long-term study in humans. *Circulation* 1999:100:1894–1900.
55. Brignole M, Menozzi C, Gianfranchi L, et al: Assessment of atrioventricular junction ablation and VVIR pacemaker versus pharmacologic treatment in patients with heart failure and chronic atrial fibrillation: a randomized controlled study. *Circulation* 1998;98:953.
56. Twidale N, Manda V, Nave K, et al: Predictors of outcome after radiofrequency catheter ablation of the atrioventricular node for atrial fibrillation and congestive heart failure. *Am Heart J* 1998;136:647.
57. Twidale N, McDonald T, Nave K, et al: Comparison of the effects of AV nodal ablation versus AV nodal modification in patients with congestive heart failure and uncontrolled atrial fibrillation. *PACE* 1998;21:641.
58. Vanderheyden M, Goethals M, Anguera I, et al: Hemodynamic deterioration following radiofrequency ablation of the atrioventricular conduction system. *PACE* 1997;20:2422–2428.
59. Marshall HJ, Harris ZI, Griffith MJ, et al: Prospective randomized study of ablation and pacing versus medical therapy for paroxysmal atrial fibrillation: effects of pacing mode and mode-switch algorithm. *Circulation* 1999;99:1587.
60. Kay GN, Ellenbogen KA, Giudici M, et al: The ablate and pace trial: A prospective study of catheter ablation of the AV conduction system and permanent pacemaker implantation for treatment of atrial fibrillation. *J Intervent Cardiol Electrophysiol* 1998;2:121.
61. Wood MA, Brown-Mahoney C, Kay GN, Ellenbogen KA: Clinical outcomes after ablation and pacing therapy for atrial fibrillation. *Circulation* 2000;101:1138–1144.

# 5

# Trials of Implantable Cardiac Defibrillators (ICDs) in Patients with Congestive Heart Failure (Nonbiventricular)

Alfred E. Buxton

As with almost every type of cardiac disease, sudden death accounts for approximately 50% of total mortality among patients with congestive heart failure (CHF), regardless of etiology. As total mortality increases with increasing severity of heart failure, so does the risk of sudden death. However, as severity of heart failure increases, the percentage of deaths accounted for by sudden death decreases.[1] This is not surprising, because patients with mild degrees of heart failure are not likely to die of nonarrhythmic causes. In evaluating the potential benefits of implantable cardiac defibrillator (ICD) therapy for patients with CHF, we are faced with the difficulty that most reports are based on heterogeneous populations with regard to the type of underlying heart disease and severity of heart failure. In addition, some studies have been limited to patients with nonischemic cardiomyopathy, whereas others have involved patients with CHF, regardless of etiology. The importance of the cause of heart failure stems from the likelihood that the mechanisms responsible for sudden death are related to the anatomic substrate causing heart failure. In addition, it is likely that the mechanisms responsible for sudden death change as disease progresses. It does seem likely that as the clinical syndrome of heart failure advances, certain common mechanisms contribute to the genesis of arrhythmias, regardless of the initial cause for heart failure. The etiology of heart failure is also important in the design and interpretation of the results of clinical trials, because patients having heart failure in the setting of ischemic heart disease have higher mortality rates than patients with nonischemic disease.[2-4]

The exact role of implantable defibrillators in patients with heart failure at this time is limited by our imperfect understanding of the mechanisms responsible for the sudden death of patients with CHF and the lack of a proven reliable test for risk stratification for patients with CHF. As a result, therapies in most studies have been assigned empirically without any mechanistic basis. We do understand that there are a number of potential pro-arrhythmic factors associated with CHF. Some of these factors are intrinsic to the condition, and these include ventricular hypertrophy and systolic dysfunction with stretch of myofibrils, which may induce arrhythmias. In addition, myocardial ischemia may play a role, and cellular damage, resulting from apoptosis, may enter into the picture. In addition, as heart failure advances, it is common to find areas of fibrosis throughout the ventricles, which may contribute to reentrant arrhythmias. Abnormalities of repolarization accompany exacerbations of heart failure and ventricular hypertrophy and may contribute to triggered arrhythmias, as do electrolyte disturbances such as hypokalemia and hypomagnesemia. In addition, elevated levels of circulating catecholamines and sympathetic tone may play a role. The extent to which these factors may influence the efficacy of the ICD to reduce mortality is unknown.

Extrinsic factors may also contribute to the genesis of arrhythmias in patients with heart failure. These include the use of inotropic agents for circulatory support, diuretic therapy, and antiarrhythmic drugs, which are often necessary to suppress symptomatic arrhythmias such as atrial fibrillation. As a result, we have seen that arrhythmias documented at the time of cardiac arrest in patients with CHF are extremely variable. Polymorphic ventricular tachycardias both with and without associated prolongation of the QT interval have been documented, as well as monomorphic ventricular tachycardias. It is important to keep in mind the possibility that monomorphic tachycardias in patients with heart failure may involve bundle branch reentry, which is curable by catheter ablation.

At this time, we have little direct data specifically delineating the efficacy of ICD therapy in patients whose primary clinical problem is symptomatic heart failure. This situation should be remedied within the next several years, when the Sudden Cardiac Death–Heart Failure Trial (SCD-HeFT) and the Defibrillators in Nonischemic Cardiomyopathy Treatment Evaluation (DEFINITE) trial are completed. However, we do have indirect evidence of the relation between efficacy of defibrillators and left ventricular (LV) dysfunction and heart failure on several levels. Secondary prevention trials, including the Antiarrhythmics Versus Implantable Defibrillators (AVID) trial and the Canadian Implantable Defibrillator Study (CIDS), compared the utility of defibrillators versus amiodarone in patients who had survived cardiac arrest or hemodynamically unstable ventricular tachycardias.[5,6] Analyses specifically relating to CHF and ejection fraction have been published from these studies. A third major randomized trial of secondary prevention, the Cardiac Arrest Study Hamburg (CASH), did not yield data specifically relating ICD effects to ejection fraction or CHF status, and it is not discussed in detail.[7] In addition, several primary prevention studies, including the Multicenter Automatic Defibrillator Implantation Trial (MADIT), the Multicenter UnSustained Tachycardia Trial (MUSTT), and the Multicenter Automatic Defibrillator Implantation Trial II (MADIT II), have analyzed the effects of ejection fraction and CHF on ICD efficacy in patients with coronary disease.[8-10] The other major primary prevention trial involving patients with coronary artery disease, the Coronary Artery Bypass Graft-Patch Trial (CABG-Patch), led to a substudy report relating ICD benefit to wall motion score and ejection fraction.[11] Finally, the Cardiomyopathy Trial (CAT) specifically evaluated the utility of the ICD in patients with nonischemic cardiomyopathy.[12] The results of these analyses are presented herein.

The AVID trial randomized 1016 patients who had survived out-of-hospital cardiac arrest or hemodynamically unstable sustained ventricular tachyarrhythmias[13] (Table 5–1). After an average follow-up of 18 months, survival among the patients randomized to ICD therapy was improved by approximately 30%

over that among patients randomized to amiodarone therapy. In the AVID trial, 42% of patients had a history of CHF prior to their qualifying episode of ventricular tachycardia (VT) or ventricular fibrillation. Forty-eight percent of patients were of New York Heart Association (NYHA) functional class I or II, and 10% were of NYHA class III. The average ejection fraction of patients in the AVID trial was 32%, and 81% of patients had coronary disease (including a prior myocardial infarction in 67%). The AVID investigators have published an analysis of the effect of ejection fraction on defibrillator efficacy.[5] Patients enrolled in the trial were divided into three groups: those having an ejection fraction less than 20%, those with an ejection fraction of 20% to 34%, and those with an ejection fraction greater than 34%. Not surprisingly, those with the lower ejection fractions were more likely to have a history of CHF: 73% of patients with ejection fraction less than 20%, 51% of those with ejection fraction 20% to 34%, and only 33% of those with ejection fraction greater than 34%. In addition, the investigators noted that VT as the presenting arrhythmia was more common in patients with an ejection fraction less than 20% (18% of patients) than in those with higher ejection fractions (13% of patients whose ejection fraction was greater than 34% had VT). When survival was analyzed, there was no difference between antiarrhythmic drug-treated and defibrillator-treated patients among those with an ejection fraction greater than 34%. In contrast, there was significantly higher survival associated with defibrillator therapy in patients whose ejection fraction was between 20% and 34% (relative risk, 1.6 at 2 years). Patients whose ejection fraction was <20% had a similar magnitude of benefit in association with defibrillator therapy, but because the numbers of patients were much smaller, statistical significance was not observed. The relative risk for antiarrhythmic therapy was 1.3 (i.e., patients having an ejection fraction less than 20% who were randomized to pharmacologic antiarrhythmic therapy had a 30% higher mortality than those randomized to ICD therapy).

**TABLE 5–1. ICD Trials Patient Characteristics**

| Trial | Number of Patients | CAD (%) | NHD (%) | NYHA Class II or III at Enrollment (%) | EF (%) |
|---|---|---|---|---|---|
| SECONDARY PREVENTION TRIALS* | | | | | |
| AVID | 1016 | 81 | 3 | 58 | 32 |
| CIDS | 659 | 82.6 | 3 | 50 | 34 |
| CASH | 288 | 73.3 | 10 | 73 | 46 |
| PRIMARY PREVENTION TRIALS | | | | | |
| MADIT | 196 | 100 | — | 65 | 26 |
| MUSTT | 704 | 100 | — | 63 | 30 |
| MADIT II | 1232 | 100 | — | 58[†] | 23 |
| CABG-Patch | 900 | 100 | — | 73 | 27 |

CAD = coronary artery disease; NHD = no structural heart disease; NYHA = New York Heart Association Functional Class; EF = left ventricular ejection fraction.
*Excludes patients randomized to propafenone.
[†]5% of patients in MADIT II were NYHA functional class IV.

The AVID investigators subsequently published a second analysis seeking to define more clearly the influence of ejection fraction as related to specific antiarrhythmic treatments (defibrillator versus pharmacologic antiarrhythmic therapy).[14] For this analysis, the patients were divided into quintiles of ejection fraction based on each treatment group. The defibrillator and antiarrhythmic drug–treated patients were well balanced with regard to prognostic characteristics, except that more patients in the ICD group were discharged while receiving beta-blockers. In this analysis, again, the total mortality among patients in the two highest quintiles of ejection fraction (constituting patients whose ejection fraction was greater than 34%) had similar survival characteristics, regardless of treatment. In the lowest quintiles of ejection fraction, survival was improved among the patients treated with defibrillators. There seemed to be more variation in survival as related to ejection fraction of patients treated with drugs than in relation to defibrillators. In other words, the baseline left ventricular ejection fraction predicted survival for drug-treated patients but not for those treated with an ICD. In a separate analysis using the endpoint of arrhythmic death, ICD-treated patients did not have any difference in outcome based on ejection fraction. However, death due to arrhythmia was associated with ejection fraction in drug-treated patients. There are several potential explanations for this, including the possibility that adverse effects of drugs are amplified in patients with lower ejection fraction fractions. It is also possible that amiodarone is more effective in patients with higher ejection fractions, either because of different arrhythmia mechanisms depending on the hemodynamic status or because it is a more effective antiarrhythmic drug for similar arrhythmias if LV function is better preserved.

The Canadian trial (CIDS) randomized 659 patients who had survived episodes of cardiac arrest, unstable VT, or syncope[15] (Table 5–2). Survival in this trial was improved by a magnitude similar to that observed in the AVID study among patients randomized to ICD therapy versus amiodarone. Fifty percent of patients in CIDS had a history of CHF prior to their qualifying arrhythmia episode. Thirty-nine percent of patients in this trial were of NYHA class I or II and 11% were NYHA class III or IV at enrollment in the trial. The mean left ventricular ejection fraction of 34% was similar to that of patients enrolled in the AVID trial. Likewise, the prevalence of coronary disease was similar to that of patients enrolled in the AVID trial (82%), and 76% of patients with coronary disease had a prior myocardial infarction. The CIDS investigators found three factors that had a significant impact on survival: increased age, reduced ejection fraction, and NYHA functional class III or IV.[6] Of note, in the CIDS study, a number of factors thought likely to influence survival were not significantly related. Specifically, gender, the presence and extent of coronary disease, and beta-blocker use did not significantly impact survival. On the basis of the three major risk factors associated with survival, the investigators then divided patients in the CIDS trial into quartiles, based on the number of risk factors present. In the three lower-risk quartiles (comprising patients having zero, one, or two risk factors), there was no significant advantage of defibrillator therapy over amiodarone therapy on overall survival. However, among patients in the highest-risk group (having all three risk factors), survival was significantly improved for those treated with defibrillators. When patients had at least two risk factors (age of 70 or more years, ejection fraction of 35% or less, and NYHA class III or IV), ICD therapy was associated with a 50% mortality reduction in comparison with amiodarone.

TABLE 5–2. ICD Trials Non-antiarrhythmic Therapy

| Trial | Beta-blocker Use in Control Patients (%) | Beta-blocker Use in ICD Patients (%) | ACE-inhibitor Use in Control Patients (%) | ACE-inhibitor Use in ICD Patients (%) |
|---|---|---|---|---|
| AVID | 17 | 42 | 68 | 69 |
| CIDS | 21 | 34 | —* | —* |
| CASH† | 0–96‡ | 0‡ | 40 | 45 |
| MADIT | 8 | 26 | 55 | 60 |
| MUSTT | 51 | 37 | 77 | 72 |
| MADIT II | 70 | 70 | 72 | 68 |
| CABG-Patch | 24 | 18 | 54 | 55 |

*The use of ACE inhibitors was not reported in the CIDS trial.
†Excludes patients randomized to propafenone.
‡The study design of the CASH trial incorporated three therapy arms: ICD, amiodarone, and metoprolol. No patient assigned to ICD or amiodarone therapy received beta-blocker; 96% of patients randomized to metoprolol received the drug.

Thus both the AVID and CIDS trials demonstrated consistent effects of ICD therapy, with relatively less benefit demonstrated among patients with higher ejection fractions. Readers should be aware of an alternative explanation for these observations that has not been fully explored. It should be noted that the follow-up duration in these studies was relatively brief. The AVID trial was stopped prematurely after an average follow-up of only 18 months, and the average follow-up in the CIDS trial was 36 months. Several prior studies have demonstrated that the frequency of ventricular arrhythmias is lower in patients with higher ejection fractions.[16-18] Thus studies with relatively brief follow-up such as those named previously are less likely to demonstrate a significant benefit of one therapy over another if the frequency of recurrent events in the study population is sufficiently low. Determining the viability of this explanation will require studies with longer follow-up.

Among the studies of primary prevention of sudden cardiac death, the MADIT study was designed to compare the ability of ICDs versus conventional therapy to reduce mortality among patients with coronary disease, myocardial infarction at least 3 weeks prior to enrollment in the trial, ejection fraction of 35% or less, spontaneous nonsustained VT, and inducible sustained VT unresponsive to procainamide[19] (see Table 5–1). Seventy-four percent of patients randomized to the conventional therapy arm received empiric therapy with amiodarone. This small trial (196 patients enrolled) demonstrated a 54% reduction in total mortality among patients treated with defibrillators after an average follow-up of 27 months (Figure 5–1). The average ejection fraction of patients enrolled was 26%. Sixty-five percent of patients were of NYHA functional class II or III, and 51% of patient were receiving treatment for heart failure at the time of enrollment in the trial. The MADIT investigators subsequently performed a separate analysis of the influence of ejection fraction and CHF on the degree of benefit from defibrillator therapy.[8] They noted higher mortality among the patients with ejection fraction less than 26% and among those with a history of congestive heart failure requiring treatment. Among the lower-risk patients with ejection fraction of 26% to 35%, there was no significant survival advantage associated with the ICD in comparison to

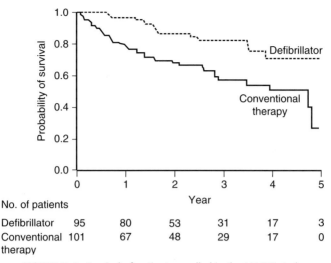

No. of patients

| | 0 | 1 | 2 | 3 | 4 | 5 |
|---|---|---|---|---|---|---|
| Defibrillator | 95 | 80 | 53 | 31 | 17 | 3 |
| Conventional therapy | 101 | 67 | 48 | 29 | 17 | 0 |

**FIGURE 5–1.** Survival of patients enrolled in the MADIT study.

conventional therapy. In contrast, among the higher-risk subset having an ejection fraction less than 26%, there was a marked improvement of survival in association with defibrillator therapy. The hazard ratio for ICD therapy in patients with ejection fraction greater than 26% was 0.5 ($P = 0.12$), whereas the hazard ratio associated with defibrillator therapy for patients with ejection fraction less than 26% was 0.27 ($P = 0.002$).

Likewise, among patients without a history of CHF, there was a nonsignificant reduction in mortality risk of 57% in association with defibrillator therapy ($P = 0.09$). In contrast, among patients with a history of CHF, there was a 70% reduction in mortality risk ($P = 0.002$).

There are several explanations for the failure to demonstrate survival benefit among the MADIT patients with higher ejection fractions and absence of CHF. First, the small number of patients enrolled (196 in total) limits the power. Ninety-five patients had no history of congestive heart failure, but 101 had a history of heart failure. Ninety-four patients had ejection fraction of 26% to 35%, versus 102 with an ejection less than 26%. When these small groups are further subdivided into the two treatment groups, one can see how difficult it might be in a lower-risk group to demonstrate survival benefit. The other explanation for the failure to demonstrate improved survival among patients without a history of heart failure and with higher ejection fractions may be similar to that noted previously regarding the AVID trial. Follow-up in MADIT was relatively brief (average of 27 months). Again, because it appears that patients with higher ejection fractions have a lower frequency of spontaneous ventricular arrhythmias, it would be more difficult to demonstrate improved survival in this group over a short-term follow-up with small numbers of patients.

The design of the MUSTT study differed fundamentally from the other studies described[20] (see Table 5–2). This trial was not designed to compare the relative efficacy of treatments to prevent sudden death. Rather, the trial was designed to evaluate the ability of electrophysiologically guided therapy to reduce the risk of sudden death for patients with documented coronary artery disease, ejection fraction 40% or less, and asymptomatic nonsustained VT (NSVT). At the time this trial was designed and initiated, several small analyses had suggested that demonstrating inducible sustained VT in patients with coronary disease and ejection fraction less than 40% without symptomatic arrhythmias was predictive of sudden death, but no large-scale controlled trial had evaluated the risks associated with inducible VT. As such, the utility of programmed stimulation as a risk-stratification test to separate patients at high versus low risk of sudden death and who might benefit from antiarrhythmic therapy was tested. In addition, patients presumed to be at high risk for sudden death on the basis of inducible sustained VT were randomized into two treatment arms: a group randomly assigned to receive no antiarrhythmic therapy and a second group treated with antiarrhythmic therapy. The latter group first underwent trials of antiarrhythmic drugs guided by serial electrophysiologic testing. If a drug was found that prevented induction of sustained VT or slowed induced tachycardia such that the patient was hemodynamically stable during induced tachycardia, the patient was treated with that drug. If at least one drug could not be found that prevented induction of sustained VT, the patient was treated with an ICD (Figure 5–2). Treatment with beta-adrenergic blocking agents and angiotensin-converting enzyme (ACE) inhibitors was strongly encouraged for all patients in the trial. After a mean follow-up of 39 months, the risk of arrhythmic death or cardiac arrest was reduced by 27% for patients randomized to electrophysiologically guided therapy ($P = 0.04$; Figure 5–3).[21] Fortuitously, equal numbers of patients randomized to electrophysiologically guided therapy were treated with antiarrhythmic drugs and ICDs. Examination of outcome revealed that all the mortality reduction associated with EP-guided therapy occurred among the ICD-treated patients. In comparison with the patients having inducible VT randomized to no antiarrhythmic therapy, ICD treatment was associated with a 76% reduction in the risk of arrhythmic death or cardiac arrest and a 55% reduction in total mortality. Although therapy was not assigned randomly, multiple analyses supported ICD therapy itself as the basis for the improved survival rate.[22]

The MUSTT investigators also analyzed the effects of CHF and ejection fraction on survival benefit associated with the ICD.[9] The median ejection fraction of patients in the MUSTT study was 30%.[21] Sixty-three percent of patients in the MUSTT study were of NYHA functional class II or III. In the MUSTT study, patients with ejection fraction less than 30% as well as those with ejection fraction 30% or greater derived significant survival benefit in association with the ICD (hazard ratio of 0.45 for patients with ejection fractions less than 30% and hazard ratio of 0.37 for patients with ejection fraction greater than 30%) ($P < 0.001$ for both groups). For patients with a history of CHF, the hazard ratio for total mortality was 0.30 in association with defibrillator therapy ($P = 0.001$). In contrast, the patients without a history of CHF did not have significant reduction in mortality in association with defibrillator therapy (hazard ratio, 0.86; $P = 0.71$). However, the numbers of patients in this comparison were small (45 defibrillator-treated patients and 85 nondefibrillator-treated patients). Of interest, although the reduction in total mortality was not statistically significant, patients with no

Round

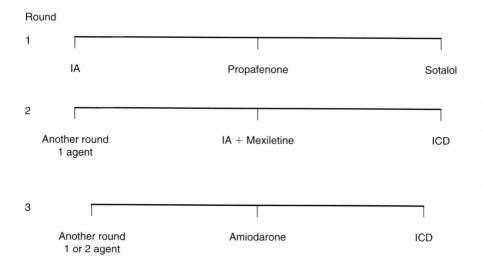

>3 Any regimen not yet chosen

**FIGURE 5–2.** Schema depicting assignment of antiarrhythmic therapy in patients enrolled in the MUSTT study having inducible VT, randomized to electrophysiologically guided therapy. Patients had to fail at least one antiarrhythmic drug trial before having an ICD implanted. Drugs were assigned randomly within each round. If a patient was randomized to a Type IA agent, the investigator chose the most appropriate drug. Amiodarone was tried after at least two other antiarrhythmic drugs had failed. All drugs (including amiodarone) were tested by programmed stimulation for effects on inducible VT.

history of CHF did experience significant reduction in the risk of arrhythmic death or cardiac arrest in association with defibrillator therapy (hazard ratio, 0.24; $P = 0.01$). It seems likely that the disparity in the degree of ICD benefit in patients with ejection fraction greater than 30% between the MADIT and MUSTT studies relates to the significantly larger size of the MUSTT study (704 patients randomized), as well as the longer follow-up in the MUSTT study (median follow-up, 39 months).

The inescapable conclusion of the results of the MADIT and MUSTT studies is that the ICD effectively reduces the mortality among patients with coronary disease who have never experienced symptomatic arrhythmia and who have inducible sustained ventricular tachyarrhythmias. Even in the highest-risk groups of patients—those having the lowest ejection fractions and CHF—mortality is reduced. However, it is important to realize that none of the studies referred to were heart failure trials. Patients were enrolled in these studies because they had characteristics identifying them to be at high risk for sudden death. Many of these patients did have heart failure, but the majority were not primarily under the care of a heart failure physician. Therefore it cannot be concluded that a large population of patients whose primary clinical problem is heart failure complicating a prior myocardial infarction will derive the same degree of benefit from ICD therapy as was observed in these studies. The screening process for enrollment in the MUSTT study (as well as the other studies) specifically targeted

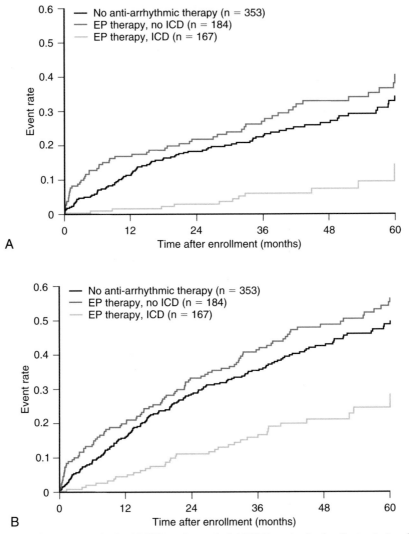

**FIGURE 5–3.** Event rates in the MUSTT study: survival, MUSTT randomized patients. *A,* Freedom from arrhythmic death or cardiac arrest. *B,* Freedom from total mortality.

patients having arrhythmia markers for sudden death risk, rather than targeting CHF patients. For example, enrollment in the MUSTT study required the occurrence of spontaneous ventricular tachyarrhythmias in patients who were hemodynamically stable and not in CHF.

The MUSTT investigators also performed a separate analysis of the relative contribution of ejection fraction and inducible VT to mortality.[23] This analysis was restricted to the 1791 patients enrolled in the trial who did not receive antiarrhythmic drugs. Patients were dichotomized into those having ejection fraction of 30% or higher versus less than 30% and those with or without inducible VT, creating four patient groups based on the possible combinations of these two factors. This analysis demonstrated that both ejection fraction and the presence of inducible VT contributed independently to mortality risk (Figure 5–4). Not surprisingly, total mortality was highest among patients who had inducible VT and ejection fraction less than 30%. Total mortality was also greater among patients with ejection fraction less than 30% and without inducible VT than among patients with ejection fraction between 30% and 40% who had inducible VT. The risk of arrhythmic death or cardiac arrest was also highest for patients who had inducible VT and ejection fraction less than 30%. However, the risk of arrhythmic death or cardiac arrest was equal for patients having ejection fraction less than 30% without inducible VT and patients with ejection fraction between 30% and 40% who had inducible VT (see Figure 5–4). This analysis also demonstrated that ejection fraction was not helpful in distinguishing how patients would die. That is, the percentage of deaths accounted for by arrhythmic events did not differ significantly between patients whose ejection fraction was less than 30% and those whose ejection fraction was 30% or higher. In contrast, the presence of inducible VT identified a group in which a significantly higher proportion of deaths were accounted for by arrhythmic events than among patients without inducible VT. This type of analysis should be helpful in decisions about how to deploy expensive technology such as ICDs in the most cost-effective manner.

The MADIT II study constituted a departure in screening/enrollment strategies in comparison with the previous primary prevention studies.[10] This study enrolled 1232 patients who had experienced myocardial infarction at least 1 month prior to enrollment who had an ejection fraction less than or equal to 30% but no specific arrhythmia risk marker, such as spontaneous nonsustained VT or inducible VT. It should be noted that the original study design also required patients to have frequent ventricular ectopy (greater than or equal to 10 PVCs/hour) or couplets or else nonsustained VT on Holter monitoring. This requirement was dropped after 23 patients had been enrolled, because many potential candidates for the trial had nonsustained VT, and when this arrhythmia was discovered investigators felt obligated to perform electrophysiologic studies. If sustained VT was induced, such patients would have been referred for defibrillator implantation, thus depriving the MADIT II of patients presumably at highest risk for sudden death. Fifty-seven percent to 60% of patients enrolled in MADIT II were NYHA class II or III, and 5% were class IV. The median ejection fraction of patients enrolled in the study was 23%. The investigators in this study, begun in 1997, achieved a far higher use of beta-blockers (70% of patients in each arm) than had been used in earlier studies, and this may well have reduced total mortality in this population. Patients were randomized to therapy with an ICD versus no antiarrhythmic therapy, and after a mean follow-up of 20 months, the investigators observed a 31% decrease in total mortality with ICD treatment (Figure 5–5). The effect of the ICD on survival was not significantly affected by the presence or absence of symptomatic heart failure or the ejection fraction at the time of enrollment in the trial. It is interesting to note that although not statistically significant, the degree of ICD benefit was less in patients with ejection fraction greater than 25% and was also less in patients with symptomatic heart failure.

The only trial reported to date that has specifically examined the role of the implanted defibrillator for primary prevention of sudden death among patients with noncoronary disease is the Cardiomyopathy Trial (CAT).[12] This trial, conducted in

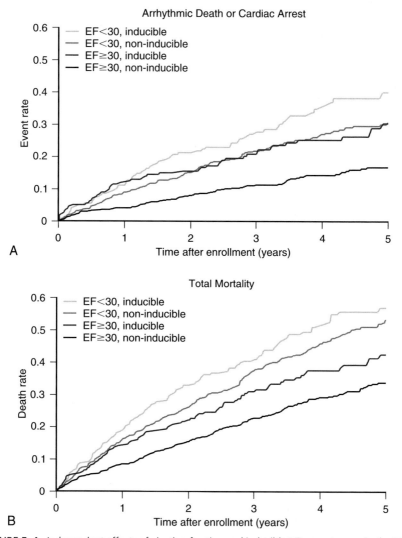

**FIGURE 5–4.** Independent effects of ejection fraction and inducible VT on outcomes in the MUSTT study: effects of ejection fraction and inducible VT on event rates. *A,* Rates of arrhythmic death or cardiac arrest. *B,* Rates of total mortality. *(Reprinted with permission from Buxton AE, Lee KL, Hafley GE, et al: Relation of ejection fraction and inducible ventricular tachycardia to mode of death in patients with coronary artery disease: an analysis of patients enrolled in the multicenter unsustained tachycardia trial.* Circulation *2002;106:2466–2472.)*

Germany, included patients with 9 months' history of symptomatic dilated cardiomyopathy, a left ventricular ejection fraction of 30% or less by angiography, and NYHA functional class II or III. Patients who had coronary stenoses greater than 70% were excluded. In addition, patients with any history of myocardial infarction, myocarditis, excessive alcohol consumption, and valvular disease were excluded, as

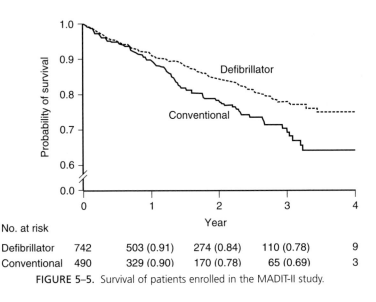

No. at risk

| | | Year | | | |
|---|---|---|---|---|---|
| Defibrillator | 742 | 503 (0.91) | 274 (0.84) | 110 (0.78) | 9 |
| Conventional | 490 | 329 (0.90) | 170 (0.78) | 65 (0.69) | 3 |

**FIGURE 5–5.** Survival of patients enrolled in the MADIT-II study.

were patients with hypertrophic cardiomyopathy. Although this trial was relatively small, including 50 patients randomized to ICD therapy and 54 controls receiving no specific antiarrhythmic therapy, it had the benefit of a mean follow-up of 5.5 years. There was no significant difference in survival between the two groups. The cumulative survival was 86% after 4 years in the ICD treatment group versus 80% in the control group ($P = 0.55$). There were no sudden deaths observed in either group during this time. The mean ejection fraction of patients in this trial was 25%. A majority (80%) of patients enrolled in the trial were male. The reasons for the low mortality observed in the trial are not clear. It was a small trial but involved reasonably long-term follow-up (more than 5 years). More than 90% of patients in each treatment group received ACE inhibitors, but only 4% received beta-blockers.

The CAT investigators made an interesting observation. Among the 50 patients randomized to defibrillator therapy, 11 received therapy for "sustained" VT. Although in each case the tachycardias were treated appropriately by the ICD, survival among patients who experienced VT was significantly worse than among those who did not develop VT (83% 6-year survival among patients without VT versus 44% 6-year survival among patients with VT). This raises the possibility that the occurrence of VT in patients with dilated nonischemic cardiomyopathy is a secondary phenomenon reflecting intrinsic deterioration of the myocardium rather than a primary phenomenon in some cases. Similar observations have been noted in reports on patients with idiopathic dilated cardiomyopathy and ICDs. Bansch et al. noted, in a retrospective analysis, that patients who developed clusters of VT had poorer survival than patients without tachycardia clusters.[24] They, too, concluded that despite appropriate antiarrhythmic therapy with the defibrillator, clusters of ventricular tachyarrhythmias could recur frequently and might be a harbinger of progressive myocardial deterioration, marking patients whose prognoses are poor. Thus it is possible that the ICD may effectively treat arrhythmias in such patients without significantly improving mortality.

Finally, it is important to note that the results of two trials currently under way are likely to influence our practice regarding utilization of ICDs in patients with heart failure and cardiomyopathy. The first, the NHLBI-sponsored Sudden Cardiac Death in Heart Failure Trial (SCD-HeFT), has enrolled 2500 patients with symptomatic heart failure (NYHA class 2 and 3) having left ventricular ejection fractions of 35% or less because of either ischemic disease or nonischemic dilated cardiomyopathy. Enrollment in this trial was completed in October 2001, and follow-up will be completed in 2003. Therapy assigned in this trial was randomized among placebo, amiodarone, and the implanted defibrillator. This is the first and only large-scale trial aimed primarily at patients with CHF. Half of the patients enrolled in this trial have coronary disease, and half have nonischemic cardiomyopathy as a cause of CHF. The second trial currently under way is the Defibrillators and Nonischemic Cardiomyopathy Treatment Evaluation (DEFINITE). This is a randomized trial comparing ICD therapy to no antiarrhythmic therapy in patients with nonischemic cardiomyopathy, reduced ejection fraction, and asymptomatic ventricular ectopy. This trial has enrolled 454 patients, and the planned minimum follow-up of 12 months will be completed in Fall 2003.

In conclusion, although subsets of patients who have coronary disease and CHF clearly gain a survival benefit from ICD therapy, the benefits of defibrillators in many other patients are not yet defined. Specifically, the role of ICD therapy for patients whose major clinical problem is CHF, especially in the setting of nonischemic dilated cardiomyopathy, is not clear. This situation may well change with the results of the ongoing trials mentioned here.

## REFERENCES

1. Stevenson WG, Stevenson LW: Prevention of sudden death in heart failure. *J Cardiovasc Electrophysiol* 2001;12:112–114.
2. Franciosa JA, Wilen M, Ziesche S, et al: Survival in men with severe chronic left ventricular failure due to either coronary heart disease or idiopathic dilated cardiomyopathy. *Am J Cardiol* 1983;51:831–836.
3. Felker GM, Thompson RE, Hare JM, et al: Underlying causes and long-term survival in patients with initially unexplained cardiomyopathy. *N Engl J Med* 2000;342:1077–1084.
4. Zannad F, Braincon S, Juilliere Y, et al: Incidence, clinical and etiologic features, and outcomes of advanced chronic heart failure: the EPICAL Study. Epidemiologie de l'Insuffisance Cardiaque Avancee en Lorraine. *J Am Coll Cardiol* 1999;33:734–742.
5. Domanski M, Saksena S, Epstein A, et al: Relative effectiveness of the implantable cardioverter-defibrillator and antiarrhythmic drugs in patients with varying degrees of left ventricular dysfunction who have survived malignant ventricular arrhythmias. *J Am Coll Cardiol* 1999;34:1090–1095.
6. Sheldon R, Connolly S, Krahn A, et al: Identification of patients most likely to benefit from implantable cardioverter-defibrillator therapy. The Canadian Implantable Defibrillator Study. *Circulation* 2000;101:1660–1664.
7. Kuck K-H, Cappato R, Siebels J, et al: Randomized comparison of antiarrhythmic drug therapy with implantable defibrillators in patients resuscitated from cardiac arrest. The Cardiac Arrest Study Hamburg (CASH). *Circulation.* 2000;102:748–754.
8. Moss AJ, Fadl Y, Zareba W, et al: Survival benefit with an implanted defibrillator in relation to mortality risk in chronic coronary heart disease. *Am J Cardiol.* 2001;88:516–520.
9. Gold M, O'Toole M, Tang A, et al: The Effect of Ejection Fraction and Congestive Heart Failure on the Benefit of Implantable Defibrillators in MUSTT (Abstract). *Pacing Clin Electrophysiol* 2000;23:II-493.
10. Moss AJ, Zareba W, Hall WJ, et al: Prophylactic implantation of a defibrillator in patients with myocardial infarction and reduced ejection fraction. *N Engl J Med* 2002;346:877–883.
11. Bigger J, The Coronary Artery Bypass Graft (CABG) Patch Trial Investigators. Prophylactic use of implanted cardiac defibrillators in patients at high risk for ventricular arrhythmias after coronary-artery bypass graft surgery. *N Engl J Med* 1997;337:1569–1575.

12. Bansch D, Antz M, Boczor S, et al: Primary Prevention of Sudden Cardiac Death in Idiopathic Dilated Cardiomyopathy: The Cardiomyopathy Trial (CAT). *Circulation* 2002;105:1453–1458.
13. The Antiarrhythmics versus Implantable Defibrillators (AVID) Investigators. A comparison of antiarrhythmic-drug therapy with implantable defibrillators in patients resuscitated from near-fatal ventricular arrhythmias. *N Engl J Med* 1997;337:1576–1583.
14. Domanski MJ, Epstein A, Hallstrom A, et al: Survival of antiarrhythmic or implantable cardioverter defibrillator treated patients with varying degrees of left ventricular dysfunction who survived malignant ventricular arrhythmias. *J Cardiovasc Electrophysiol* 2002;13:580–583.
15. Connolly S, Gent M, Roberts R, et al: Canadian Implantable Defibrillator Study (CIDS): A randomized trial of the implantable cardioverter defibrillator against amiodarone. *Circulation.* 2000;101:1297–1302.
16. Bansch D, Castrucci M, Bocker D, et al: Ventricular tachycardias above the initially programmed tachycardia detection interval in patients with implantable cardioverter-defibrillators: incidence, prediction and significance. *J Amer Coll Cardiol* 2000;36:557–565.
17. Freedberg NA, Hill JN, Fogel RI, et al: Recurrence of symptomatic ventricular arrhythmias in patients with implantable cardioverter defibrillator after the first device therapy: implications for antiarrhythmic therapy and driving restrictions. *J Am Coll Cardiol* 2001;37:1910–1915.
18. Raitt MH, Dolack GL, Kudenchuk PJ, et al: Ventricular arrhythmias detected after transvenous defibrillator implantation in patients with a clinical history of only ventricular fibrillation: Implications for use of implantable defibrillator. *Circulation* 1995;91:1996–2001.
19. Moss AJ, Hall WJ, Cannom DS, et al: Improved survival with an implanted defibrillator in patients with coronary disease at high risk for ventricular arrhythmia. Multicenter Automatic Defibrillator Implantation Trial Investigators. *N Engl J Med* 1996;335:1933–1940.
20. Buxton AE, Fisher JD, Josephson ME, et al: Prevention of sudden death in patients with coronary artery disease: the Multicenter Unsustained Tachycardia Trial (MUSTT). *Prog Cardiovasc Dis* 1993;36:215–226.
21. Buxton AE, Lee KL, Fisher JD, et al: A randomized study of the prevention of sudden death in patients with coronary artery disease. *N Engl J Med* 1999;341:1882–1890.
22. Lee KL, Hafley G, Fisher JD, et al: Effect of Implantable Defibrillators on Arrhythmic Events and Mortality in the Multicenter Unsustained Tachycardia Trial. *Circulation* 2002;106:233–238.
23. Buxton A, Hafley G, Lee K, et al: Relation of ejection fraction and inducible ventricular tachycardia to mode of death in patients with coronary artery disease. *Circulation* 2002;106:2466–2472.
24. Bansch D, Bocker D, Brunn J, et al: Clusters of ventricular tachycardia signify impaired survival in patients with idiopathic dilated cardiomyopathy and implanted cardioverter defibrillators. *J Am Coll Cardiol* 2000;36:566–573.

# 6

# Anatomy and Implantation Techniques for Biventricular Devices

Seth Worley • Angel Leon • and Bruce L. Wilkoff

The technical challenges involved in delivering cardiac resynchronization therapy (CRT) are significant. There is no one technique, singular approach, magic set of tools, or particular training that has been proven to provide a superior result. There are many hundreds of physicians implanting left ventricular (LV) leads with varieties of backgrounds and little consensus but lots of passion and conviction as to how to approach this evolving therapy. This chapter discusses a variety of techniques that will likely be obsolete in the near future. However, they represent the result of significant experience, failure, and success. This chapter includes the techniques, experiences, and biases of the physicians at the Lancaster, Emory, and Cleveland Clinic Foundation hospitals, which will provide some contrasts in views and approaches that are identified in the text.

Implanting LV pacing leads to deliver CRT involves the following steps (Table 6–1): obtaining venous access, inserting leads into the right atrium and right ventricle, locating and entering the coronary sinus (CS), selecting a target LV vein, advancing the pacing lead to the targeted site, and removing the implantation tools. An effective technique for implantation of LV pacing leads requires an understanding of the anatomy of the failing heart and the coronary veins and the combination of standard pacing lead insertion skills with techniques common to diagnostic cardiac catheterization and interventional cardiology. Integrating knowledge of cardiac anatomy with an understanding of the variety of available diagnostic cardiac catheterization tools and familiarity with maneuvers utilized in advancing catheters over guide wires can allow the implanter to safely and effectively provide CRT for patients with congestive heart failure (CHF) and conduction system disease.

## Planning the Operation

### Left or Right Shoulder Venous Access

One can choose to implant CRT systems using either right or left subclavian access. Each method has its advocates. Implanters in Europe popularized and gained

**TABLE 6–1. LV Implant Procedure Summary**

1. Locate the coronary sinus ostium (CS OS).
2. Establish a stable platform in the CS from which to work.
3. Fully define the coronary venous anatomy with occlusive CS venography.
4. Based on the CS venograms, select a lateral wall coronary vein (target vein) for left ventricular (LV) lead placement. Selection is based on vein origin and its course on the lateral wall of the left ventricle.
5. Select an LV pacing lead based on the size and course of the target vein.
6. Determine a method of delivery based on the target vein characteristics, including size, origin from the CS (proximal, mid, distal), initial angle of take off from the CS, and subsequent course.
7. Select the appropriate shape and size directional catheter/guide for the target vein, if needed.
8. Place the LV pacing lead on the lateral wall of the left ventricle. This may require advanced guide wire techniques (buddy wire), better support for the pacing lead (add a directional guide through the CS platform), or percutaneous coronary venous angioplasty (PCVA) with or without stenting.
9. Test the LV pacing lead to ensure adequate thresholds (<3V at 0.5 msec) and lack of phrenic pacing.
10. Remove the directional guide (if used) and the CS platform without disrupting LV lead position.

proficiency with the right subclavian approach. Advantages cited for this preference include the ability to rotate imaging equipment to the left anterior oblique view without interfering with surgery and the ability to cannulate the CS ostium (OS) easily. The majority of implanters in the United States and those in our three centers prefer left shoulder access. Advocates of this approach suggest that the left subclavian approach provides a more natural route for the curved guiding catheters to follow from the subclavian vein to the CS OS. Furthermore, the ability to seat the guiding catheter deep in the CS to provide stability during venography and lead advancement appears greater from the left subclavian access site. Access from the right subclavian introduces an additional challenge to CS catheterization by requiring the guiding catheter to make two right-angle turns in opposite directions. The catheter has to turn from the subclavian into the superior vena cava and then make another turn in the opposite angle from the right atrium to the CS OS. Implanters at Emory approach the right and left shoulder approach with the same initial choice of equipment and guide catheter selection. The availability of various guide catheter curves and straight guide catheters that can be advanced over a deflectable electrophysiology mapping catheter provides the implanting physician with an array of tools, so that when the initial approach fails to find the CS OS, switching to a different tool increases the likelihood of success. Experienced implanters eventually develop proficiency with either approach, and operator preference usually reflects the initial experience during the individual's learning curve. The successful LV lead implanter needs to perfect the approach from either shoulder, particularly when having to upgrade pre-existing pacing or defibrillating systems to CRT.

## Upper-Extremity Venography

Obtaining venous access for LV lead implantation begins with the insertion of a peripheral access line into a large arm or forearm vein on the side selected as the implantation site, prior to beginning the surgical preparation of the patient. Peripheral venous access for contrast injection enables subclavian venography that helps localize the cephalic and subclavian veins during a difficult puncture. Performing venography prior to a new implantation is a reasonable option; subclavian venography is not done prior to every case. However, one should strongly consider subclavian venography prior to a procedure for upgrading an existing system to CRT by addition of only an LV lead. The venogram can demonstrate asymptomatic subclavian vein thrombosis (Figure 6–1) or difficult, tortuous anatomy associated with scarring from previous insertion of pacing leads.[1]

Asymptomatic subclavian vein thrombosis may be present in 10% to 15% of patients with multiple chronically implanted pacing  leads. Once the venogram demonstrates a patent subclavian vein, the implanter can proceed with confidence that the selected site can provide adequate access for multiple lead insertions during a new implantation or for addition of an LV lead to a previously implanted pacing or defibrillating system. Appropriate venous access for a new CRT device implantation provides access for three pacing or defibrillating leads; a right atrial (RA) pacing/sensing lead; the right ventricle pacing or defibrillating lead; and the LV lead delivery system. The implanter can opt to make three separate direct axillary or subclavian punctures or a cephalic cutdown for one or both of the right heart leads, combined with a separate puncture for the LV lead. Use of the cephalic vein for all three leads presents a challenge, because movement of one lead may dislodge the other when the vessel contains three leads. Whether one opts for the triple puncture or the combined subclavian/cephalic method, creating a separate access site for the LV lead delivery system, prevents inadvertent dislodgement of the RA and right ventricular (RV) leads during manipulation of the guide catheter or, worse,

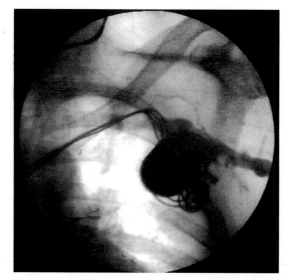

FIGURE 6–1. Injection of contrast into a left antecubital vein opacifies the axillary and subclavian vein demonstrating an obstruction in a patient with two chronically implanted leads.

dislodgement of the LV lead while having to reposition one of the right heart leads near the end of the implantation procedure.

## Lead Implantation Order

Virtually all patients selected to receive CRT have underlying intraventricular conduction system disease; most have a left bundle branch block (LBBB) pattern of activation. Rotation, advancement, and manipulation of the guide catheter within the right atrium in an attempt to enter the CS often advances the catheter into the right ventricle, where it strikes the RV septum at a site near the specialized conduction system. Trauma to the right bundle branch in a patient with pre-existing LBBB often produces high-degree atrioventricular (AV) block and asystole. If temporary pacing through temporary femoral catheters or transthoracic stimulation does not provide adequate rate support, prolonged asystole may prove catastrophic. However, the presence of the RV lead provides emergency RV pacing through an external pulse generator. Therefore insertion of the RV lead should precede insertion of the LV guiding catheter system. Should instrumentation with a guiding catheter inadvertently traumatize the right bundle branch during attempts to enter the CS, backup demand ventricular pacing allows the operator to proceed with the implantation safely and without interruption. Insertion of the RA lead prior to the LV lead eliminates the need to manipulate leads in the pocket or in the central circulation after LV lead insertion. The RA lead implantation can occur either before or after the LV lead implantation, at the discretion of the operator. However, if the LV lead implantation fails, leaving the RA and RV leads in place eliminates the need to insert them when the patient undergoes thoracoscopic or thoracotomy implantation of the LV lead as an option to failed transvenous implantation. The surgeon implanting the LV lead needs to tunnel the LV lead only to the subcutaneous pocket containing the RA and RV leads, where all can be connected to the pulse generator.

# Cannulation of the Coronary Sinus (Lancaster)

Transvenous placement of the LV epicardial lead requires cannulation of the coronary sinus by the pacing lead, which is facilitated by cannulation by a sheath or catheter that serves as a work station. This can be done by multiple techniques. Both the contrast-based and electrography-based catheter techniques will be described in detail.

Contrast-based cannulation of the CS is a two-step process:

1. Locate the CS OS.
2. Advance the sheath or guide into the CS.

## Finding the Coronary Sinus Ostium

Regardless of whether contrast is used, it is important to understand the anatomy surrounding the coronary sinus and the effect of torque on a catheter in the area of the CS.

## Anatomy Surrounding the Coronary Sinus Ostium: Making It Work for You

Successful location of the CS OS is facilitated by a complete understanding of the anatomy around the CS OS. In Figure 6–2 the structures that have an impact on locating the CS are demonstrated.

The key to easy, rapid location of the CS OS is to use the eustachian ridge and thebesian valve to direct the catheter toward—not away from—the OS. On the basis of the anatomy demonstrated in Figures 6–2 and 6–3, it is clear that a catheter approaching the CS OS along the inferior posterior wall of the right atrium (see Figure 6–3A) will be deflected away from the OS by the eustachian ridge and thebesian valve. However, if approached from the posterior superior tricuspid annulus (see Figure 6–3B), the eustachian ridge and thebesian valve will direct the catheter tip into the OS. Therefore the catheter must be directed from the posterior superior tricuspid annulus inferiorly toward the right atrium to enable utilization of the eustachian ridge and thebesian valve to guide the tip of the catheter toward the OS. A properly shaped guide must be capable of approaching the CS OS from the posterior superior tricuspid annulus.

### Effect of Torque on a Catheter in the Area of the Coronary Sinus

*Directing a Catheter into the Coronary Sinus Using the Eustachian Ridge and Thebesian Valve*

As is illustrated in the previous section, it is easier to enter the CS OS from the posterior superior tricuspid annulus by using the eustachian valve and thebesian

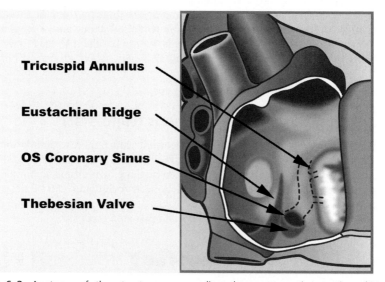

**FIGURE 6–2.** Anatomy of the structures surrounding the coronary sinus ostium (CS OS). The eustachian ridge protrudes into the right atrium from the posterior wall of the right atrium. The eustachian ridge is more prominent inferiorly near the inferior vena cava. The OS is located behind the eustachian ridge as the CS is approached from the right atrium. The thebesian valve protrudes from the posterior wall of the right atrium below the CS and forms the inferior boundary of the OS. The OS is located behind the thebesian valve as the OS is approached from below. The posterior inferior tricuspid annulus forms the boundary of the OS on the right.

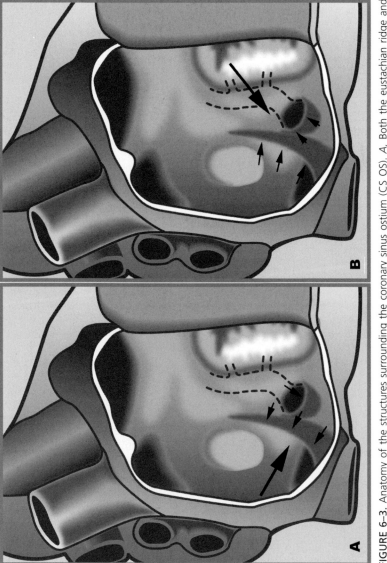

FIGURE 6–3. Anatomy of the structures surrounding the coronary sinus ostium (CS OS). *A*, Both the eustachian ridge and thebesian valve (*small arrows*) block entrance to the CS OS as it is approached from the atrium along the inferior posterior wall (*large arrow*). *B*, Both the eustachian ridge and thebesian valve (*small arrows*) direct the tip of the guide into the CS OS as it is approached from the posterior superior tricuspid annulus (*large arrow*).

valve to direct the catheter into the OS. But how can this catheter direction be accomplished? Figure 6–4 demonstrates the effect of counterclockwise torque on the tip of a braided guide. If counterclockwise torque is applied to a braided guide, the tip is initially directed posteriorly until it contacts the heart. As more torque is applied, the heart limits the posterior direction of the tip. The additional torque directs the tip inferiorly and toward the right atrium. The shape and position of the braided guide are adjustable through the application of counterclockwise torque.

If the tip of the guide is above the CS on the tricuspid annulus when torque is applied, it will be directed posteriorly and inferiorly toward the right atrium into the CS. However, if the guide is at or below the CS as torque is applied, the tip will move inferiorly away from the CS. For counterclockwise torque to be effective in finding the OS, the initial tip position must be superior and on the RV side of the OS. As an aside, clockwise torque will direct the tip of the guide's anterior away from the OS.

## A Guide Shape to Cannulate the Coronary Sinus with Use of the Eustachian Ridge and Thebesian Valve

Using the eustachian ridge and thebesian valve to direct the guide into the OS requires the guide to be positioned above the CS on the tricuspid annulus. The natural rest position of many of the available guide shapes places the tip of the guide at or below the CS in the right atrium (Figure 6–5). Counterclockwise torque directs the guide inferiorly and posteriorly away from the OS. The addition of a "proximal curve" to the guide (Figure 6–6) places the tip above the CS on the tricuspid annulus or in the right ventricle rather than in the right atrium. Counterclockwise torque directs the "proximal curve" guide inferiorly, posteriorly, and toward the right atrium into the OS.

## Catheters with a "Proximal Curve"

A catheter with a "proximal curve" can be created in a variety of ways, as illustrated in Figures 6–7 and 6–8. In Figure 6–7, a proximal curve is added to an 8-F multipurpose guide.

A proximal curve is introduced by running the Cyber guide between the thumb and forefinger from proximal to distal, starting 5–7 inches from the tip of the catheter, similar to shaping a pacing stylet. When a proximal curve is added to a multipurpose 1 Cyber guide, the tip is too short to reach the tricuspid annulus. The Cyber guide responds well to shape changes applied by hand. Attempts to add a proximal curve by hand to other guides frequently results in collapse of the lumen.

As shown in Figure 6–8, a "proximal curve" shape is available or can be created in a variety of ways. Many operators report success with the combination of an 8-F multipurpose guide and deflectable electrophysiology catheter. The curve created by this combination is illustrated in Figure 6–8D. Other operators describe the use of a 5-F or 6-F multipurpose catheter within the 7-F multipurpose guide. The shape resulting from this combination is illustrated in Figure 6–8E. The Guidant version of the "proximal curve" guide (CS-W) is demonstrated in Figure 6–8C. A SafeSheath-CSG/Worley with the "proximal curve" is demonstrated in Figure 6–8A. However, application of torque to the peel-away SafeSheathCSG/Worley-STD does not result in the tip deflection required for easy CS cannulation. Figure 6–8B illustrates a modified SafeSheathCSG/Worley-STD in which torque control is added and shape is retained by the addition of a preshaped 8-F multipurpose 2 Cyber guide and amputating 2.5 cm from the tip of the SafeSheath.

*Text continued on page 128*

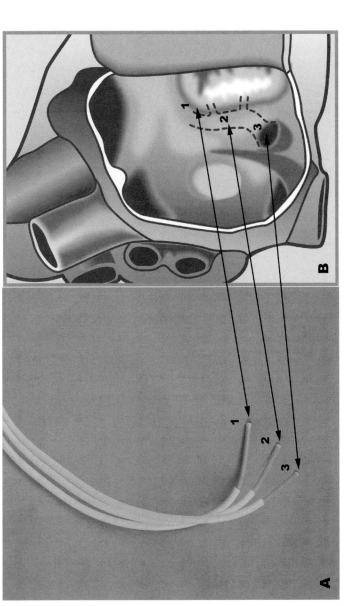

FIGURE 6-4. Effect of counterclockwise torque applied to a braided guide inside a peel-away sheath. *A,* Three positions of a guide with progressive application of torque are superimposed. (*1*) Initial counterclockwise torque at the hub of the guide directs the tip of the guide back. (*2*) With additional counterclockwise torque the guide tip can no longer move back. The torque thus directs the tip of the guide down and to the left. (*3*) As more counterclockwise torque is added, the tip of the guide continues to move down and to the left. In *2* and *3* the proximal section of the guide lifts off the surface (out of the plane of the illustration). *B,* A drawing of the area of the coronary sinus ostium demonstrates the relative position of the tip of the guide as torque is applied assuming an initial position on the posterior superior tricuspid annulus.

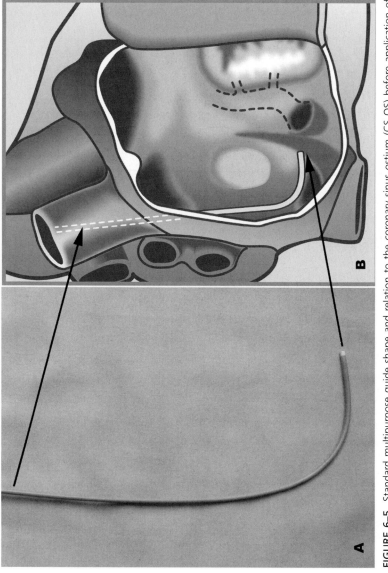
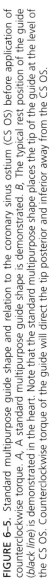

**FIGURE 6–5.** Standard multipurpose guide shape and relation to the coronary sinus ostium (CS OS) before application of counterclockwise torque. *A,* A standard multipurpose guide shape is demonstrated. *B,* The typical rest position of the guide (*black line*) is demonstrated in the heart. Note that the standard multipurpose shape places the tip of the guide at the level of the CS OS. Counterclockwise torque of the guide will direct the tip posterior and inferior away from the CS OS.

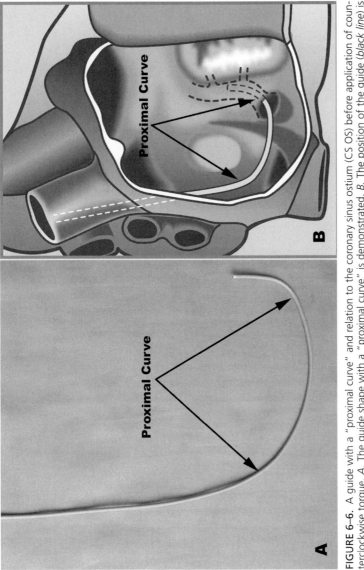

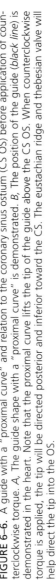

FIGURE 6-6. A guide with a "proximal curve" and relation to the coronary sinus ostium (CS OS) before application of counterclockwise torque. A, The guide shape with a "proximal curve" is demonstrated. B, The position of the guide (black line) is demonstrated in the heart. Note that the proximal curve lifts the tip of the guide above the CS OS. When counterclockwise torque is applied, the tip will be directed posterior and inferior toward the CS. The eustachian ridge and thebesian valve will help direct the tip into the OS.

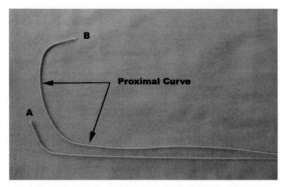

**FIGURE 6–7.** Straight (*A*) and "proximal curve" added (*B*) to a Boston Scientific Medi Tech Multipurpose 2 Cyber Guide (Catalog No. 15-290).

With the introduction of the braided core (Figure 6–9*A*), it is no longer necessary to use the reshaped 8-F CyberGuide to provide torque control for the SafeSheath CSG/Worley.

### Locating the Ostium of the Coronary Sinus with a Guide and Contrast Injection

When using contrast to locate the OS of the CS, cannulation of OS is often separate from advancing the guide deeper into the vessel. Each step may be easy or

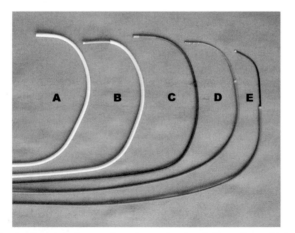

**FIGURE 6–8.** "Proximal curve" shapes that places the tip of the catheter high on the tricuspid annulus to facilitate coronary sinus access. (*A*) SafeSheathCSG/Worley-STD. (*B*) Modified SafeSheathCSG/Worley-STD (2.5 cm cut from tip and 8-F Cyber multipurpose 2 guide inserted). (*C*) Guidant CS-W shape. (*D*) Medtronic 6216 guide with deflectable catheter. (*E*) Medtronic 6216 guide with 5-F multipurpose catheter.

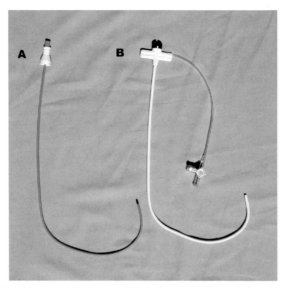

**FIGURE 6–9.** Updated Pressure Products SafeSheathCSG/Worley with braided inner core (A) to provide torque control for the peel-away sheath with hemostatic valve (B). The braided inner core has a soft radiolucent tip to facilitate placement in the coronary sinus.

difficult, depending on the anatomy. The two steps frequently flow together when the CS is easy to cannulate. However, the steps are independent. On occasion it may be difficult to locate the OS of the CS but easy to advance the catheter once the OS is located. Conversely, it may be easy to locate the OS, but advancing the catheter may require additional manipulation and the use of a support wire, as demonstrated in Figure 6–10.

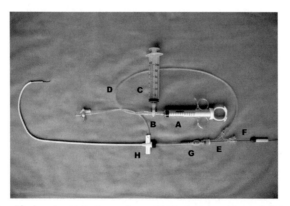

**FIGURE 6–10.** Simplified contrast injection system with Y-adaptor, guide, and glide wire. (A) Injection syringe. (B) Three way stopcock. (C) Reservoir syringe. (D) Eight-inch extension tubing. (E) Touhy-Borst Y-adaptor with hemostatic valve. (F) Terumo angled tip 0.035-inch glide wire with steering handle. (G) Boston Scientific Cyber 8-F 55-cm multipurpose 2 guide (proximal curve shaped by hand). (H) Pressure Products SafeSheathCSG/Worley STD.

## Locating the Ostium of the Coronary Sinus

The variable location of the CS OS (Figures 6–11 and 6–12) in patients with CHF explains why it can be difficult to find, even with contrast. The location of the OS varies because of the combination of cardiac rotation, cardiac dilation, and distortion from previous open heart surgery (OHS). As viewed on the fluoroscopy screen in the anterior-posterior (AP) view, the OS can be to the right or left of the spine, as seen in Figure 6–11. In addition, the OS may be high or low relative to the floor of the tricuspid annulus, as seen in Figure 6–12. Systematic use of contrast injection with an understanding of the anatomy (Figures 6–13 to 6–19) allows the operator to quickly recognize where the catheter tip is relative to the coronary sinus OS. The direction of the catheter can then be adjusted toward the OS.

## Anatomy Surrounding the Coronary Sinus Ostium, as Defined by Contrast Injection

The right ventricle, tricuspid annulus, eustachian ridge (valve of the inferior vena cava), thebesian valve (valve of the CS), OS of the CS, and subeustachian space are all important structures to recognize when exploring for the CS OS with contrast. The use of contrast injection through the guide defines the anatomy of the CS area and indicates where the catheter tip needs to be directed. In Figure 6–13 the tip of the guide is across the tricuspid annulus and directed posteriorly with 20–30 degrees of counterclockwise torque. A 2-ml puff of contrast outlines the trabeculae and confirms the location of the guide in the right ventricle.

In Figure 6–14, additional counterclockwise torque directs the tip inferiorly and toward the right atrium. Trabeculae confirm the guide is still in the right ventricle. In Figure 6–15 the contrast trapped between the tricuspid valve and posterior wall of the right ventricle outlines the tricuspid annulus. In Figure 6–16, the tip of the guide is in the right atrium near the fossa. In Figure 6–17, the tip of the guide enters the CS OS.

Figures 6–18 and 6–19 demonstrate the subeustachian space, another important landmark defined by contrast. Recognizing the angiographic appearance of the subeustachian space allows the operator to adjust the position of the guide. When the guide is in the subeustachian space, it is too low and on the atrial side of the CS OS. The tip of the guide must be directed superiorly and advanced across the tricuspid valve into the right ventricle. This can be accomplished by withdrawing the guide 1 cm, applying 20 degrees of clockwise torque to orient the tip toward the tricuspid valve, and then advancing the guide into the right ventricle. If the tip of the guide remains in the right atrium, a wire may be advanced through the Touhy-Borst and out the tip of the guide into the right ventricle. Once the wire is in the right ventricle, the guide is advanced over the wire into the right ventricle.

In summary, the procedure for quickly finding the CS OS with contrast is to start with a "proximal curve" braided guide (see Figures 6–7 and 6–8) that directs the tip superiorly and then to proceed as follows: (1) Advance the guide across the tricuspid annulus into the right ventricle. (2) Apply 20 degrees of counterclockwise torque to the hub of the guide, directing the tip to the posterior superior tricuspid annulus. (3) Confirm location with 2-ml contrast injection. (4) Apply an additional 20–40 degrees of counterclockwise torque, watching the tip of the guide for inferior deflection. (5) As the tip of the guide walks inferiorly and toward the right atrium in response to the torque, inject 2-ml puffs of contrast to visualize the structures demonstrated in Figures 6–13 to 6–19. (6) On the basis of the contrast-visualized

*Text continued on page 140*

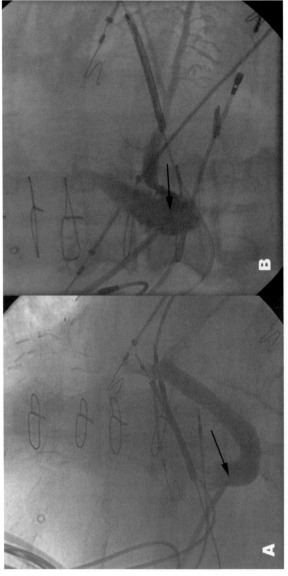

FIGURE 6–11. Anterior-posterior coronary sinus (CS) angiography where it was difficult to advance the guide. A, The hook shape of the proximal CS makes it difficult to advance the guide (arrow). B, A large posterior vein catches the tip of the guide (arrow), preventing it from advancing into the vertically oriented CS. In both cases, without contrast, the operator would be unaware that the tip of the guide was at or beyond the CS ostium. Contrast not only confirms location but also outlines why it is difficult to advance the catheter.

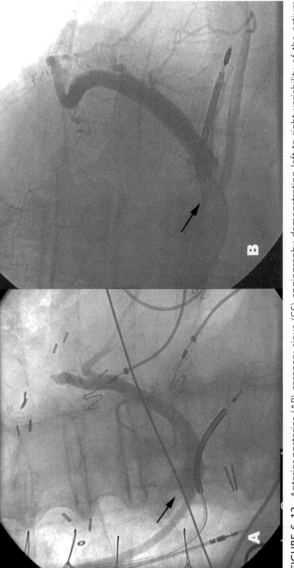

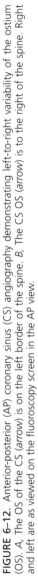

**FIGURE 6-12.** Anterior-posterior (AP) coronary sinus (CS) angiography demonstrating left-to-right variability of the ostium (OS). *A,* The OS of the CS (*arrow*) is on the left border of the spine. *B,* The CS OS (*arrow*) is to the right of the spine. Right and left are as viewed on the fluoroscopy screen in the AP view.

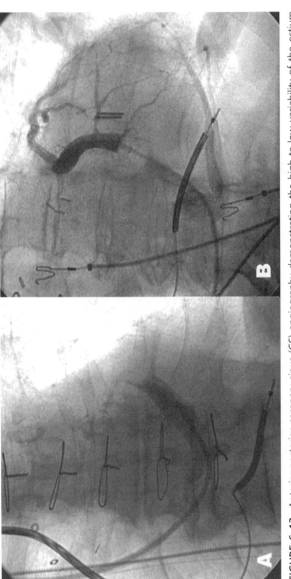

**FIGURE 6–13.** Anterior-posterior coronary sinus (CS) angiography demonstrating the high-to-low variability of the ostium (OS). *A,* The CS OS is high relative to the floor of the tricuspid valve. *B,* The CS OS is low. In both panels the floor of the tricuspid valve is defined by the pacing lead.

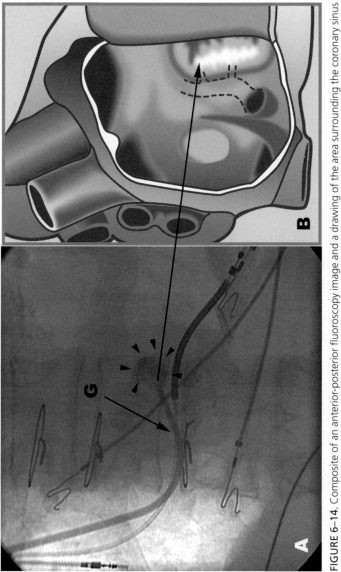

**FIGURE 6–14.** Composite of an anterior-posterior fluoroscopy image and a drawing of the area surrounding the coronary sinus ostium. *A,* The guide (*G*) is rotated 20–30 degrees counterclockwise, placing the tip of the guide posterior and superior to the pacing lead. A 2-ml puff of contrast outlines the trabeculae (*arrowheads*), confirming that the tip of the guide is in the right ventricle. *B,* The location of the tip of the guide from *A* is indicated on the drawing of the heart (*long arrow*).

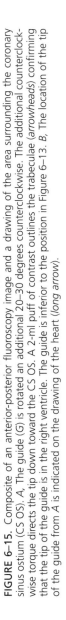

**FIGURE 6–15.** Composite of an anterior-posterior fluoroscopy image and a drawing of the area surrounding the coronary sinus ostium (CS OS). *A,* The guide (*G*) is rotated an additional 20–30 degrees counterclockwise. The additional counterclockwise torque directs the tip down toward the CS OS. A 2-ml puff of contrast outlines the trabeculae (*arrowheads*) confirming that the tip of the guide is in the right ventricle. The guide is inferior to the position in Figure 6–13. *B,* The location of the tip of the guide from A is indicated on the drawing of the heart (*long arrow*).

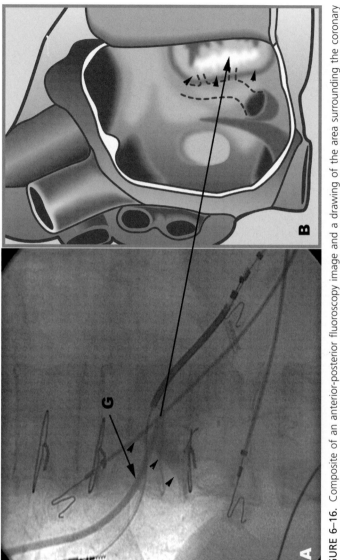

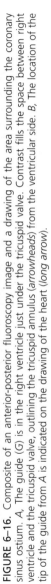

**FIGURE 6–16.** Composite of an anterior-posterior fluoroscopy image and a drawing of the area surrounding the coronary sinus ostium. *A,* The guide (*G*) is in the right ventricle just under the tricuspid valve. Contrast fills the space between right ventricle and the tricuspid valve, outlining the tricuspid annulus (*arrowheads*) from the ventricular side. *B,* The location of the tip of the guide from *A* is indicated on the drawing of the heart (*long arrow*).

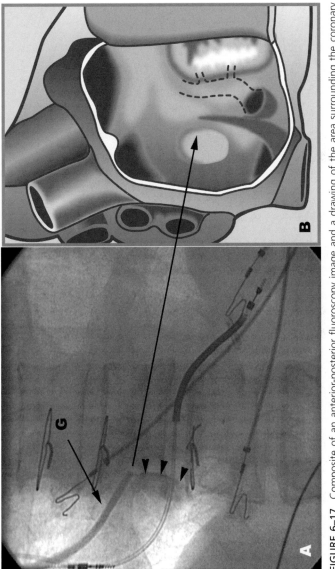

FIGURE 6–17. Composite of an anterior-posterior fluoroscopy image and a drawing of the area surrounding the coronary sinus ostium. A, A linear stream of contrast without trabeculae (arrowheads) is formed with a 2-ml contrast injection. The position of the pacing lead and the lack of trabeculae confirm the position of the guide in the right atrium. B, The location of the tip of the guide from A is indicated on the drawing of the heart (long arrow).

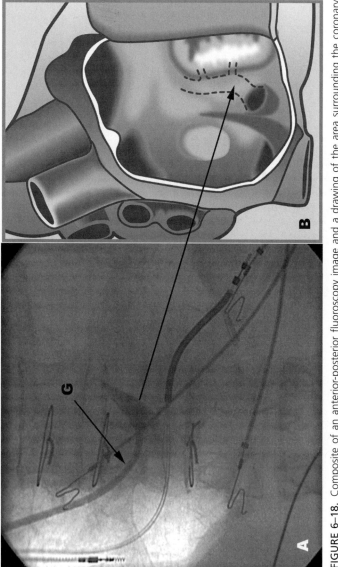

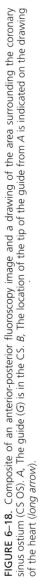

**FIGURE 6–18.** Composite of an anterior-posterior fluoroscopy image and a drawing of the area surrounding the coronary sinus ostium (CS OS). *A,* The guide (*G*) is in the CS. *B,* The location of the tip of the guide from *A* is indicated on the drawing of the heart (*long arrow*).

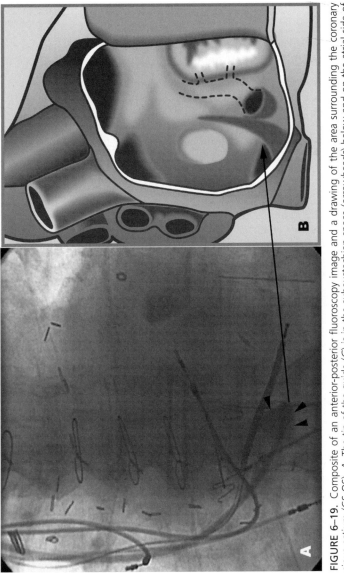

**FIGURE 6–19.** Composite of an anterior-posterior fluoroscopy image and a drawing of the area surrounding the coronary sinus ostium (CS OS). *A*, The tip of the guide (*G*) is in the subeustachian space (*arrowheads*) below and on the atrial side of the CS OS. Contrast outlines the subeustachian space. *B*, The subeustachian valve is the curved linear "wall" at the tip of the long arrow. The location of the tip of the guide from *A* is indicated on the drawing (*long arrow*).

anatomy, the guide can be advanced or withdrawn, or more or less torque can be applied to direct the tip into the OS.

### What Makes it Hard to Find the Coronary Sinus Ostium?

The two most common anatomic variants that make it difficult to locate the CS OS include the high CS and the huge right atrium.

### The High Coronary Sinus Ostium

The most difficult OS to find can be the high CS. As illustrated, the CS in Figure 6–12*A* is well above the usual location illustrated in Figure 6–12*B*. Exploring the CS area from high to low with a guide that has a proximal curve (See Figures 6–7 and 6–8) will make it more likely that the high CS is located. Given the trajectory of catheters placed from below, the high CS may explain why some physicians report finding a difficult CS from the leg.

### The Huge Right Atrium

When the right atrium is extremely large, as in patients with permanent atrial fibrillation (AF) or massively dilated right heart structures, the catheter tip usually ends up in the right atrium below the tricuspid valve, even when a guide with a proximal curve is used. Unless the shape of the catheter is changed significantly, the tip will flail about aimlessly in the right atrium. A 2-ml injection of contrast will confirm that the tip is in the right atrium, not the right ventricle, by the lack of trabeculae (see Figure 6–17). A guide wire through the Touhy-Borst of the Y-adapter and out the tip of the guide can help to get the tip of the guide into the right ventricle. Alternatively, an enlarged guide with a proximal curve specifically designed for the massive right atrium may be selected. Figure 6–20 demonstrates the larger curve required for guide entry in patients with large right atria, particularly in patients with AF.

### What Makes it Hard to Advance a Sheath or Guide into the Coronary Sinus?

Several variables affect the ease of advancement. These include the following:

1. A proximal vein branch that catches and misdirects the tip of the guide.
2. The initial angle of approach from the right atrium to the CS OS.
3. The thebesian.
4. A vertical CS.
5. A sigmoid CS.
6. CS stenosis from previous surgery.
7. Mid-CS valve.
8. Double OS CS.

If the sheath/guide is difficult to advance, it is first important to establish why. Inject 1–2 ml of contrast into the OS in the left anterior oblique (LAO) and right anterior oblique (RAO) view to establish the nature of the problem. Often this maneuver immediately suggests a solution to the problem. For example, the tip of

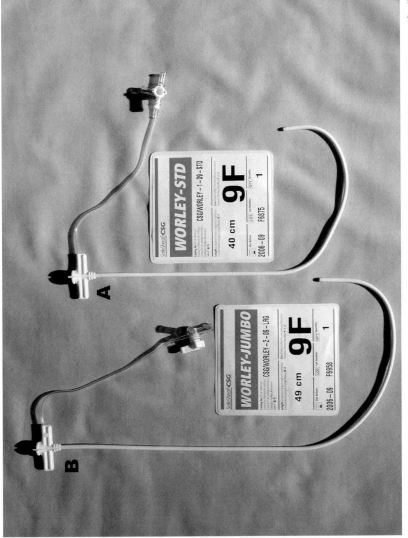
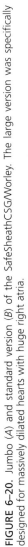

**FIGURE 6–20.** Jumbo (A) and standard version (B) of the SafeSheathCSG/Worley. The large version was specifically designed for massively dilated hearts with huge right atria.

the guide may be caught in a venous branch. Simply withdrawing the guide a few millimeters and adding additional torque may free the tip and allow the guide to advance (Figure 6–21).

## Tortuous Coronary Sinus

The ability to track a catheter or sheath over a wire into the CS is dependent on the flexibility of the guide as well as the wire. In some cases where the CS is very tortuous, a stiff guide wire (Amplatz 0.035-inch Extra Support) will not advance. In this case a 0.035-inch Glide wire may advance. However, the stiff wire provides more support once in place. On some occasions an 8-F guide may be too stiff to track

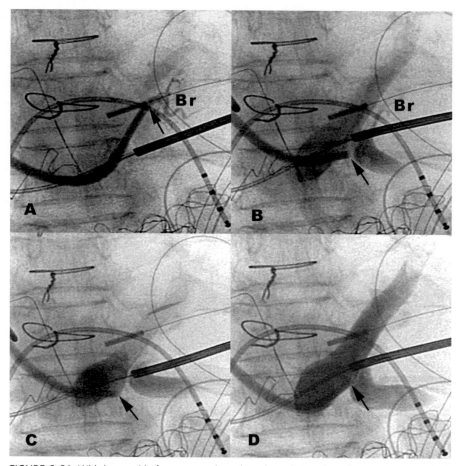

FIGURE 6–21. Withdraw guide from venous branch and re advance into the coronary sinus (CS). A, The tip of the guide (arrow) is in a venous branch (Br) of the posterior lateral vein. B, The tip of the guide (arrow) is withdrawn back into the posterior lateral vein with counterclockwise torque. The branch (Br) is still visible. C, The tip of the guide (arrow) is back in the CS. Additional counterclockwise torque is added. D, The tip of the guide is advanced beyond the ostium of the posterior lateral vein into the CS. With limited experience the entire procedure is accomplished in a single motion with 3–5 ml of contrast.

over a wire. By starting with the thinnest, most flexible catheter first and then advancing the next catheter over that, you can get the next larger catheter over that. For example, a Glide wire followed by a 5-F to 6-F multipurpose guide, followed by an 8-F guide, followed by a 9-F sheath may be required in some cases. In cases such as this the importance of establishing a stable CS platform from which to work is abundantly clear. Figures 6–22 to 6–25 demonstrate various obstacles to guide advancement.

## Electrography- and Contrast-Guided Coronary Sinus Cannulation (Emory)

Inserting a guide catheter into the CS provides a platform for performing contrast venography to delineate the cardiac venous anatomy and for advancement of the LV pacing lead to the desired location. Experienced implanters have independently developed a variety of techniques for approaching the challenges of CS catheterization. One can classify the approaches to CS catheterization into two general categories: the angiographic approach and the electrophysiologic (EP) approach. The angiographic approach utilizes techniques and equipment native to coronary catheterization and interventional cardiology to manipulate catheters to locate the ostium of the CS. Manipulation and reshaping of preformed guiding catheters alone or in conjunction with standard diagnostic catheters allow engagement of the ostium of the CS. Manipulation of the guide catheter includes the application of torque to rotate the catheter, reshaping the catheter with the right atrium to achieve the desired orientation or shape, and inserting a diagnostic angiographic catheter into the guide catheter to create a different three-dimensional orientation to successfully approach the CS ostium. Advancing a guide wire into the CS after engagement allows for the guide catheter or the combination of a diagnostic catheter-within-the guide catheter, to advance over the wire into a stable position 4–5 cm into the body of the CS.

The EP approach to CS catheterization utilizes tools more familiar to implanters who map cardiac chambers with steerable catheters, who use intracardiac recordings to confirm the anatomy position of a catheter, or those with little experience with diagnostic cardiac catheterization and interventional cardiology techniques. Inserting a steerable mapping catheter into a straight or preformed guide catheter allows the implanter to find the CS by changing the curve of the mapping catheter and gently advancing it until it follows the familiar contour of the CS. Fluoroscopic visualization, usually in the left anterior oblique projection, confirms the position within the CS. Advancement of the guide catheter over the mapping catheter then places the guide in position for venography and lead advancement. When necessary, connecting the mapping catheter to an electrophysiology recording system allows the implanter to identify the position of the catheter tip by analyzing the morphology of the intracardiac electrogram.

### *Congestive Heart Failure Alters Coronary Sinus Anatomy*

Regardless of the approach one takes to finding the CS, having a thorough understanding of the anatomic changes seen in the failing heart increases the likelihood of successful CS catheterization. RA enlargement, upward rotation of the long axis of the heart, posterior rotation of the short axis, and the increasing diameter of the mitral annulus that combine to change the position of the CS ostium relative to

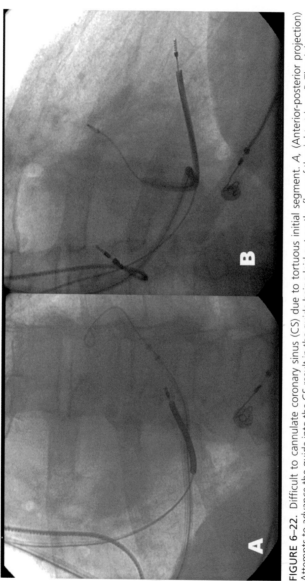

**FIGURE 6–22.** Difficult to cannulate coronary sinus (CS) due to tortuous initial segment. *A,* (Anterior-posterior projection) Attempts to advance the guide into the CS result in the guide being laid out on the floor of the right atrium. *B,* The right anterior oblique projection demonstrates that the forces are directed from left to right initially rather than up into the CS. Application of torque to the catheter to provide a straight approach can resolve the problem. Reviewing the line of the guiding catheter into the CS in various projections is important for understanding how to adjust the torque to keep the catheter as straight as possible as it is advanced.

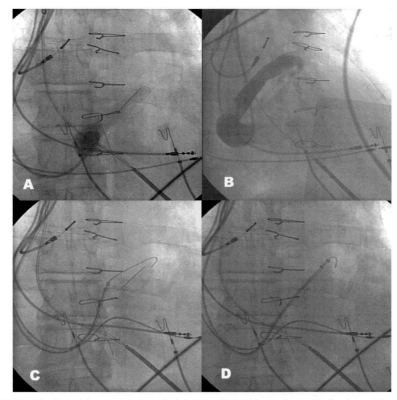

**FIGURE 6–23.** Sigmoid coronary sinus (CS) in a patient with previous mitral valve repair: use of guide wire to advance the catheter into the CS. *A,* The tip of the guide rests at the ostium (OS) but will not advance into the CS. *B,* Contrast injection in the right anterior oblique projection reveals the sigmoid shape of the proximal CS. *C,* A J-tip guide wire is advanced out the tip of the guide deep into the CS. *D,* The guide wire is held taut and the guide is advanced over the guide wire deep into the CS. Several important points are demonstrated in sequence. First, without contrast, the operator would not be aware that advancing into the CS rather than finding the CS was the problem. Contrast also demonstrated the nature of the anatomic variant, which provides a potential solution (use of a guide wire). Advancing the guide wire through the sigmoid section of the CS is possible because the guide provides support for the wire as it is advanced. Once in place deep in the CS, the wire provides a track to advance the wire. It is important to hold the wire taut as the guide is advanced over the wire.

the typical fluoroscopic landmarks are used to identify cardiac structures during cardiac procedures.[2] An exaggerated eustachian ridge or enlarged subeustachian space within the right atrium creates a physical barrier to CS entry. Strictures, tortuous segments, and valves within the CS and its tributaries prevent advancing catheters or guide wire to desirable positions that allow positioning of leads into target veins. Reviewing the echocardiogram prior to the implantation procedure alerts the implanter of unusual RA enlargement or anatomy. Brief fluoroscopic inspection of the cardiac silhouette at the start of the implantation may demonstrate the degree of cardiomegaly or cardiac rotation, the presence of anatomic markers such as right coronary artery calcifications, and the lucent adipose pad marking the AV groove that may help target the entry site into the CS.

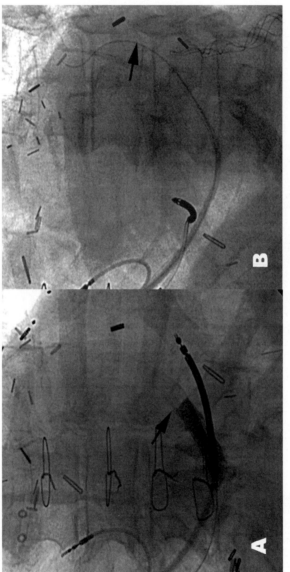

FIGURE 6–24. Valve near the coronary sinus ostium (CS OS) prevents the guide from advancing. A, The anterior-posterior projection demonstrating the valve (arrow). B, The left anterior oblique projection with the glide wire beyond the valve. The guide would not advance despite normal take off of the CS. Manipulation of the guide at the valve did not allow the guide to cross the valve. A 0.035-degree angled Terumo glide wire was advanced through the hemostatic valve in the Y-adapter and out the tip of the guide. Manipulation of the glide wire at the valve allowed it to cross.

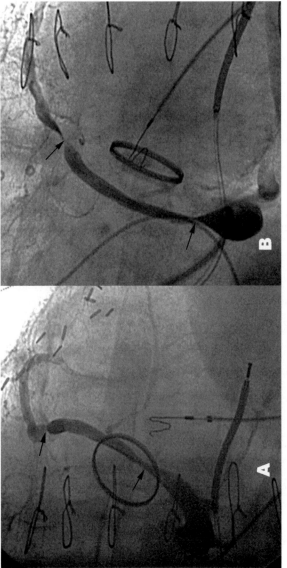
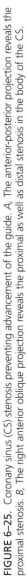

**FIGURE 6–25.** Coronary sinus (CS) stenosis preventing advancement of the guide. *A,* The anterior-posterior projection reveals the proximal stenosis. *B,* The right anterior oblique projection reveals the proximal as well as distal stenosis in the body of the CS.

Small-volume injections of contrast material from the tip of the guiding catheter sometimes help identify the CS ostium. However, contrast "puffing" can introduce potentially nephrotoxic doses to a patient with compromised cardiac output. A review of cardiac cineangiograms obtained prior to the implantation procedure sometimes provides a general guide as to the position of the CS in the right atrium. Visualization of contrast entering the atrium during the levo-phase after coronary injection may help locate the CS.

### Catheter Manipulation

Successful catheterization of the CS involves entry into the CS from the inferior aspect of the right atrium, with the guide catheter directed upwardly and posteriorly to find the ostium. Trying to enter the CS with a shallow-curve guiding catheter while approaching the ostium from above often leads to difficulty or failure. Manipulation of preformed guiding catheters with tips curved to varying degrees may locate the CS ostium. Counterclockwise rotation of the preshaped guide catheter directs the guide posterior in the atrium. Should the guiding catheter enter the right ventricle, withdrawal of the catheter while applying counterclockwise pressure should also cause the catheter to take the desired approach to the CS ostium. Remodeling of the right atrium interferes with successful CS cannulation. When standard maneuvers with the preformed guiding catheters fail to find the CS ostium, using diagnostic coronary catheters inserted into the guiding catheters provides additional three-dimensional flexibility to locate the CS. Inserting a multipurpose (MP), left internal mammary (LIMA), or Amplatz (AL-3) catheter in the commercially available CS guiding catheters can help reach the CS in markedly abnormal right atria (Figure 6–26).

The combination of each diagnostic catheter within the guide catheter creates a variety of catheter shapes that can target the CS in patients with abnormal RA anatomy. The catheter-within-a catheter technique allows the insertion of a guide wire within the diagnostic catheter to enhance the flexibility of the system to engage the CS. Also, use of diagnostic catheters within the guide catheter permits injection of contrast material to aid in identifying the location of the CS OS. Alternative approaches to finding the CS OS include manipulation of deflectable electrophysiology mapping catheters within the guiding catheter and recording intracardiac electrograms to identify the CS OS. In cases where the implanter encounters great difficulty locating the ostium, left coronary angiography during the implantation procedure may provide a guide to the OS. Intracardiac ultrasound may also assist in locating the CS OS. However, one should use these modalities judiciously. Failure to visualize or enter the OS after numerous attempts with guiding catheters, deflectable electrophysiology catheters, or a telescoping catheter-within-a-catheter suggests that another attempt on a different day or by another implanter may be the prudent step.

### Advancing the Guide Catheter into the Coronary Sinus

When the guide catheter engages the CS OS, advancement of the guide-catheter 3–4 cm into the CS provides adequate stability for introduction of balloon venography catheters or a pacing lead into the CS and cardiac veins (Figure 6–27).

Advancing the guide catheter into the CS over a soft-tip guide wire (0.032–0.036 inch diameter) reduces the likelihood of mural trauma. Loading a guide wire into the guiding catheter before inserting into the central circulation facilitates

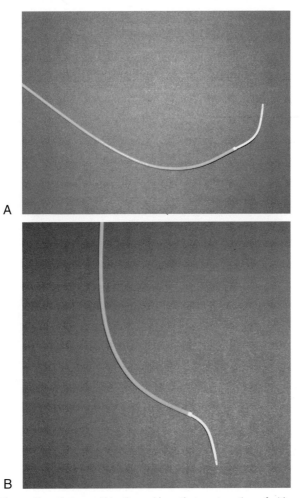

**FIGURE 6–26.** Diagnostic catheters within the guide catheters. Insertion of either a multipurpose (MP-A2), left internal mammary (LIMA), or Amplatz (AL-3) catheter into a standard guide catheter increases the flexibility of the guide catheter system to locate the coronary sinus (CS) in patients with difficult anatomy. The MP within the guide can target the CS in a very large atrium when pointing the MP up (*A*), or can directly cannulate a posterior or postero-lateral vein when directing the MP down (*B*).

*Continued*

its passage into the right atrium, provides a way to confirm that the guiding catheter has entered the CS by advancing the wire ahead of the catheter after engagement, and provides a guide for seating the catheter within the CS and reducing the risk of dissection (Figure 6–28).

Once the guiding catheter sits at least 3–4 cm within the CS, one can remove the guide wire and insert the balloon-tip catheter into position for contrast venography. Valves either near the ostium of the CS (eustachian valves) or well within the CS (valve of vieussens) may obstruct proper entry of the guide catheter and guide wire into the desired position.

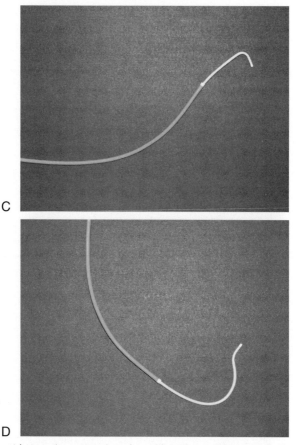

**FIGURE 6–26, cont'd.** Inserting a LIMA into the guide catheter allows subselective entry into veins that enter the CS at very acute angles (C). When encountering markedly enlarged right atria, use of the AL-3 within the guide directs the tip of the combined catheters into the CS (D).

## Eustachian Valve

The eustachian valve forms a flaplike cover over the CS ostium; the valve represents the more posterior extension of the eustachian ridge within the right atrium. A large eustachian valve may prevent the guide catheter from engaging the CS OS, particularly when one tries to approach the ostium beginning from the superior aspect of the right atrium moving down to the CS. The eustachian valve acts like a roof, covering the entry to the CS. Approaching the CS with the guide catheter pointing up and posterior from the floor of the right atrium often avoids the obstruction created by the valve. The valve of Vieussens, commonly found near the site of entry of the posterolateral LV vein into the CS, interferes with proper advancement of the guide catheter, the guide wire, or pacing leads into the CS. When encountering a valve of Vieussens, crossing the valve with the 0.035 inch guide wire may open the valve and allow catheter advancement without damage to the valve and potential dissection (Figure 6–29).

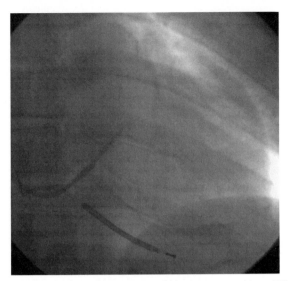

FIGURE 6–27.  The guide catheter position 4–5 cm within the coronary sinus (CS) provides a stable platform for insertion of a venogram catheter and for pacing lead insertion. Leaving the guide catheter within the first segment of the CS may result in dislodgement of the catheter during lead insertion.

One may choose to pass a smaller-diameter guide wire (0.025 inch) through the balloon venogram catheter deep into the CS over which to safely advance the balloon catheter across strictures, curves, or valves found in the CS. One should take care not to disrupt or tear valves within the CS. Forcing a guide catheter or guide wire into the valve often tears or perforates the CS. Aggressive advancement of a rigid mapping catheter into a CS valve may also traumatize the valve. Upon encountering resistance to advancement of a catheter within the CS, injection of a small amount of contrast usually reveals the presence of a valve, stricture, or kink in the vessel. Gentle advancement of the guide catheter just short of the point of an obstruction allows injection of a small amount of contrast under low pressure. Defining the cause of the obstruction allows the implanter to select either a coated wire, a 0.025 guide wire, or a diagnostic angiographic catheter for crossing the obstruction with care. Once the guide wire crosses, advancing a flexible diagnostic catheter such as the MP across the obstruction usually facilitates advancement of the guide catheter

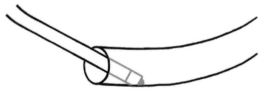

FIGURE 6–28.  Insertion of the guide catheter inferiorly into the coronary sinus (CS) directs the balloon catheter into the wall of the vessel and may lead to dissection or vascular trauma by the balloon catheter or pacing lead. Seating the guide catheter in a coaxial orientation to the CS prevents vascular trauma.

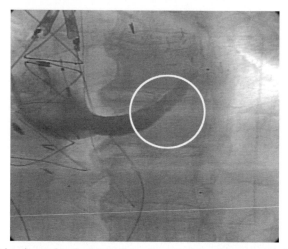

**FIGURE 6–29.** Valves located in the posterolateral aspect of the coronary sinus (CS) often present an obstacle to advancement of balloon catheters or pacing leads. One should approach these valves with care, preferably by passing small-diameter guide wires ahead of a balloon or guide catheter to avoid dissection at the site of the valve.

deep into the CS. Advancing the flexible diagnostic catheter or the balloon venography catheter may straighten a tortuous segment. Sequential advancement of a small guide wire, then a diagnostic catheter, followed last by the guide catheter, avoids the abrupt transition from a guide wire to a large-diameter catheter that may catch the CS wall with the edge of the guide catheter. The guide catheter reaches the desired position within the CS when the tip advances to the lateral aspect of the CS. Injection of 2–3 cc of contrast through the catheter confirms the position and allows detection of any mural trauma or dissection. Ruling out a small tear or dissection of the CS prior to full-injection venography reduces the probability of injecting a large contrast load into the extravascular space that may compromise the patient or stain the tissue around the CS that prevents visualization enough to jeopardize the implant. Once the "proof shot" confirms proper position within the CS, proceed to venography.

## Coronary Sinus Venography

Injection of radiographic contrast material into the coronary venous system can delineate all potential target veins, valves, strictures, collateral connections, and other specific anatomic details that permit optimal placement of LV pacing leads (Figure 6–30).

The risks of venography include dissection, balloon inflation in small-caliber vessels that can explode the vein, allergic reaction to contrast, and nephrotoxicity from excessive administration to the compromised patient. One can also perform venography by injecting contrast material through the guide catheter into the CS (Figure 6–31).

However, the large bore of the guide catheter requires injection of a large volume of contrast in order to fill the catheter and then opacify the CS. Also, the lack of a balloon at the tip of the guide catheter prevents occluding CS blood flow and

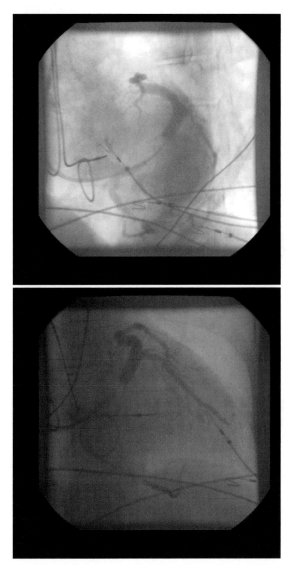

**FIGURE 6–30.** Biplane venography. Injection of contrast after balloon inflation illustrates all cardiac veins, the point of entry of each vein into the coronary sinus, second-order tributaries into the veins, and collateral connections between the major veins.

produces suboptimal venography. Some CS guide catheters incorporated a balloon near the tip of the guide. The occlusive guide catheter design limits the ability to occlude the CS at various sites that may be necessary for optimal venography. The preferred approach to coronary venography utilizes a catheter inserted through the guide catheter for positioning anywhere along the course of the CS for injection of contrast with or without occluding CS blood flow. The commonly used venogram catheters measure 4–6 F in diameter, have a single lumen, and have an inflatable

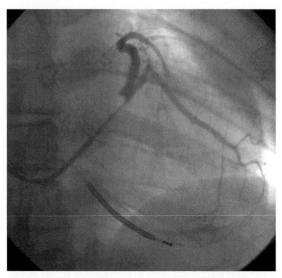

**FIGURE 6–31.** Contrast injection through the guide catheter without balloon inflation may provide adequate anatomic information for lead insertion. One can adequately fill moderate-size left ventricular veins without the need for occlusion, but without occluding coronary sinus blood flow, opacification of all the venous tributaries is unlikely.

balloon located about 1 cm from the tip. Balloon inflation at the tip of the catheter within the CS blocks blood flow and permits injection of contrast into the entire venous tree directly or indirectly through collateral venous channels. Low-pressure injection of 10 cc of contrast material reduces the chance of vascular trauma. Diluting the contrast with saline (50%) decreases the risk of nephropathy and excessive osmolar loads to the patient with CHF. Avoiding overinflation of the balloon in a CS with small diameter or in a tributary vein reduces the likelihood of exploding the vessel during contrast injection.

## Image Projections

Adequate venographic technique consists of acquiring and storing images in at least two radiographic planes (AP/LAO or RAO/LAO) to provide the optimal anatomic roadmap for advancement of guide wires and pacing leads into the targeted LV site (Figure 6–32).

The venogram should demonstrate all possible cardiac venous targets, the site at which each LV vein enters into the CS, and the course of each vein and its tributaries, from base to apex (Figure 6–33).

A venogram in the LAO projection at 30–45 degrees with slight cranial or caudal angulation generates excellent views of the LV veins as they enter the CS (Figure 6–34).

The LAO venogram also removes overlap seen in the AP view between anterior/septal veins and anterior-lateral veins. However, the LAO view usually foreshortens the view of the body of the tributary vein. Therefore a venogram in another view should demonstrate clearly the LV vein and its tributaries for targeting specific pacing lead

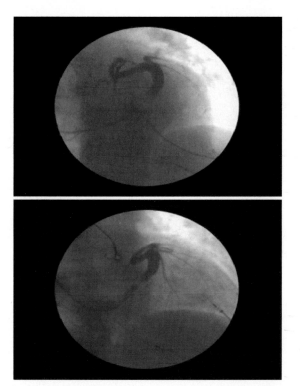

FIGURE 6–32. Performing venograms in multiple planes removes overlap of potential target veins. An image in the anterior-posterior plane (*top*) fails to distinguish between a lateral vein and the great cardiac vein. Taking another venogram in the left anterior oblique projection removes the overlap between the two veins, and shows a desirable target vein draining the lateral left ventricular wall (*bottom*).

locations inside the vein. Fluoroscopy in the AP or RAO 15- to 30-degree projection best visualizes the course of LV veins from the CS to the apex of the ventricle. Venography in two views, LAO (35–45 degrees) and AP or RAO (15 degrees), provides the implanter with the adequate anatomic information necessary for successful LV lead advancement. The LAO view facilitates entry into the cardiac vein from the CS; the AP or RAO guides advancement within the LV vein to the target site. Extending the fluoroscopic acquisition for a few seconds after contrast injection allows time for the contrast to reach all venous tributaries through collateral flow. Opacification of collaterals to posterior and posterior-lateral LV veins demonstrates potential target veins that would otherwise go unnoticed during injection of contrast beyond the point at which those veins enter the CS. Normal physiology dictates that all of the LV myocardium requires venous drainage. The inability to identify venous drainage from a large segment of the LV implies that venography failed to detect the tributary from that segment or collateral flow from one segment to a vein draining an adjacent segment or that failure to occlude the CS led to suboptimal contrast injection. Failure to utilize venography to guide LV lead implantation can diminish the chance of a successful implantation. One may fortuitously find LV veins without obtaining a venogram simply by probing for CS tributaries with a guide wire. However, the

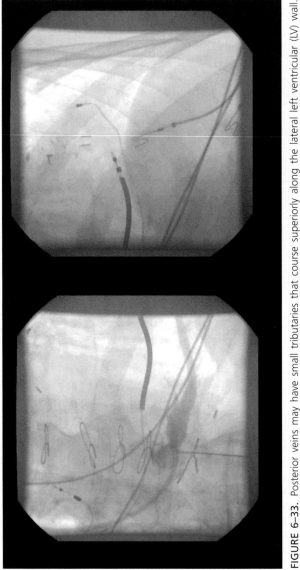

**FIGURE 6–33.** Posterior veins may have small tributaries that course superiorly along the lateral left ventricular (LV) wall. Locating the insertion of the posterior vein (*left*) and the small tributaries that reach the LV free-wall provide an adequate target site for LV lead implant (*right*) in the absence of adequate primary target veins along the lateral wall.

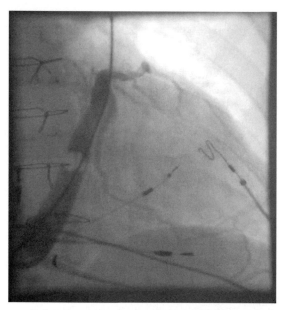

**FIGURE 6–34.** Demonstrating the angle of entry of the target left ventricular (LV) vein into the coronary sinus (CS) is crucial to successful lead insertion. Entry of LV veins into the CS at acute angles presents obstacles to LV lead insertion. The presence of strictures calls for selection of alternate veins or venoplasty to open access through obstructed veins.

advantages of proper venography greatly outweigh its risks to the patient. Venography provides a roadmap to primary and secondary venous targets, should the primary target vein yield poor pacing thresholds or lie too close to the phrenic nerve.

## Cardiac Venous Anatomy

Cardiac venous anatomy varies greatly, perhaps more so than the anatomy of coronary arteries. We would classify LV venous drainage into four general types based upon the site along the mitral annulus where the posterior, posterior-lateral, and lateral LV veins enter the CS. The course of the anterior cardiac vein around the anterior aspect of the intraventricular groove and the aortic root follows a fairly consistent pattern in most individuals. The angle at which LV veins enter the CS varies greatly, ranging from very shallow (120–160 degrees) to very acute (30–60 degrees) angles with respect to the CS (see Figure 6–34). The most acute angles of entry usually occur along the lateral and high-lateral CS, with the less acute angles usually along the posterolateral aspect of the AV groove. Superimposing a clock over the mitral annulus facilitates a nomenclature to describe the anatomic site where LV veins enter the CS as viewed by fluoroscopy at LAO 45 degrees. The suggested nomenclature assigns the 7 o'clock position to the CS ostium and an 11 o'clock position to the junction of the anterior wall and septum.

The most commonly encountered coronary venous drainage pattern parallels the typical left-dominant coronary artery anatomy. The posterior interventricular vein enters the CS within 1–2 cm of the ostium (6 o'clock position). Occasionally the posterior interventricular vein enters the right atrium through what appears to be a separate ostium. The posterior interventricular vein courses below the intraventricular septum and often receives divisions draining the posterior and lateral segment of the left ventricle. The posterolateral vein enters the CS near the point where the CS begins its upward course along the free-wall aspect of the mitral annulus (4–5 o'clock positions). The lateral vein usually enters the CS near the midpoint of the free-wall of the left ventricle (2–3 o'clock positions). The CS becomes the great cardiac vein as it courses across the anterior mitral annulus and around the aortic root (12 o'clock position) before descending over the intraventricular septum toward the cardiac apex as the anterior cardiac vein. As the anterior cardiac vein courses to the apex, the anterolateral vein draining the high-lateral LV free-wall enters into the upper segment of the anterior cardiac vein. Injection of contrast at the lateral CS may not demonstrate any lateral vein draining the lateral LV wall. In this situation collateral flow usually reveals the presence of a large posterolateral vein with divisions that parallel the CS slightly below the AV groove and serve as venous drainage of the LV free-wall. This type of posterolateral vein may have a number of posterior-lateral and lateral divisions not seen during brief injections within the CS that also travel up the mid-lateral wall of the left ventricle. Contrast injection through a catheter selectively inserted into the posterolateral vein trunk demonstrates all the possible divisions of the trunk that can serve as target veins. Occasionally, a single trunk may leave the CS at or near the 3 o'clock position and give superior and inferior divisions that serve as the lateral vein, posterolateral vein, and anterolateral vein (Figure 6–35).

The posterior interventricular vein maintains its separate entry into the CS. Rarely, one may encounter a variety of anomalous CS and LV venous patterns, including

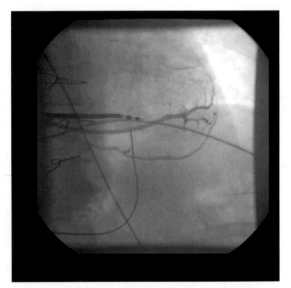

**FIGURE 6–35.** A large posterolateral venous trunk enters the coronary sinus and drains the large aspect of the left ventricular (LV) free-wall. Absence of any lateral or anterolateral veins should herald the presence of such a posterolateral trunk. Proper positioning of the venogram balloon should demonstrate this access point to the lateral LV veins.

persistent left superior vena cavae that drain directly into the CS, persistent anterior drainage from the great cardiac vein to the right atrium, and multiple veins draining the left ventricle at any one segment along the CS.

An anatomic description of coronary venous anatomy based upon flow through the vessel designates the proximal end of the vein as that near the capillary bed, with the distal portion entering the CS. Any coronary vein may demonstrate tortuous segments or multiple points of confluence along its course to the CS. The most distal segments of the veins, as they enter the CS, usually contain the most tortuous segments. The proximal segments, near the ventricular apex, show confluence of small veins to form the main vein as it approaches the AV groove. The diameter of LV veins also varies from barely visible, small veins to a large posterolateral vein or lateral vein with a diameter exceeding 4 mm. Venography often uncovers extensive collateral channels that connect the posterior interventricular vein , posterolateral vein, lateral vein , and antero-lateral veins. The extent of collateral circulation in the venous circulation greatly exceeds that observed in coronary arteries. One may frequently pass a guide wire from the posterolateral vein to the anterolateral vein through one of the channels. The presence of rich collateral connections between the main LV veins produces greater access to potential pacing sites along the left ventricle from different LV veins along the CS. The ability to use collateral veins to reach a desired pacing site may salvage an otherwise unsuccessful implantation, when anatomic barriers prevent antegrade insertion of a pacing lead to the desired site (Figure 6–36).

### Stylet-Driven Lead Insertion (Emory)

The design of the available stylet-driven leads incorporates a curve near the distal part of the electrode intended to facilitate entry into LV veins or promote fixation within the target vein. Insertion of a less-compliant, straight stylet into the lead usually straightens the distal curve enough to facilitate advancement through the guiding catheter and into the CS. Once inside the CS, the implanter advances the lead slightly beyond the entry point of the targeted vein. Withdrawal of the straight stylet allows the lead tip to assume its designed curve, and with the application of torque to steer the lead, the tip enters the vein. Once the lead tip enters the vein, advancement of the lead should place it at the desired location within the LV vein. Ideally, one should advance the lead to a site in the vein that places the pacing electrode at the midpoint between the AV groove and cardiac apex. The curved segment at the end of the pacing lead could impair movement of the lead to a desired position within a small caliber or tortuous vessel. Inserting a compliant stylet into the lead straightens the distal segment without dislodging the lead tip from the target vein, and allows further advancement of the lead down the vein. Withdrawal of the stylet once the lead reaches the desired site in the target vein allows the curve to form, and fixes the lead within the vein. Use of the straight stylet technique to passively enter a LV vein works best when there is a shallow angle between the CS and the target vein. Using a straight stylet limits the degree of control one can transmit to the tip of the pacing lead. Encountering severe angles, tortuous veins, or small caliber LV veins makes the passive/straight stylet approach less likely to succeed. The alternative approach to advancing stylet-driven leads into LV veins involves bending the distal 1–2 cm of the stylet at an angle that corresponds to the angle of entry of the target LV vein into the CS. The proper venogram should illustrate the angle of entry of LV veins into the CS. Bending the stylet provides the ability to steer

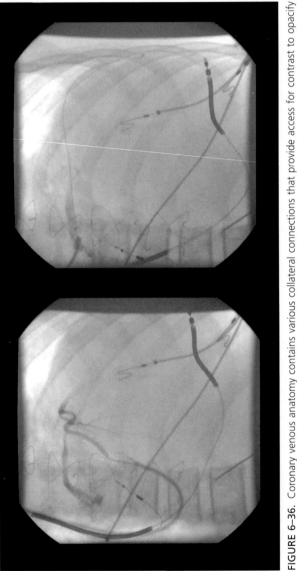

**FIGURE 6–36.** Coronary venous anatomy contains various collateral connections that provide access for contrast to opacify the entire venous anatomy from a number of injection points along the coronary sinus. One may also use a collateral connection to advance a pacing lead from the posterior vein to the lateral wall when poor anatomy prevents direct entry.

the lead tip into the desired vein by turning the stylet knob and delivering the torque directly to the lead tip. Instead of passively allowing the lead to enter the target vein passively by withdrawing the stylet, this approach actively uses the shaped stylet to guide the lead tip into the vein. Once in the tributary vein, removal of the stiff, shaped stylet and insertion of a compliant, straight stylet allows advancement of the lead to the desired position in the same manner as in the passive stylet approach. Generally stylet driven leads have a larger diameter, and are less compliant than over-the-wire pacing leads. These two characteristics make stylet-driven leads more difficult to insert into small-caliber LV veins, but may provide advantages when used in very large LV veins, by making them fixate better and less likely to dislodge.

## Over-The-Wire Insertion Techniques (Emory)

The development of the over-the-wire pacing lead technology provides the ability to maneuver thin guide wires into small and tortuous cardiac veins. Advancing a flexible and small diameter pacing lead over the guide wire allows the implanter to target many more potential pacing sites within the coronary venous circulation. Over-the-wire lead delivery may facilitate targeting the ideal cardiac vein, manipulate the lead into a second-order tributary in order to achieve optimal lead stability, avoid stimulation of the left phrenic nerve, and optimize LV stimulation thresholds. Over-the-wire lead insertion incorporates tools and techniques developed for interventional cardiology. The tools include preshaped guide catheters, a family of guide wires, each with unique characteristics, and leads that share properties of angioplasty balloons but contain pacing electrodes for LV stimulation. The implanting physician should understand how to select and shape guide wires, the maneuvers utilized to advance leads over guide wires, and the how forces applied to the guide wires and leads can dislodge guide catheters from the CS.

The guide catheters available for over-the-wire technique do not differ from those used for stylet driven leads. However, the manufacturers of guide catheters have increased the variety of guide catheters available in order to meet the anatomic challenges posed by the remodeled heart, from straight guide-catheters intended for advancement over steerable EP mapping catheters, to guide catheters with traditional diagnostic shapes, such as Amplatz curves. The guide wires designed for interventional cardiology include wires with a spectrum of diameters, flexibility, points of transition between relatively flexible and nonflexible elements, lubricious coatings, and materials. The variety in characteristics for guide wires used in LV pacing lead insertion need not be as extensive as those needed for interventional cardiology. Most LV lead implants require only a medium-weight guide wire (0.014 in diameter) with a transition 5–10 cm from the tip. Occasionally, a heavy weight wire, with a transition point close to the tip can facilitate passage of a lead through tortuous veins by straightening some of the curves before pacing lead advancement. Newly developed guide wires offer a compromise between the stiff, heavy wires and the floppy or middleweight wires.

Bending the distal 3 mm of the wire 40–60 degrees creates the ability to steer the tip of the wire into a target vein. Rotating a torque-delivery device attached to the wire steers the guide wire tip toward the target vein. The guide wire should protrude 1–4 cm ahead of the lead. One can load the wire into the pacing lead and insert them together through the guide catheter into the CS. Advancing the lead closer to the tip of the guide wire provides additional support to the wire. The combination of wire advancement and rotation guides the wire into the LV vein. Alternatively, one can insert the guide wire alone into the guide catheter for advancement of the "naked" guide wire into a cardiac vein. Once the wire advances to the distal segment of the vein, "back loading" the lead over the guide allows the lead to advance to the target site. Inserting the lead and wire together into the guiding catheter allows advancement of the guide wire ahead of the lead, and advancement of the combined system out of the guiding catheter. Rotation of the guide wire tip while referring to the stored venogram aims the wire toward the desired tributary vein. Regardless of the method used to insert the guide wire into the CS, once the guide wire enters the targeted vein, advancement of the wire into the distal segment of the vein provides a stable platform for over which the lead tracks into the vein to reach the desired position for the pacing electrode. Ideally, once in the targeted vein, advancing the guide wire as far as possible into the LV vein provides the greatest stability. The ability of the pacing lead to "track" over the guide wire increases directly with the stiffness of the wire. Advancing the lead while simultaneously retracting the wire (the "push-pull" technique) promotes advancement of the lead within a vessel. Having inserted sufficient guide wire that extends beyond the target site allows retraction of some of the guide wire during lead advancement. Failure to insert enough guide wire length can cause inadvertent retraction of the guide wire out of the vein during the "push-pull" approach. When a lead advances into a vessel of small enough caliber to prevent further advancement, a final "push-pull" of the lead and wire wedges the lead tip into the small caliber vessel. Inserting the wire into second-order tributary veins moves the electrode tip away from a large caliber vein that may otherwise not create the lead the desired stability. The over-the-wire technique also permits movement of the pacing electrode to multiple sites within one vein, or to easily select alternate veins when one encounters unacceptably high stimulation thresholds or extra-cardiac stimulation during LV pacing.

## LIMA Catheter Use

Acute angles at the entry of veins into the CS may prevent advancement of the guide wire far enough into the vein to allow the lead to track into position. Advancing the lead in this situation often pulls the guide wire back into the CS and out of the LV vein. One can overcome this problem in two ways. Inserting a diagnostic catheter (6Fr LIMA) into the guide catheter and selectively engaging the targeted vein with the LIMA catheter provides access to the vein for inserting a stiff or heavyweight guide wire deep into the vein. The heavyweight wire will provide a track for the lead to follow, often diminishing the acuity of the angle between the vein and CS. Removing the LIMA catheter without dislodging the guide wire allows back loading of the lead over the wire into the vein. This maneuver requires careful attention to the guide wire and the guiding catheter during the removal of the LIMA catheter and advancement of the pacing lead. Placing a sterile, covered table perpendicular to the patient's shoulder provides a work station for safely removing the catheter and loading the lead. Removing the LIMA catheter without simultaneously feeding guide wire into the catheter will pull the guide wire out of position. Failure to fix the wire to prevent excessive wire advancement during lead insertion will push the guide catheter out of the CS. Fixing the guide wire to a stationary point and removal of all slack from the wire prior to lead insertion increases the likelihood of success. An alternative to using the LIMA catheter within the guide catheter involves using an angioplasty wire conduit (transit tube) inserted into the LV vein. The conduit allows advancement of the wire into the LV vein in a manner similar to the LIMA catheter.

Introduction of excessive lengths of guide wire or a pacing lead into the LV vein will push the guide catheter out of the CS when the wire or vein meets an obstruction or reaches the end of the vein. If the guide catheter falls out of the CS, it will drag the guide wire and lead out with it. The common reflex response is to advance the guiding catheter into the CS, but in this circumstance that move will dislodge the catheter, LV lead, and guide wire. The way to reseat the catheter involves retraction of the excessive guide wire/lead that created the problem. One must make this correction quickly to prevent guide catheter dislodgement.

Coronary veins may contain tortuous segments, strictures, or severe angles that block advancement of the guide wire or pacing lead (Figure 6–37).

If the first choice in guide wire does not enter the vein, reshaping the tip, or switching to another wire with a transition of different length may provide a better outcome. When the guide wire tip loses its shape or becomes damaged, one should change the wire. If the wire enters a vein, but cannot cross a tortuous segment or a stricture, advancing the lead closer to the tip of the wire provides greater support to the wire. If the wire fails to cross, leaving the lead as far in the vein as possible, removing the wire, and reinserting a new, stiffer wire, may cross the difficult segment. Leaving the lead within the vein prior to wire removal prevents the need of having to enter the vein from the CS again. Crossing a difficult segment with the guide wire often creates an adequate track for the lead to follow. However, advancement of the guide wire does not guarantee successful lead insertion.

Failure to cross a stricture or a tortuous segment of vein, or the absence of veins with large enough caliber to accept pacing leads could force selection of an alternate site for pacing lead insertion. The venous anatomy in most patients offers at least two potential sites for LV pacing. Occasionally, no site may provide adequate pacing, leading to a failed transvenous implantation.[3] Use of heavyweight guide wires,

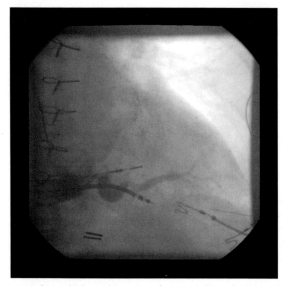

**FIGURE 6–37.** Acute angles or kinks within veins often complicate lead insertion. Crossing these segments with rigid guide wires allows for pacing leads to track across the tortuous segments.

catheter-within-a catheter technique, and proper venogram technique will produce excellent results in most cases. Venous strictures, and veins of inadequate caliber, may respond to balloon venoplasty techniques and lead to successful introduction of LV leads (Figure 6–38).

The combined total of CRT device implantations at Emory University exceeds 900 cases. The overall success rate of transvenous LV lead implantations in our laboratories exceeds 93%, with a 97% success rate over the past two years after the adoption of the over-the-wire approach. We have utilized venoplasty in three cases. The implanting cardiologist with experience using interventional techniques may view venoplasty as another tool to approach difficult cases. However, the need for resorting to venoplasty to achieve success has not been fully determined in controlled studies. An evaluation of the extraordinary measures to achieve successful LV lead implantation needs to consider the incremental cost of equipment and the potential hazard to the patient. Some transvenous LV implantations will fail, creating the need for a surgical procedure to implant LV leads via thoracoscopy or thoracotomy.[4] Alternative access to LV lead implantation after failure of the transvenous approach include open thoracotomy, video-assisted thoracoscopy (VAT), and robotic insertion of LV leads.[5]

### Occlusive Coronary Sinus Venography

At least two-view occlusive CS venography is essential to proper LV lead placement. Unless this is performed, the target vein anatomy will not be fully understood. Figure 6–39 illustrates a case in which the AP venogram made it seem

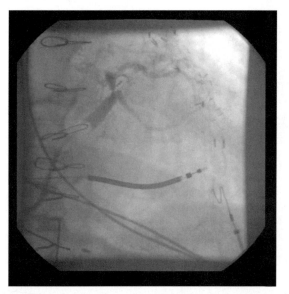

**FIGURE 6–38.** Epicardial fibrosis following cardiac surgery commonly constricts the coronary sinus (CS) or its tributaries. Strictures along the CS prevent advancement of pacing lead, requiring either venoplasty to relieve the obstruction or selection of an alternative route for left ventricular lead insertion.

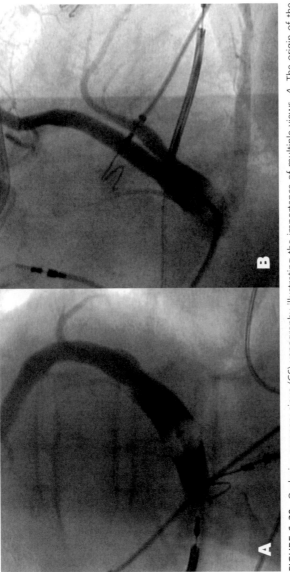

FIGURE 6–39. Occlusive coronary sinus (CS) venography illustrating the importance of multiple views. A, The origin of the lateral wall target vein appears to be mid-CS. B, The right anterior oblique (RAO) view reveals that the origin is close to the CS ostium. Time was lost trying to advance a left ventricular pacing lead into the vein until repeat venography in the RAO view revealed the proximal origin of the vein.

as if no further contrast was required. After more than an hour of unsuccessful lead manipulation, additional CS venogram angles were obtained, revealing the proximal takeoff and parallel course of the target vein. Once the anatomy was understood the lead was quickly placed (Figure 6–40).

The variable anatomy of cardiac veins does not present the only challenge to the physician implanting an LV lead. Acquired abnormalities in the LV veins can present obstacles to LV lead implantation. Epicardial fibrosis due to pericarditis, surgical intervention, or external radiation may greatly affect venous anatomy and present an impediment to successful resynchronization. Median sternotomy for coronary bypass surgery appears to be the most common cause of epicardial fibrosis in patients referred for LV lead implantation. Postoperative pericarditis may constrict cardiac veins and completely block them, creating collaterals with excessive tortuosity that prevent lead insertion. The distal anastomosis of vein grafts to native arteries may inadvertently suture the adjacent coronary vein, rendering it useless for LV lead

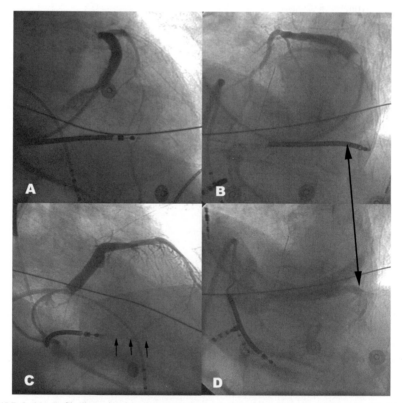

**FIGURE 6–40.** Defibrillator lead in target vein. *A,* No lateral wall target vein is identified in the anterior-posterior projection. The defibrillation lead is placed in the mid–right ventricular (RV) septum. *B,* Again, no lateral wall target veins are identified; however, the location of the defibrillator lead is unusual for the midseptum. *C,* The right anterior oblique projection reveals that the defibrillator lead is in a large, lateral wall target vein, not the RV septum as was originally thought. *D,* The defibrillator lead is removed from the lateral wall vein. The left anterior oblique projection now reveals the target vein.

insertion. Large myocardial infarction, producing scarring in the capillary bed, may close off venous drainage in infracted segments. Infectious (viral) pericarditis, postoperative mediastinitis, and external radiation therapy for Hodgkin's or other malignancy may also produce fibrosis around the heart. Extensive scarring may leave the patient with narrow and tortuous coronary venous anatomy not amenable to pacing lead insertion. Scarring may obstruct the main venous channel and open collateral channels that may be too small or tortuous to accommodate lead insertion.

## Effect of Prior Mitral Valve Replacement

The most challenging cases arise in the setting of prior mitral valve repair or replacement, presumably because of the distortion of the CS and associated venous structures when the valve is repaired or replaced. Figure 6–41 demonstrates the tortuous vein segments frequently seen in such patients.

Venous tributaries of the CS that drain the free-wall of the left ventricle appear to provide the best conduit for LV pacing lead insertion. Leaving a pacing lead within anterior cardiac vein or posterior interventricular vein does not provide effective CRT; from those sites the LV lead stimulates the septum, with little change in the delay until the wavefront reaches the lateral LV wall.[6] Inserting LV pacing leads with the pacing electrode in the anterolateral vein, lateral vein , or posterolateral vein provides the most effective cardiac resynchronization. Implanters can choose between large-diameter, stylet-driven leads and smaller-diameter, over-the-wire leads for LV venous pacing. Implanters at Emory utilize over-the-wire leads in over 95% of cases, reserving the stylet-driven leads for when we encounter very large LV veins in which one cannot stabilize the smaller, over-the-wire lead, thus posing an increased risk of lead dislodgement.

## Responders and Nonresponders

Proper placement of the LV lead on the lateral wall of the left ventricle is critical to successful resynchronization therapy. Figure 6–42 is the typical post implantation chest radiograph of a "responder." Note that the LV and RV leads are maximally separated on the lateral chest radiograph. Figure 6–43 shows the lateral chest radiographs of two patients who did not respond to resynchronization. We consistently find the lateral chest radiograph essential in evaluating patients who do not respond, despite successful LV lead placement. Placement of the LV lead anterior surface is now clearly recognized as inadvisable and may worsen LV function. Figure 6–43A is the lateral chest radiograph of a nonresponder, whose lead was placed in the anterior interventricular vein. Patients with a lead in this position are not expected to respond. However, Figure 6–43B shows the lateral chest radiograph of a patient who did not respond, despite lateral wall lead placement. Note that the tip of the LV pacing lead is closer to the RV pacing lead than the ideal position, seen in Figure 6–42B.

## Contrast or No Contrast to Cannulate the Coronary Sinus

The noncontrast method of CS cannulation is familiar to many operators who typically use the combination of a deflectable electrophysiology catheter inside a multipurpose guide (see Figure 6–8D). Electrograms may or may not be recorded. However, as noted previously, finding the OS and placing a catheter in the CS can

*Text continued on page 171*

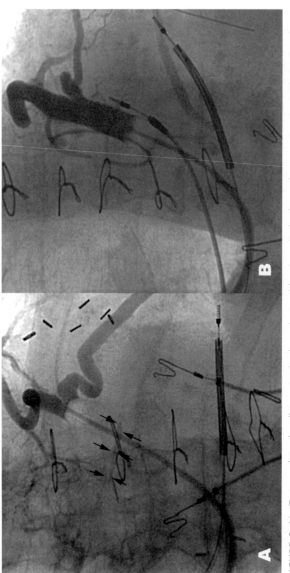

**FIGURE 6–41.** Tortuous lateral wall target veins in patients with prior mitral valve replacement/repair. A, The patient has a St. Jude mitral valve (arrows). B, The patient has a mitral ring placed. In both cases the lateral wall target vein is tortuous resulting in difficult lead delivery.

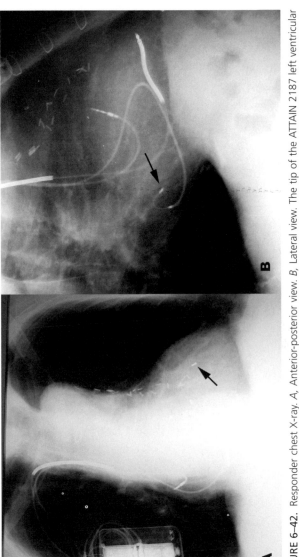

**FIGURE 6–42.** Responder chest X-ray. *A,* Anterior-posterior view. *B,* Lateral view. The tip of the ATTAIN 2187 left ventricular (LV) pacing lead is indicated by the arrow. In the lateral view the LV lead is located directly posterior, at a maximal distance from the right ventricular lead.

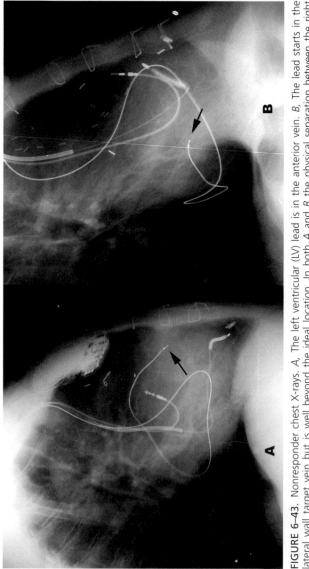

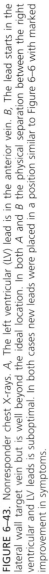

FIGURE 6–43. Nonresponder chest X-rays. A, The left ventricular (LV) lead is in the lateral wall target vein but is well beyond the ideal location. In both A and B the physical separation between the right ventricular and LV leads is suboptimal. In both cases new leads were placed in a position similar to Figure 6–6 with marked improvement in symptoms.

be quite difficult in patients with CHF who present for resynchronization therapy. The limitations of both the contrast and noncontrast method are outlined below.

## Limitations of the Noncontrast Method

1. The catheter must advance out into the CS to confirm location. The noncontrast method assumes (incorrectly) that if the tip of the catheter is in the OS it will advance easily from the OS into the CS. Without contrast, the operator recognizes only that the tip of the catheter was in the OS once the catheter advances into the CS. Confirmation that the catheter has advanced into the CS is best appreciated in the LAO projection. However, even by monitoring electrograms, the operator may have no idea that he or she is or was in the OS if the catheter does not advance into the CS. Figure 6–11 demonstrates two cases in which it was easy to find the OS with contrast but difficult to advance the catheter beyond the OS.

Without contrast injection, the operator would not recognize that the tip of the catheter was in the OS of the CS and could spend hours continuing to look. A simple puff of contrast reveals that the tip of the catheter is in the CS OS but will not advance. In many cases where the operator has difficulty, the problem is not finding the CS OS but advancing the catheter beyond the OS. The problem is not apparent unless contrast is used. Working in the LAO projection to confirm that the catheter has advanced into the CS to confirm location increases radiation exposure.

2. The catheter does not provide anatomic landmarks to assist in locating the OS. With the noncontrast method, the catheter does not provide the anatomic landmarks provided by contrast injection to help guide the operator toward the CS OS. For example, the operator may spend hours looking for the CS, not recognizing that the tip of the catheter is only a few millimeters from the OS. In this situation a 2-ml puff of contrast will reveal the location of the OS and allow the operator to adjust the trajectory of the catheter accordingly. Recording electrograms does not provide the same type of information.

## Limitations of the Contrast Method

Transient renal insufficiency can result from contrast. Proper preparation of the patient essentially eliminates the risk of even temporary dialysis. The concern over renal insufficiency may greatly exceed the actual risk. Details and references are provided at the end of the chapter.

# Telescoping Delivery System (Lancaster)

The need for a telescoping system stems from the fact that the catheter shape best suited for rapid, easy CS access may not be appropriate for delivering the wire/lead to the target vein. In approximately 50% of cases the lead/guide wire advances easily into the target vein. Figure 6–44 demonstrates a case in which the pacing lead easily advances onto the epicardial surface of the left ventricle through the lateral wall target vein. However, in many cases the angioplasty wire/LV lead will not advance, because of either an angulated takeoff or a tortuous vessel, beyond the ostium of the target vein. Figure 6–45 demonstrates lateral wall target vein anatomy that is frequently encountered during a biventricular implantation procedure. As you can see, the target veins do not line up in the same direction as

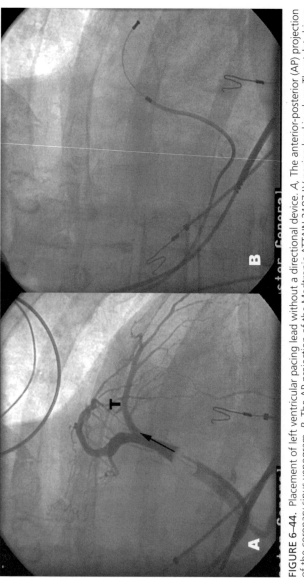

**FIGURE 6-44.** Placement of left ventricular pacing lead without a directional device. *A,* The anterior-posterior (AP) projection of the coronary sinus venogram. *B,* The AP projection of the Medtronic ATTAIN 2187 LV pacing lead in place. The stylet-driven lead easily advances into the lateral wall target vein (*T*) without the need for a telescoping system. The takeoff of the target vein lines up with the sheath. The forward vector of the lead is not degraded by the need to change direction to enter the target vein. In addition there are no twists, turns, or stenotic segments in the vein after the origin.

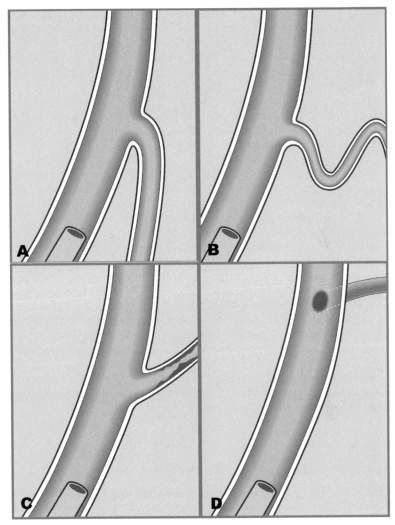

**FIGURE 6–45.** Difficult target vein anatomy. *A,* An acutely angulated target vein. *B,* A tortuous target vein. *C,* A stenotic target vein. *D,* A target vein with a posterior takeoff remote from coronary sinus ostium (CS OS). In all panels, the CS access sheath is located just inside the CS OS. If a traditional one-component approach is taken, the wire must be advanced from the sheath into the target vein without any additional equipment. Given the anatomic variants demonstrated, wire insertion without a second component (*directional device*) is difficult or impossible regardless of the type of pacing lead. However, if a two-component approach is applied (create a *telescoping system* by the addition of a *directional device*), these anatomic variants are easily addressed.

the sheath that rests in the CS. In fact, the best shape for CS access may actually direct the wire or pacing lead away from the target vein. In cases such as this, many fruitless hours may be spent trying to overcome what represents a mechanical impossibility. In these cases, an additional component specifically designed to address the target veins is needed. Conceptually, a telescoping system breaks the delivery of the pacing lead down into two independent but interrelated steps, with separate equipment for each step. First you have equipment to get into the CS, and second, you have equipment to direct the lead out of the CS into the lateral wall target onto the LV epicardial surface. By breaking the process into two steps the equipment design is specific to that step. The dedicate equipment is labeled as follows:

1. *CS platform:* Equipment designed to gain and maintain access to the CS.
2. *Directional device:* Equipment designed to deliver the wire/lead to the lateral wall target vein.

A telescoping delivery system has several advantages over a sheath alone, which include the ability to insert and remove a variety of leads and directional devices into the CS through the "CS platform" without the need to repeatedly cannulate the CS. In addition, the CS platform provides support for the wire/lead while the inner directional catheter/guide is removed.

A telescoping system for the biventricular pacing implantation procedure has two components: (1) the "outer sheath" or CS platform and (2) the directional device. The outer sheath is designed for rapid CS access, stability in the CS, and ease of removal. It serves as the platform for the telescoping system. The directional device is inserted into the CS through the CS platform to direct the angioplasty wire or lead into the target vein. The directional device is designed to selectively cannulate the target vein. Together, the CS platform and the directional device provide the support and direction necessary to advance the wire or pacing lead onto the lateral wall of the left ventricle.

In order to describe a telescoping system we must first define the terminology. It is important to understand what is meant here by the terms sheath, introducer, directional catheter, and directional guide.

## Definitions

### Coronary Sinus Platform (Outer Sheath/Introducer)

For the purposes of this discussion, sheath and introducer are used synonymously. In the context of a telescoping system the sheath serves as a stable conduit between pectoral area and the CS for the *directional device*. In this role the sheath becomes the CS platform for the telescoping system. When referring to the size of a sheath or introducer it is important to remember that the French size refers to the internal diameter, whereas the French size of guides and catheters refers to the external diameter. Guides and catheters are designed to be placed in the body through a sheath or introducer. For example, a 7-F catheter/guide fits through a 7-F introducer/sheath.

### Directional Device (Catheter or Guide)

The directional device fits within the *CS platform*. The internal diameter of the directional device and the size of the pacing lead determine whether we refer to the directional device as a *directional catheter* or *directional guide*. The advantage of a directional guide over a directional catheter is explained at the end of this section.

## Directional Catheters

When the internal diameter of the directional device is large enough to deliver only the angioplasty wire, it is referred to as the *directional catheter.* As part of a telescoping system, the *directional catheter* is placed in the CS through the *outer sheath (CS platform).* It provides direction, support, and a low-friction environment for an angioplasty wire. Various shaped directional catheters are used depending on the venous anatomy. Recall that the French size of a catheter refers to the outer diameter. The internal diameter of all 6-F (outer diameter; OD) and smaller catheters are too small for the available pacing leads.

## Directional Guides

When the internal diameter of the directional device is large enough to deliver the pacing lead, it is referred to as the *directional guide.* As part of a telescoping system, the directional guide is placed in the CS through a sheath. It provides direction, support, and a low-friction environment for a pacing lead or an angioplasty wire. Various shaped directional guides are used depending on the venous anatomy. Recall that the French size of a guide refers to the outer diameter. The internal diameter of most 7-F (OD) interventional guides are large enough to deliver the Medtronic ATTAIN 4193 LV lead. The internal diameter of some 8-F (OD) interventional guides are large enough to deliver the Medtronic ATTAIN 2187 LV lead and the Guidant EASYTRAK LV pacing lead. The internal diameter of all 9-F (OD) interventional guides is sufficient for both Medtronic ATTAIN leads and the Guidant lead.

### *Coronary Sinus Platform: The Outer Sheath*

The first step in deploying a telescoping system is to establish a stable platform in the CS from which to work and maintain CS access throughout the procedure. The *CS platform* provides support for the wire/lead or *directional device* as you work to implant the lead. The physical requirements of the *CS platform* are as follows:

1. Easy to place in the CS.
2. Stable within the CS.
3. Does not kink.
4. Does not dislodge the LV pacing lead as it is removed.

(See Figures 6–46 to 6–50)

### *Directional Device for Selective Target Vein Cannulation*

The *CS platform/outer sheath* not only provides a stable platform in the CS from which to work, but it also directs and supports the angioplasty wire and/or LV pacing lead (wire) between the subclavian vein and the CS. However, once the wire/lead is in the CS, it must be advanced out of the CS onto the lateral wall of the left ventricle through a venous branch referred to as the target vein. To understand the importance of the *directional device* it is useful to consider how a wire moves within the support tubing of a directional device (sheath/guide/catheter) versus how the same wire moves along the same path in a vein without support tubing. As long as a wire is within the support tubing of the CS platform or directional device it is

*Text continued on page 180*

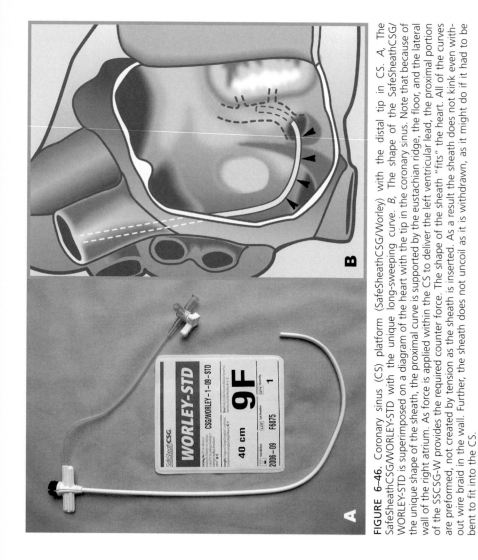

**FIGURE 6-46.** Coronary sinus (CS) platform (SafeSheathCSG/Worley) with the distal tip in CS. *A,* The SafeSheathCSG/WORLEY-STD with the unique long-sweeping curve. *B,* The shape of the SafeSheathCSG/WORLEY-STD is superimposed on a diagram of the heart with the tip in the coronary sinus. Note that because of the unique shape of the sheath, the proximal curve is supported by the eustachian ridge, the floor, and the lateral wall of the right atrium. As force is applied within the CS to deliver the left ventricular lead, the proximal portion of the SSCSG-W provides the required counter force. The shape of the sheath "fits" the heart. All of the curves are preformed, not created by tension as the sheath is inserted. As a result the sheath does not kink even without wire braid in the wall. Further, the sheath does not uncoil as it is withdrawn, as it might do if it had to be bent to fit into the CS.

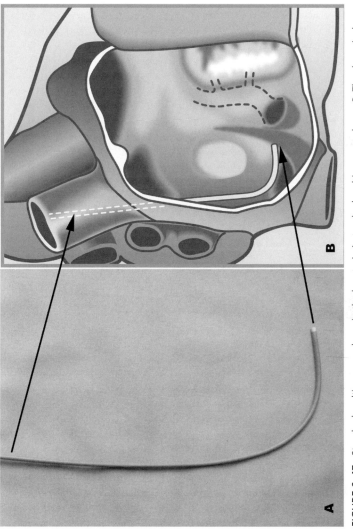

**FIGURE 6–47.** Standard multipurpose shape in the heart. *A,* A standard multipurpose shape. *B,* The shape is shown superimposed in a diagram of the heart with the tip at the level of the coronary sinus (CS). To place the sheath in the CS, the shape must be re-formed using another catheter or the endocardial surface of the heart. Once in the CS, the guide is under tension supported by the tip within the CS. If the walls of the sheath were not supported by a wire braid, they would possibly kink. Note that because there is no proximal curve, the guide does not rest in the right atrium or on the eustachian ridge.

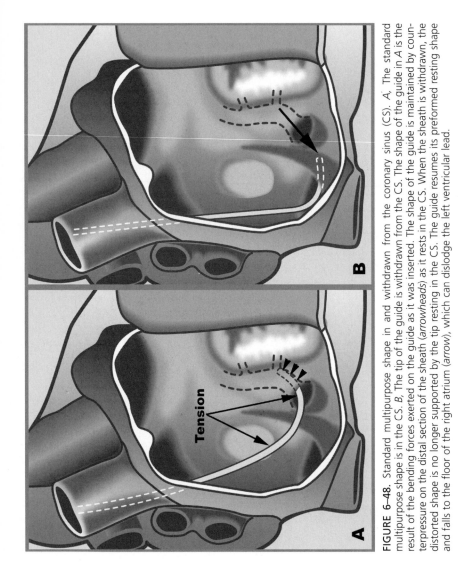

**FIGURE 6–48.** Standard multipurpose shape in and withdrawn from the coronary sinus (CS). *A,* The standard multipurpose shape is in the CS. *B,* The tip of the guide is withdrawn from the CS. The shape of the guide in *A* is the result of the bending forces exerted on the guide as it was inserted. The shape of the guide is maintained by counterpressure on the distal section of the sheath (*arrowheads*) as it rests in the CS. When the sheath is withdrawn, the distorted shape is no longer supported by the tip resting in the CS. The guide resumes its preformed resting shape and falls to the floor of the right atrium (*arrow*), which can dislodge the left ventricular lead.

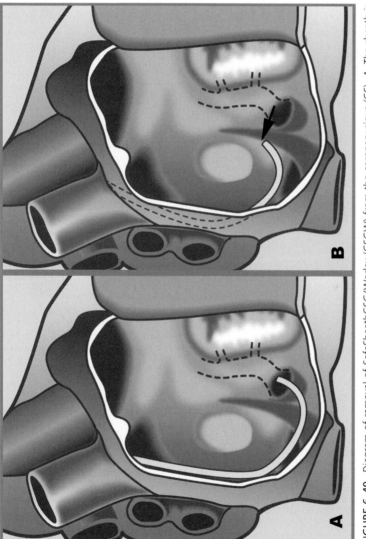
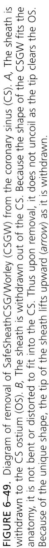

FIGURE 6–49. Diagram of removal of SafeSheathCSG/Worley (CSGW) from the coronary sinus (CS). A, The sheath is withdrawn to the CS ostium (OS). B, The sheath is withdrawn out of the CS. Because the shape of the CSGW fits the anatomy, it is not bent or distorted to fit into the CS. Thus upon removal, it does not uncoil as the tip clears the OS. Because of the unique shape, the tip of the sheath lifts upward (arrow) as it is withdrawn.

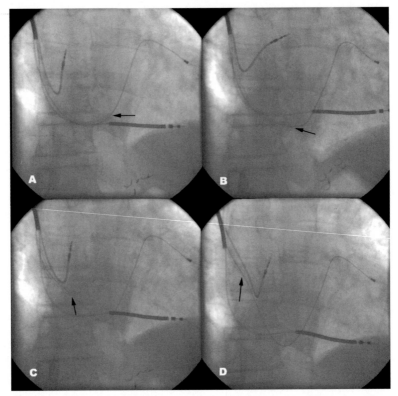

**FIGURE 6–50.** Example of removal of SafeSheathCSG/Worley (SSCSG-W) from the coronary sinus (CS). *A,* The sheath is in the CS with the tip (*arrow*) just inside the ostium (OS). *B,* The tip of the sheath (*arrow*) is withdrawn to just beyond the CS OS. Note that the tip of the sheath is at the level of the CS OS. *C,* The sheath is withdrawn further. Note that the tip of the sheath (*arrow*) is now well above the CS. *D,* The sheath is withdrawn still further. The tip of the sheath (*arrow*) distorts the shape of the lead slightly. Note that the left ventricular lead remains in place in the target vein. Because of its shape, the SSCSG-W does not drop to the floor of the right atrium as it is removed from the OS, as occurs with more traditional shapes.

in a low-friction environment where the direction is controlled by the wall of the tubing. The tubing also provides axial stability for the wire. However, as soon as the wire exits the tubing the direction, axial support and low-friction environment are lost. Direction is then controlled by the venous anatomy. The further the wire extends from the support tubing the lower the stability. To better understand the physics of the situation, consider the six functions the support tubing of the directional device can provide individually:

1. Wire direction.
2. Preservation of the force of the initial forward vector.
3. Preservation of the ability to manipulate the tip of the wire.
4. Axial stability.
5. Guide support.
6. Straightening tortuous veins.

## Wire Direction

In 50% of cases the direction taken by the wire as it exits the CS platform is not appropriate for the target vein. The support tubing of the directional device (sheath/guide/catheter) can be used to aim the wire in the desired direction, a direction that may not be possible through manipulation of the wire alone. Figure 6–51 is a diagram demonstrating the use of a directional catheter to insert a wire into a target vein that is in the opposite direction of the wire as it enters the CS. Remember from the definitions, that the internal diameter of the directional catheter is only large enough for an angioplasty wire whereas the internal diameter of a directional guide is sufficient to deliver the LV lead directly. Various preformed shapes are used to direct the wire depending on the coronary venous anatomy. Figure 6–52 is a photograph of a variety of preformed catheter shapes used in interventional radiology that we have found useful as *directional catheters* to aim the angioplasty wire into the target vein. Note that all the major companies produce similar shapes. Some but not all of theses shapes are also available in the cardiac catheterization laboratory as well. However, the catheter length of interventional radiology (55–65 cm) is much easier to deal with at the shoulder than the length used in cardiology (90–100 cm). At the time this chapter was being written, there were no directional catheters or guides available that are specifically designed for selective cannulation of CS target veins. Pressure Products is in the process of developing directional guides specifically designed to access the target veins in the CS. However, interventional radiology also has several guide shapes that are suitable and readily adapted to use for biventricular pacing. The 55- to 65-cm length of the radiology guides is also ideal. When approaching selective target vein cannulation, the operator may choose to use a directional guide that to deliver the pacing lead directly (7-F to 9-F external diameter depending on the lead) or choose to use a directional catheter to deliver the angioplasty wire and do an exchange (4-F to 6-F external diameter).

## Preservation of the Force of the Initial Forward Vector

The force of the initial forward vector is defined as the force applied to the wire by the operator at the shoulder as she/he pushes the wire. The force of the final forward vector is defined as the force at the tip of the wire that allows it to advance. Friction or obstruction acting along the length of the wire degrades the initial forward vector. The initial and final forward vector are similar in magnitude as long as the wire is in a low-friction environment along a straight line, such as in a support tubing. Once outside the support tubing the initial forward vector may be degraded by the high-friction environment in the veins. Resistance to forward progress of the lead is a function of three factors; vessel turns, vessel size, and presence of a focal stenosis. For a wire to continue to advance the force of the forward vector applied at the shoulder must overcome the resistive forces along the length of the wire without buckling. Advancing the LV pacing lead out of the CS onto the lateral free-wall of the left ventricle also requires the lead to move forward in a direction selected by the operator.

## Degradation of the Forward Vector from Change in Wire Direction

As the wire is advanced from the shoulder to the CS, the CS platform serves as support tubing for the wire providing a low-friction environment. The wire easily

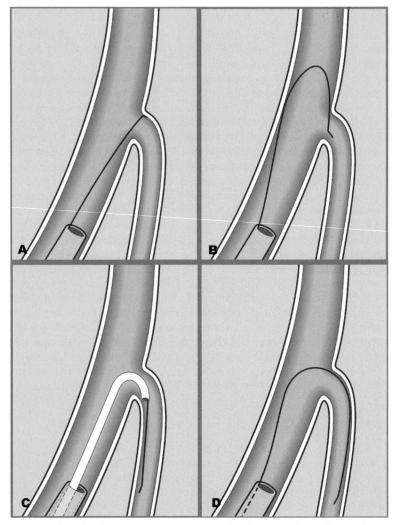

FIGURE 6–51. *"Directional catheter"* for acutely angulated target vein. *A,* The angioplasty wire approaches an acutely angulated target vein. *B,* The wire buckles into the coronary sinus (CS) as it is advanced. *C,* The wire is directed into the target vein with a directional catheter. *D,* The directional catheter is removed, leaving the wire in place. The direction of the target vein is in the opposite direction of the wire as it exits the CS platform into the CS. It is physically impossible to redirect the wire down the target vein without an additional piece of equipment: the *directional device.* With a properly shaped directional device in the target vein, the wire is easily redirected. In this example the directional device only delivered the angioplasty wire; thus we refer to it as a directional catheter. If it delivered the pacing lead directly, we would refer to it as a directional guide.

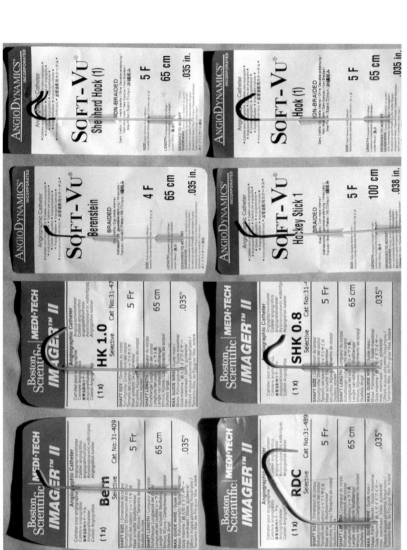

**FIGURE 6–52.** Directional catheters available from various companies. A variety of shapes are available from the interventional radiology division of large catheter companies. The shapes demonstrated here are more useful than most cardiac shapes. In addition, the 65-cm length used in radiology is more appropriate for our use. The shorter length is easier to manipulate and does not require an exchange length angioplasty wire.

negotiates twists and turns between the shoulder and the CS within the support tubing without significant loss of the forward force or control. Once the wire exits the CS platform into the CS it is no longer supported. When a wire changes direction outside the support tubing, the forward vector is broken down into two components, the displacement vector and the residual forward vector. The residual forward vector is the component of the initial forward vector that advances the wire/lead in the desired direction. The displacement vector is the component of the initial forward vector that follows the original direction of the wire as it exits the sheath. When the displacement vector exceeds the residual forward vector, the wire is displaced rather than advanced by additional force. Each time the direction of the wire is changed within a vein the forward vector is degraded by the displacement vector. The number of times the wire changes direction and the magnitude of the change in direction of each turn determines the residual forward vector. Whether a wire continues to move outside the support tubing depends on how much of the initial forward vector is lost to the displacement vector at each turn. The frictional forces that redirect the wire from the original course not only degrade the magnitude of the forward vector but also impair the ability of the tip of the wire to be manipulated through the addition of torque at the shoulder. Figure 6–53 is a diagram in which the takeoff of the target vein is along the same line as the sheath. Little if any of the initial forward vector is lost as the lead enters the target vein. The lead passes easily without the need for a directional catheter/guide. Figure 6–54 is a diagram of the breakdown of the forward vector as the direction is changed considerably from the direction of the sheath in the CS. Because the wire must change direction significantly to enter the target vein, the displacement vector is larger and the initial forward vector is degraded further than in Figure 6–53. Figure 6–55 is diagram of the breakdown of the forward vector as the wire essentially reverses direction. The displacement vector is larger than the forward vector. It is physically impossible to direct the wire down into the target vein without a directional device, as discussed in Figure 6–51. Even if the wire is advanced into the vein with a directional device the forward vector will be severely degraded by the friction between the wire and the vein at the acute angle turn.

## Degradation of the Forward Vector by High Resistance

The force of the initial forward vector is also degraded by high-resistance situations along a straight line. As long as the wire remains in the support tubing without kinks there is little loss of the forward vector. However, once the lead is in the venous anatomy it may encounter high resistance from diffusely small or stenotic target vein segments.

### *Directional Catheter vs. Directional Guide*

As mentioned previously, the internal diameter of the directional device determines whether the lead can be advanced directly through the device (directional guide) or whether it must be removed first (directional catheter). The pros and cons of directional catheters and directional guides are discussed in the next section.

## Directional Catheter for Wire Delivery Only

The option of using a directional catheter to place an angioplasty wire only applies for over-the-wire pacing leads. The advantage of placing the angioplasty wire

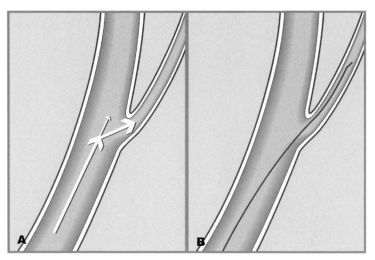

**FIGURE 6–53.** Minimal degradation of forward vector (<45 degrees). *A,* The wire requires little change in direction to enter the target vein. The forward vector before the turn and the residual forward vector after the turn are almost equal. The wire is minimally displaced from the original direction. *B,* The wire is in the target vein. The wall of the vein (*arrow*) redirects the wire. The friction between the wire and the wall of the vein reduces the forward vector and impedes movement of the tip when torque is applied at the shoulder. Because the direction of the wire was only minimally changed, there is minimal friction between the wire and vein to degrade the forward vector or reduce torque control.

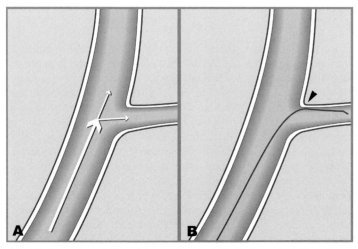

**FIGURE 6–54.** Moderate degradation of forward vector (45–90 degrees). *A,* The wire must change direction considerably to enter the target vein. The initial forward vector is divided into equal residual forward and displacement vectors. *B,* The wire is in the target vein. The wall of the vein redirects the wire. The friction between the wire and the wall of the vein (*arrows*) reduces the forward vector and impedes movement of the tip when torque is applied at the shoulder. Because the direction of the wire is changed considerably, there is more friction between the vein and the wire to degrade the forward vector and reduce torque control.

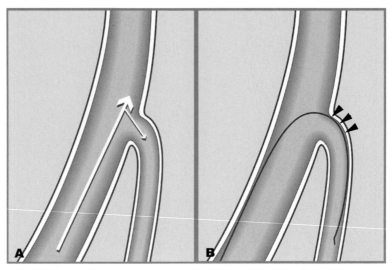

**FIGURE 6–55.** Severe degradation of forward vector (>90 degrees). *A,* The wire must reverse the initial direction to enter the target vein. The initial forward vector is divided into a small residual forward and a large displacement vector. *B,* The wire has been placed in the target vein with a directional catheter. The wall of the vein redirects the wire. The friction between the wire and the wall of the vein (*arrows*) degrades the forward vector and impedes movement of the tip when torque is applied at the shoulder. Because the direction of the wire is changed markedly, there is more friction between the vein and the wire. The greater the change in wire direction, the more force applied at the shoulder is lost to friction when redirecting the tip of the wire/lead into the target vein. The residual forward vector is far less than the original forward vector. In this case, the residual forward vector may be too small to advance the wire.

then removing the directional catheter is that it requires a smaller diameter catheter. In addition, the catheter does not need to be cut away once the lead is in place. However, removing the directional catheter and leaving the wire in place in the target vein can be difficult. Occasionally the position of the wire in the target vein is lost in the process. Figure 6–56 is a diagram that depicts the pitfalls of removing a directional catheter while retaining the angioplasty wire in place. Note that if too much or too little wire is advanced as the catheter is withdrawn the wire will be dislodged from the target vein. This process is particularly cumbersome when a standard 100-cm cardiology diagnostic catheter is used as the directional catheter because an exchange length (300-cm) angioplasty guide wire is required. When a 65-cm catheter from interventional radiology is chosen, the exchange process can be accomplished using a standard length (192-cm) angioplasty guide wire. A further disadvantage of removing the directional catheter is that there is nothing to support the lead as it tracks over the wire. The wire alone may not provide enough support to redirect the over-the-wire in cases in which there is a sharp curve or small stenotic vessel. Figure 6–57 is a diagram of what happens when trying to advance an over-the-wire pacing lead into an acutely angulated target vein. The angioplasty wire is first placed with a directional catheter then removed, leaving the wire in place. As the pacing lead starts the turn into the target vessel there is friction between the vein and the lead that pulls the wire up out of the target vein and the wire dislodges. A directional guide will alleviate the problem.

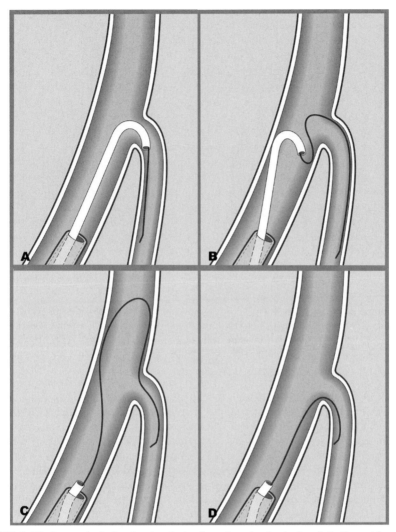

**FIGURE 6–56.** Removal of directional catheter from target vein. In Panel *A*, the guide wire is inserted into the target vessel using a preshaped 4-F to 6-F OD (outer diameter) directional catheter. *B*, The wire is advanced and the catheter is withdrawn out of the target vein into the coronary sinus (CS). *C*, Too much wire is advanced and a loop of wire forms in the CS distal to the target vein. Advancing the wire further will create a larger loop in the CS and pull the wire further out of the target vein. *D*, Not enough wire is advanced as the catheter is removed. The tip of the wire is pulled back proximally in the target vein and the wire is taut. From this diagram it is clear that great care must be taken to advance just enough wire as the catheter is removed.

## Directional Guide for Direct Lead Delivery

When the internal diameter of the *directional device* is large enough to accommodate the pacing lead it is referred to as the *directional guide* of the telescoping system. An interventional guide with an internal diameter of 0.078 inches

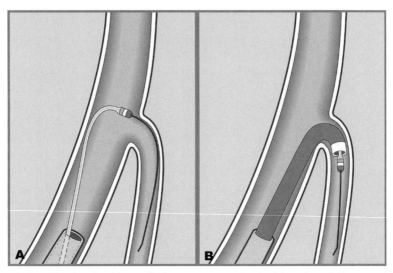

FIGURE 6–57. Directional guide required to support pacing lead insertion. *A,* An over-the-wire pacing lead is advanced toward the target vein. The wire must be under just the right amount of tension as the pacing lead turns the corner into the target vein. However tension on the angioplasty wire pulls the tip out of the vein. The angioplasty wire does not provide adequate support for the acute angle. The wire and lead pull out of the vein. *B,* The pacing lead is advanced over the wire within a directional guide into the target vein. The lumen of the directional guide helps direct the lead into the target vein. Minimal support is required from the wire.

(2 mm) or greater is large enough to deliver a Medtronic 4193 ATTAIN lead directly into the target vein. All 7-F OD interventional guides have sufficient ID to accommodate the 4193 ATTAIN LV lead. The 2187 ATTAIN requires a guide with an internal diameter of 0.088 inches (2.2 mm) or greater. Some 8-F OD (Cordis Vistabritetip) and all 9-F OD interventional guiding catheters have an adequate internal diameter. Once the directional guide is coaxially seated in the target vein the hub of the guide is cut off before the lead is inserted. Once the lead is in the target vein, the guide is cut away using the Medtronic cutters from a Solotrak or ATTAIN sheath (Figures 6–58 and 6–59).

## Preservation of the Ability to Manipulate the Tip of the Wire

As long as the wire remains in the unkinked support tubing the tip of the wire is easily directed by the application of torque at the shoulder. However, once outside the support tubing the frictional force between the wire and vein that results from either changes in wire direction or small and/or stenotic vein segments not only degrade the initial forward vector applied at the shoulder; they also impede manipulation of the tip of the wire. When the operator applies torque at the shoulder to redirect the tip of the wire, the rotational movement is resisted at all the sites of friction along the length of the wire. The ability of the operator to direct the tip of the wire is severely degraded. If the wire remains in the low-friction support tubing without kinks (sheath/guide/catheter) torque control is not lost (see Figures 6–56 and 6–60).

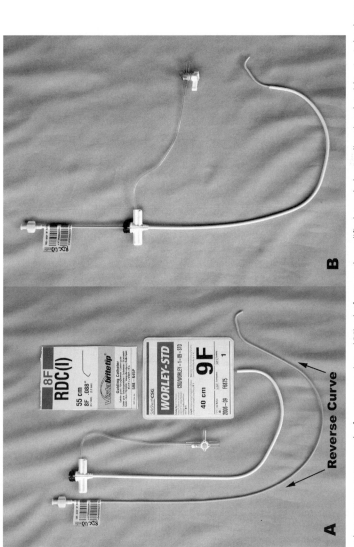

**FIGURE 6–58.** Telescoping system composed of coronary sinus (CS) platform and modified renal shape directional guide. *A*, A back-curved 8-F Cordis Vistabritetip RDC(1) and SafeSheathCSG/Worley (SSCSG-W) are shown side by side. *B*, The directional guide is inserted into the CS sheath. Note that the curve placed on the body of the guide is in the opposite direction of the curve at the tip. When inserted into the SSCSG-W, the tip curve points outward toward the target veins, reducing the amount of torque required in the CS. The internal diameter of the 8-F Cordis Vistabritetip guide is large enough to deliver the following leads: Medtronic ATTAIN OTW 4193 LV Pacing Lead; Medtronic ATTAIN 2187 LV Pacing Lead; and Medtronic CapSure SP 4023 pacing lead. The hub of the guide must be cut off before the lead is inserted into the guide. Once the lead is in place and thresholds confirmed, the guide is cut away using the cutter from a Medtronic Solotrack Introducer.

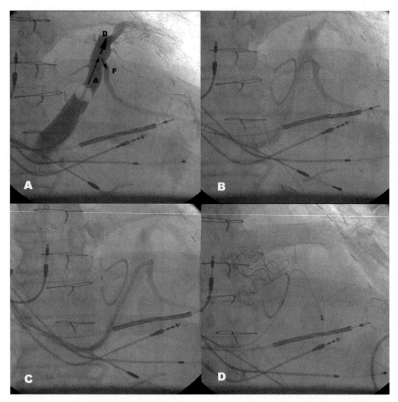

FIGURE 6–59. Acutely angulated lateral wall target vein. *A,* Anterior-posterior coronary sinus (CS) venogram. *B,* A 5-F hook catheter is in the target vein. *C,* An 8-F Cordis Vistabright Tip RDC(1) catheter is in the target vein. *D,* The ATTAIN 4193 lead is in the target vein. Without a directional catheter it is impossible to advance any angioplasty wire into the target vein. The axial vector (*arrow A*) of the lead/wire as it exits the sheath is in the opposite direction as the required forward vector (*arrow F*). The displacement vector (*arrow D*) is the dominant force. The 5-F hook directional catheter (*B*) points the wire into the target vein. However, the wire alone does not provide sufficient support to counteract the displacement vector. Attempts to advance the ATTAIN 4193 into the target vein dislodged the wire as the lead turned into the target vein. An 8-F Cordis Vistabright Tip directional guiding catheter is inserted into the target vein (*C*). The 8-F directional guide reorients the axial vector into the target vein. The lead advances onto the lateral wall of the left ventricle.

## Axial Stability

When the operator initially advances the wire at the shoulder the forward vector moves the wire ahead through the sheath into the CS. Resistance encountered at the tip of the wire will tend to cause the wire to bend or buckle. As more forward force is applied at the shoulder there is a greater tendency to buckle. Two factors determine how much force can be applied before a wire will buckle; the axial stability (stiffness) of the wire itself and the support around the wire. For example, an angioplasty wire may have little if any axial stability of its own. If the wire is contained within support tubing, the axial stability of the wire is amplified by the axial stability of the support tubing. As long as the wire is within the walls of the tubing it will not buckle (see Figures 6–54 and 6–61).

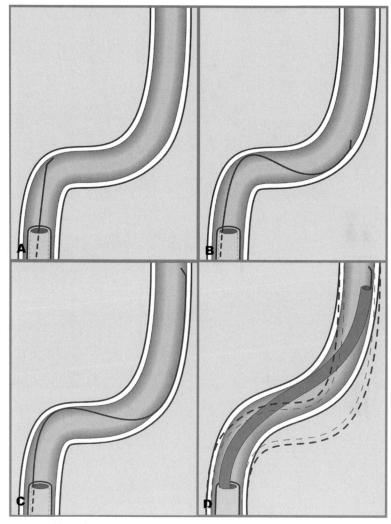

**FIGURE 6–60.** Effect of support tubing on wire manipulation in a venous structure. *A*, The wire encounters a turn in the vein after it exits the sheath. *B*, The first bend in the vein redirects the tip of the wire perpendicular to the original direction. As the wire is advanced there is friction between the wire and the vein with loss of forward force. Some of the forward force applied at the shoulder is lost to friction at the first turn. A degree of torque control is also lost. *C*, The wire is advanced beyond the second bend in the vein. There is further loss of forward force and torque control due to friction between the vein and the wire. *D*, A directional device (*black tube*) is advanced beyond the curved vein segment. The directional device straightens the vein (*dotted lines* indicate the original position of the vein), as well as providing a low-friction environment for the wire. In this example the directional device provides 3 of the 5 functions of the support tubing: (1) preservation of the initial forward vector force (the forward vector is not degraded by friction between the vein and the wire in the two areas where the direction of the wire is changed) because the support tubing partially straightens the vein and provides a low-friction environment to redirect the wire tip; (2) preservation of the ability to manipulate the tip of the wire (there is no longer friction in the two areas where the wire changes direction); and (3) straightening the vein.

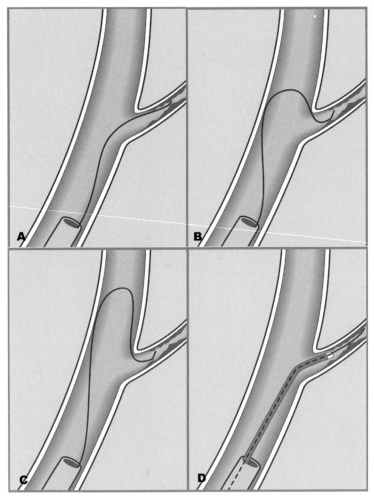

**FIGURE 6–61.** Axial stability of a wire enhanced by a directional catheter to cross a stenotic lesion. *A,* The wire is easily directed into the target vein without loss of the initial forward vector; however, the wire encounters the resistance of a stenotic vein segment and stops moving forward. *B,* Additional force is applied at the shoulder in an attempt to cross the stenotic segment. The wire does not have sufficient axial stability (stiffness) to transmit the added force to the tip and starts to buckle. *C,* As more forward force is applied at the shoulder, the wire buckles further and the tip pulls out of the vein. *D,* The wire is supported within the directional catheter, which is inserted into the target vein. The axial support provided by the catheter allows the additional forward force applied at the shoulder to be transmitted directly to the stenosis without buckling the wire. As long as the guide is not displaced, the entire forward force applied at the shoulder will be directed at the stenosis. In addition to axial stability, the catheter provides "back support." The size stiffness and shape of the directional device determines the amount of back support. In cases of extreme narrowing, the directional catheter may be displaced out of the target vein when the wire is advanced. Directional catheters with a shape that allows the back of the catheter to rest on the wall of the CS are less likely to be displaced. The size, stiffness, and back support provided by the directional device, in addition to the intrinsic axial stability of the wire, determine whether the wire will advance across the stenosis.

## Guide Support

In simple terms, guide support refers to how much the directional device resists being pushed back out of the target vein by attempts to advance a wire into the target vein. The greater the guide support provided by the directional device the more it resists being pushed out of the target vein as the wire is advanced. When the wire exits the directional device forward progress may be resisted by a small, tortuous or stenotic vein segment. If the operator attempts to advance the wire against the resistance it may advance, or if the resistance is excessive the directional device may be displaced backwards out of the ostium or the wire may buckle. Whether the directional device is displaced or the wire buckles depends on the axial stability of the wire and the guide support. The guide support provided by the directional device is determined by the shape, composition, wall thickness, and French size of the support tubing. In general, a 9-F directional device will provide more guide support than an 8-F directional device with the same shape and composition. Wire-braided directional devices have greater guide support than unbraided devices of the same size. The *wall thickness* of the directional tubing also impacts on the guide support; the greater the wall thickness, the greater the support. The shape of the guide in the CS can have a major impact on guide support. If the *shape* of the directional device places the back of the curve against the wall of the CS it will provide far more support than the same guide with a different shape. This concept is demonstrated in Figures 6–62 to 6–65.

## Straightening Tortuous Veins

The directional device's vein-straightening effect is demonstrated in Figure 6–64. Using the support tubing of the directional device to straighten a tortuous vein segment is usually accomplished by first placing a wire through the vein segment and then advancing the directional device over the wire. The ease with which the operator can advance the support tubing over the wire depends on the support provided by the wire and the French size, flexibility, and shape of the directional device. First consider wire support. In general, the thicker and stiffer the wire, the greater support. Thus a "floppy" 0.014-inch angioplasty wire provides little support, whereas a 0.035-inch Amplatz extra support wire will provide much greater support. However, a stiff wire is more difficult to advance through a tortuous vein segment and a softer wire, such as a Terumo Radiofocus Glidewire may need to be accepted at least initially. Once the wire is through the tortuous vein segment the support tubing is advanced over the wire. Here the stiffness and size and shape of the directional device impact on whether it can be advanced. In some cases a 9-F direction Guide will advance through a tortuous vein segment over a standard 0.035-inch wire with little difficulty. In other cases it is difficult to advance even a 4-F directional device. In difficult cases a series of larger French size catheters can be advanced progressively over the wire. For example, if the goal is to advance a 9-F guide through a tortuous vein segment it may be necessary to first advance a 5-F (or 4-F) catheter over the wire. While the 5-F catheter and wire are kept in place, a 7-F catheter is advanced over the 5-F catheter. Finally, with the wire and the 5-F and 7-F catheter kept in place, the 9-F is advanced over the 5-F to 7-F catheter combination. The takeoff angle of the target vein and then shape of the 9-F directional guide will have an impact on how easily this can be accomplished. If the tortuous target vein has a right-angle takeoff, then it may be difficult to advance a guide unless it also has a right angle (Figure 6–62).

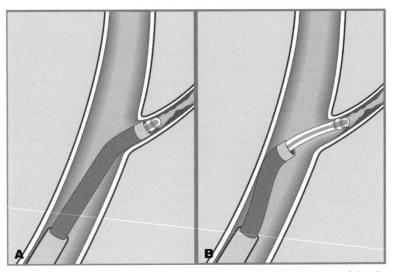

**FIGURE 6–62.** Directional guide shape that provides little support. *A,* The shape of the directional guide helps direct the pacing lead into the target vein. *B,* The directional guide is displaced as the operator attempts to advance the pacing lead against the resistance of the stenosis. The axial support provided by the guide to the pacing lead at the site of the stenosis is lost as the guide is displaced. Without the axial support provided by the directional guide the pacing lead will tend to buckle as the operator attempts to advance the lead.

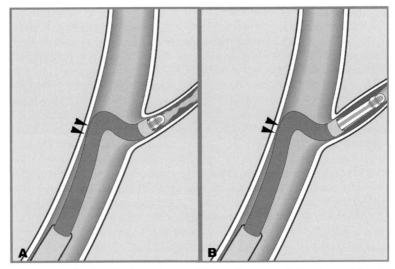

**FIGURE 6–63.** Directional guide shape that provides good support. *A,* The shape of the directional device places the proximal curve against the wall of the coronary sinus (CS) when the tip is in the target vein. *B,* The pacing lead is advanced through the stenotic lesion. The support provided by the directional device resting against the CS allows the pacing lead to be advanced through the stenotic vein segment. The axial support provided by the guide is maintained at the site of stenosis as the pacing lead exits the guide.

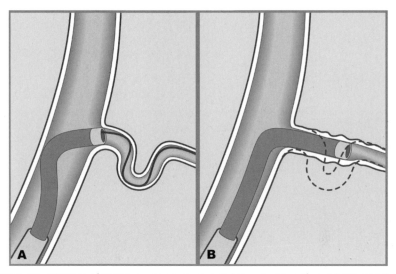

FIGURE 6–64. Diagram of tortuous vein segment straightened with preformed directional guide. *A*, The tortuous vein segment is demonstrated with a wire advanced through the segment and the hockey stick preformed directional guide at the ostium of the target vein. *B*, The vein segment is straightened by a preformed the directional guide advanced over a guide wire. Note that when selecting the shape of the preformed directional device, the angle of take off as well as the length of any tortuous segment is important. Tortuous vein segments can also be straightened with an angioplasty wire, as described in PTCA techniques.

Until recently, using a telescoping system required a fair amount of improvisation on the part of the operator. The ideal guide for a telescoping system would be pre-shaped to fit into the CS through a stable platform. In addition, the hub of the guide would be hemostatic and would not need to be cut away until satisfactory lead position is achieved. Figure 6–66 is the new Pressure Products version of a directional guide with a hemostatic hub that can be broken away when lead placement is confirmed. In addition, the back curve is added during manufacture to key to the shape of the SafeSheathCSG/Worley sheath.

## Additional Telescoping Techniques

Once inside the CS itself, barriers to successful advancement of guide wires and leads into the target veins include severe angles at which veins enter the CS, tortuous segments within the veins, and the caliber of the veins themselves. Proper shaping of the guide wire tip, providing adequate guiding catheter support to the lead/wire system, and venograms that define venous entry into the CS provide the best chance of successful over-the-wire lead advancement. When a vein enters the CS at a very acute angle (>120 degrees), the guide wire may not enter the vein easily, or cannot advance to a distal stable site in the vein, or the lead may not track across the acute angle and actually dislodge the wire. The following approach deals with the problem with veins entering at acute angles: Insert a 6-F LIMA into the guiding catheter positioned in the CS beyond the target vein, utilize the distal hook of the LIMA to engage the vein by pulling the LIMA back to the insertion point. Once the LIMA engages the vein

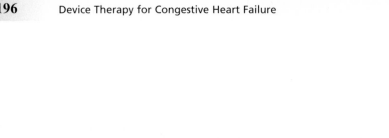

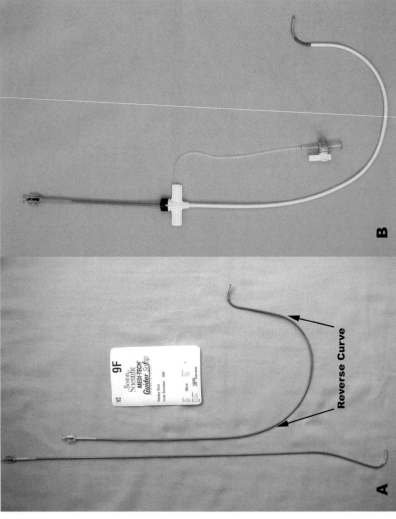

**FIGURE 6–65.** Telescoping system composed of coronary sinus platform and modified hockey stick shape directional guide. *A*, Boston Scientific 9-F Guider Softip Hockey Stick guide is shown straight and modified with the reverse curve to fit in the SafeSheathCSG/Worley. *B*, The hockey stick guide with reverse curve added is inserted into the 9-F SafeSheathCSG/Worley. Note the reverse curve directs the tip of the guide in the direction of the target veins as it emerges from the sheath. The longer snout of the hockey stick is better suited for straightening tortuous veins than the renal shape shown in Figure 6–15.

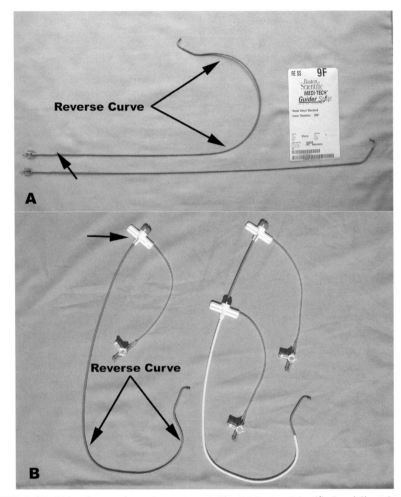

**FIGURE 6–66.** Old and new telescoping system. *A,* The 9-F Boston Scientific Renal Short Standard guide is illustrated straight as it comes out of the box and with the reverse curve added. The hub is not hemostatic or removable and must be cut off prior to inserting the lead. The guide can be cut away but is not designed for cutting. *B,* The new directional guide from Pressure Products is illustrated as it comes out of the box and inserted into the matching SafeSheathCSG/Worley homeostatic peel-away sheath. During manufacture, the reverse curve is added to the guide to fit the shape of the sheath. The hub of the guide is hemostatic and can be broken away after the lead is in place.

(confirmed by contrast injection), pass a heavyweight angioplasty through the LIMA into the most distal segment of the target vein. Remove the LIMA, leaving the guide wire in place. The heavyweight wire will straighten much of the angle and curves in the vein. Have the LV lead prepared, and back load the lead through the wire into the target vein. The back-load technique requires that the implanter fix the guide wire in space to prevent advancement of the wire during lead advancement. Pushing the wire into the vein will dislodge the guiding catheter from the CS. Only quick removal of the excess guide wire (and sometimes the LV lead as well) will reseat the guiding catheter at the proper position. The common reflex response attempts to advance the guiding catheter into the CS, but in this circumstance will dislodge the catheter, LV lead, and guide wire.

## Miscellaneous Techniques

### Electrically Acceptable Positioning

The criteria that identify an ideal LV pacing site include anatomic position along the LV free-wall, maximal RV to LV electrode separation, stimulation at a LV site with the latest local activation, where a local electrogram falls in the most distal part of the surface QRS complex on electrocardiography (ECG), absence of phrenic nerve stimulation, and a stable lead position. Data from the numerous clinical trials of CRT systems have not been able to discriminate which segment of the free-wall (lateral, anterolateral, posterolateral, or apical) provides the greatest hemodynamic benefit during CRT. Acceptable LV stimulation thresholds vary from what is commonly accepted for RV and atrial stimulation. The implanter may readily accept thresholds of up to 3 V at 0.5 msec pulse duration in order to deliver CRT to the patient with CHF when multiple sites along the LV veins fail to yield lower energy thresholds. When encountering high stimulation threshold at an otherwise desirable anatomic LV lead position, measuring thresholds at a variety of pulse duration settings (0.5–1.5 msec) to generate a strength duration curve for the left ventricle can identify the optimal device output settings. Often, LV pacing at higher pulse width lowers capture threshold to within an acceptable range of pulse generator energy output. The tradeoff between successful LV pacing and decreased pulse generator duration should favor delivery of therapy to the patient who responds to CRT over concerns for pulse generator duration.

Stimulation of the phrenic nerve as it courses along the lateral wall of the heart produces diaphragmatic stimulation during LV pacing. LV leads positioned within posterior or posterior-lateral veins may directly stimulate the left hemidiaphragm. Intermittent diaphragmatic stimulation, even at high outputs during lead testing, should encourage repositioning of the LV lead. Often, when the patient sits or stands after the procedure, the diaphragmatic threshold drops, and even intermittent stimulation becomes unacceptable. Reprogramming the device output may not alleviate diaphragmatic stimulation. Persistent diaphragmatic stimulation requires lead repositioning. Correcting the problem during the initial implantation procedure reduces the need for reoperation.

### Removing the Sheath System

All catheter manipulation utilized to achieve an acceptable LV lead position occurs through the delivery system. Upon obtaining an acceptable lead position the operator must remove the implant delivery system without dislodging the LV lead. The available techniques for removing the guiding catheter from the CS include longitudinal slitting of the catheter, removal of the catheter over the lead while stabilizing the lead through a relatively stiff wire kept in the lead, and breakage and peeling away of a catheter scored along its long axis. Unintentional advancement of the lead during removal of the guiding catheter will introduce redundancy of the lead into the venous system and potentially dislodge the tip of the lead. Inadvertent advancement of the lead occurs during slitting when the implanter pushes the slitting tool forward into the guiding catheter, instead of fixing it in space and drawing the guiding catheter into the blade. Advancement of the finishing wire within a lead pushes the lead, whereas removing the guiding catheter over the lead creates an analogous problem. When the lead tip reaches a "dead-end" within the target vein, either maneuver introduces excessive lead into the patient. A loop may form in the CS, in the right atrium, or in the subclavian or innominate vein. If a loop of lead prolapses into the tricuspid annulus, blood flow will push the lead into the right ventricle and pull the lead tip out of the CS. Pushing the lead into the subclavian vein while pulling the peel-away guiding catheter out of the patient may produce the same unintended effect. One can diminish the probability of lead dislodgement during guiding catheter removal by fixing the cutter on the patient's shoulder or other stable structure. Fixing the position of the finishing wire in space, or on a table positioned perpendicular to the patient's shoulder may prevent excessive movement of the lead during guiding catheter removal. Interrupted or stuttering motion of the lead during cutting, removal of the guiding catheter over the lead, or breaking and peeling of the sheath can transmit the force to the lead and promote dislodgement. Securing the sewing collars tightly after removal of the stylet or finishing wire from the LV lead diminishes the risk of further dislodgement.

*Troubleshooting.*

The leading causes of failed LV lead implantation include failure to locate the CS OS or advance the guiding catheter to a stable position and poor LV vein anatomy. Persistent phrenic nerve stimulation, CS dissection or perforation, and unacceptable stimulation thresholds lead to failure less often. Table 6–2 lists the causes of failed implantation in a collection of large clinical trials of CRT.

## Testing for Viability and Phrenic Pacing Before Lead Placement

Before making the effort to insert a pacing lead into the target vein, it is useful to know where phrenic pacing will be found and to get a rough estimate of myocardial viability. This can be accomplished by using an angioplasty wire as a test pace system. Any angioplasty wire with an uncoated tip (Luge, *not* ChoicePT) can be used as a unipolar test system. However, because the length of the exposed tip is 3–5 cm, pacing is not very specific unless the tip is covered up to the last 5 mm with insulation. The 3-F Cordis Transit Infusion catheter (REF 600-350A) can be used as insulation to cover the wire, except at the tip. Alternatively, the SiteFinder guide wire (Figure 6–67) may be used. The SiteFinder is insulated with a lubricious coating, except at the proximal and distal 5 mm.

#### TABLE 6–2.  **MIRACLE: Reasons for Unsuccessful Lead Placement**

| | |
|---|---|
| Unable to access coronary vein | 14 |
| Unable to obtain distal location | 13 |
| Dislodgement/unstable position of LV Lead | 10 |
| Elevated LV pacing threshold | 4 |
| Cardiac vein vessel too small | 2 |
| Phrenic nerve stimulation | 1 |
| Inadequate sensing | 1 |
| Heart block | 1 |

Total of 43 subjects unsuccessfully implanted. Reasons are not mutually exclusive.

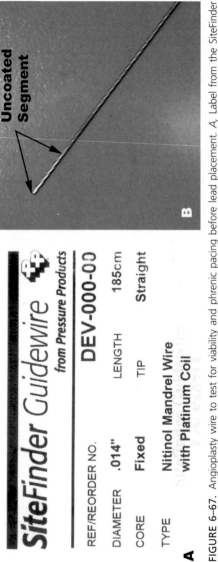
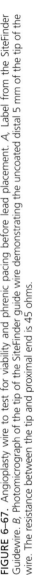

FIGURE 6–67. Angioplasty wire to test for viability and phrenic pacing before lead placement. A, Label from the SiteFinder Guidewire. B, Photomicrograph of the tip of the SiteFinder guide wire demonstrating the uncoated distal 5 mm of the tip of the wire. The resistance between the tip and proximal end is 45 ohms.

# Angioplasty Techniques for Cardiac Resynchronization (Lancaster)

Most physicians implanting CRT systems have a background in Electrophysiology and Pacing (EP). As a result, they may be reluctant to utilize contrast and learn techniques they consider the province of the interventional cardiologist. However, all aspects of EP have become more interventional over the last several years. Unless the EP physician is willing to embrace the use of interventional techniques, the optimal implementation of biventricular pacing will remain a frustrating issue that may be relegated to a surgical epicardial approach in a significant number of patients. Utilization of balloon angioplasty techniques to insert a LV pacing system is essential to achieving a high success rate and uncompromising lead position. It is useful to learn the full range of angioplasty techniques, including stent placement to optimize the chance of a successful implant. At first it seems a bit odd to learn theses techniques but remember that many of the leads are delivered over an angioplasty wire.

## The Buddy Wire Technique

In the Telescoping System section of the chapter we describe the use of the support tubing of the directional device to straighten tortuous target veins and provide a low-friction environment for lead placement. An alternative and sometimes complimentary interventional method is referred to as the "buddy wire technique." Here one angioplasty wire (the buddy wire) is used to straighten the tortuous or looped vascular segment to allow a second wire (the tracking wire) or device to pass more easily. Why does it work? Recall that when attempting to deliver a lead through a tortuous vein, the friction generated at each of the curves as the lead changes direction reduces the forward vector. The sharper the curve the more the lead must change direction, creating more friction between the lead and the vein. The buddy wire is used to straighten the vein to reduce the loss of the forward vector. The vein is straightened by advancing a wire far enough into the vein that the stiff segment of the wire is in the tortuous area. Remember that angioplasty wires have a floppy distal segment followed by a more proximal stiff segment. The ability to advance the stiff part of the wire through the tortuous vein segment requires a stable CS platform; otherwise the sheath will be displaced rather than the wire advancing. In many cases the axial stability provided by a directional device is required to prevent the wire from buckling in the body of the CS as the wire is advanced. After the stiff segment of the stiff wire straightens the vein it is left in place and the lead is delivered using either a stylet or over a second wire (tracking wire). The stiff segment of the wire used to straighten the vein should be stiffer than the stiff segment of the tracking wire. In angioplasty terms the straightening wire should be an extra support wire (e.g., Choice PT Extra Support or Platinum Plus ST), whereas the tracking wire should be a floppy wire (e.g., Choice PT Floppy). Figure 6–68 is a diagram of the buddy wire technique.

Figure 6–69 is a case example using a buddy wire to deliver a stylet driven lead. The directional guide (9-F Boston Scientific Guider Softip RESS) is inserted into the CS through the CS platform (SafeSheathCSG/Worley) and rests in the OS of the target vein. The direction guide provides preservation of the forward vector, direction, axial stability, and guide support for both the straightening wire and pacing lead. In Figure 6–69*A*, the distal soft segment of a Boston Scientific Choice PT Extra

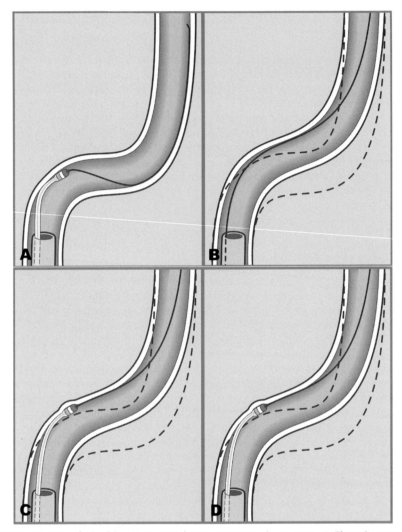

**FIGURE 6–68.** Use of a buddy wire to straighten a tortuous vein segment. *A,* The vein segment is too tortuous to allow the lead to advance over the wire. *B,* A "stiff" angioplasty wire (buddy wire) is advanced beyond the tortuous segment, straightening the vein. *Dotted lines* indicate the course of the vein prior to being straightened by the buddy wire. *C,* The pacing lead is delivered over a second wire, the tracking wire. The tracking wire is not taut enough; thus the progress of the pacing lead is impeded by friction between the vein and the lead. *D,* Tension is applied to the tracking wire, centering the lead in the vein and reducing friction. It is important to keep as much tension on the tracking wire as possible to keep the lead centered in the vein without pulling the wire out.

Support wire is advanced through the loop in the target vein. Because the tip of the stiff wire is soft, it does not straighten the vein. In Figure 6–69*B*, the wire is advanced further into the vein until the stiff segment of the wire is through the loop which straightens the vein. Without the support of the direction guide the stiff segment of the buddy wire would not advance through the resistance of the vein loop. In Figure 6–69*C*, the

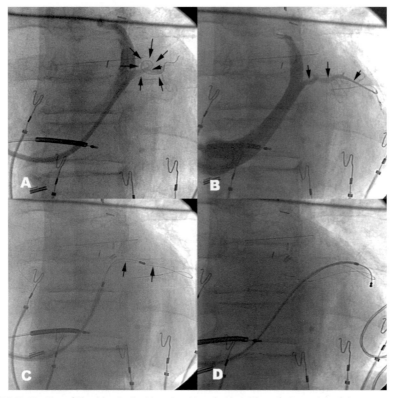

**FIGURE 6–69.** Use of "buddy wire" with stylet-driven lead. *A,* The soft tip section of the extra support angioplasty wire is advanced into the target vein. The wire forms a loop (*arrows*) as it follows the vein. The vein is outlined with a contrast injection delivered through the 9-F Guider Softip RESS directional guide catheter, which is in place in the ostium of the target vein. *B,* Using the support of the directional guide, the angioplasty wire is advanced deep into the target vein. The stiff segment of the wire (*arrows*) straightens the loop in the proximal portion of the vein. *C,* The stylet-driven Medtronic ATTAIN 2187 left ventricular pacing lead is advanced into the loop segment of the target vein. The stiff segment of the angioplasty wire (*arrows*) keeps the vein straight. *D,* The 2187 lead is advanced beyond the vein loop with the assistance of the directional guide and the "buddy wire."

ATTAIN 2187 LV pacing lead is also advanced through the directional guide into the target vein. Because the buddy wire removed the loop in the vein, the stylet driven lead can be advanced into the target vein. As the operator applies force at the shoulder to the stylet-driven lead the directional guide supports and directs the advance of the pacing lead. In Figure 6–69*D*, the 2187 lead is well beyond the loop in the vein. Once the buddy wire is removed, pacing thresholds assessed and phrenic pacing ruled out, the directional guide is cut away using the 6-F cutter from a 7-F or 9-F Medtronic Solo-Trak KR lead introducer.

### Balloon Venoplasty of the Subclavian Vein

Balloon dilation of the subclavian vein is a good place to start for EP/pacing physicians to gain comfort and familiarity with the venoplasty procedure. There is a large population of patients with pre-existing devices in need of resynchronization. In this setting, it is not uncommon to encounter occlusion or high-grade stenosis in the subclavian vein. In the past, EP/pacing physicians typically dealt with this issue via the use of progressively larger dilators. Although effective the process can be time consuming and lead manipulation is often difficult due to residual stenosis. Difficult lead manipulation due to a residual subclavian stenosis may prevent successful LV lead placement. The most efficient way to deal with a subclavian stenosis is simple venoplasty. Figure 6–70 illustrates a typical example. The patient developed worsening CHF after receiving a dual chamber defibrillator. He required ventricular pacing support. The wire for the sheath would not advance from the site of axillary access. The venogram revealed a high-grade stenosis in the subclavian vein. A Teflon-coated 0.035-inch angled Terumo Glidewire was manipulated across the stenosis but the sheath would not advance. The stenosis was dilated with a 6-mm by 4-cm balloon delivered over the Terumo Glidewire. Figure 6–70*B* (angioplasty of a stenotic subclavian vein) demonstrates the balloon at 12 atm. Once the balloon was inflated to 16 atm the stenosis was relieved and the 9-F sheath (11-F OD, 9-F ID) passed easily. In similar cases we have advanced two 9-F sheaths after venoplasty, using a retained guide wire.

On occasion a stenotic lesion in the main body of the CS or the lateral wall target vein prevents placement of the LV pacing lead. In other cases the target vein may be too small or even occluded, preventing access to the desired area on the LV epicardial surface. Percutaneous coronary venoplasty (PCV) is a safe and effective alternative to failure or accepting a less desirable target vein. At Lancaster we have performed PCV procedures in 62 of 600 patients since our first BIV case in 1999. Initially, we used PCV as a last resort. As we became comfortable with the safety and efficacy of the procedure, utilization increased. The importance of specific lateral wall target veins to successful resynchronization further increased our utilization of PCV. In the 62 cases we have performed, there have been no related complications. The majority (79%) had prior OHS. The overall success, defined as the ability to pass the lead beyond the stenosis, is 68%. Despite the relatively low success rate the use of PCV has increased our implantation success, defined as placement of the lead on the lateral wall of the left ventricle by 6.8%.

Analysis of our failed cases revealed the potential solutions as follows:

1. Highly tortuous or folded veins do not respond to PCV. They are best approached initially by placement of a directional guide through the area or the use of the "buddy wire" technique. Failing this, stent implantation can be used to straighten the vein allowing the lead to pass.
2. Stenotic lesions that do not open with a conventional noncompliant balloons (e.g. PowerSail or equivalent) inflated to 20 atm will respond to high pressures (up to 25 atm) delivered by an ultra noncompliant balloon (e.g., NC Monorail or equivalent).
3. Persistent stenosis (as evidenced by a continued indentation in the balloon) responds to the Cutting Balloon and may be used in selected cases with prior OHS.

Improved success with PCV will further increase the absolute success of the transvenous approach to cardiac resynchronization close to 100%.

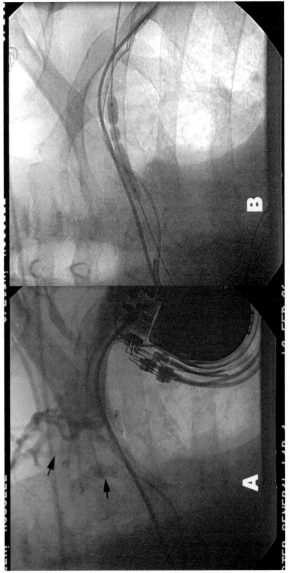

**FIGURE 6–70.** Venoplasty of a stenotic subclavian vein. *A,* The subclavian vein stenosis is seen at the site of the patient's previously implanted defibrillator leads. Collateral filling distal to the stenosis *(arrows)* is seen. *B,* A 6-mm by 40-mm balloon is inflated at the site of stenosis. Despite the stenosis seen in *A,* it was possible to pass a 0.035-inch angled Glidewire across the stenosis. The balloon was then advanced over the Glidewire and inflated to 16 atm, relieving the stenosis and allowing for easy passage of a 9-F sheath (9-F ID [inner diameter], 11-F OD [outer diameter]). Subsequent pacing lead manipulation in the coronary sinus was not hindered by the stenosis.

## Angioplasty of the Main Body of the Coronary Sinus

On occasion a fixed stenosis in the main body of the CS in a patient with prior OHS prevents CS cannulation despite the techniques described in the CS access and cannulation section. Balloon venoplasty can be used to relieve the stenosis and thus permit lead placement. The most difficult part of the procedure may be advancing the angioplasty wire beyond the stenosis. To get the wire past the stenosis it is useful to use a multipurpose directional catheter (4-F to 6-F), inserted through the CS platform to provide wire support and direction. In addition, puffs of contrast through the directional catheter help to identify a potential opening through which to direct the wire. Finally, once the wire is past the stenosis, the directional catheter is advanced beyond the stenosis over the wire and contrast injected to confirm that the wire is in the CS (not in the tissue surrounding the vein) before proceeding to balloon dilation (Figure 6–71).

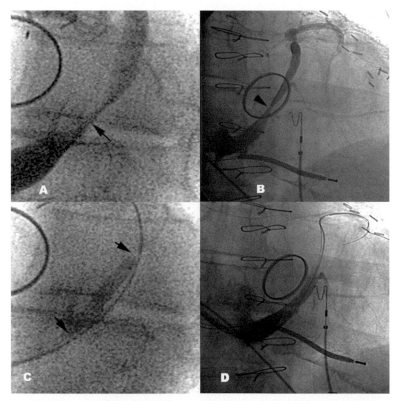

**FIGURE 6–71.** Balloon angioplasty of the body of the coronary sinus (CS). *A,* The stenosis is seen in the left anterior oblique projection. *B,* The stenosis is seen in the anterior-posterior projection. The first lateral wall target vein is seen at the 2 o'clock position on the mitral valve ring. *C,* The 4-mm balloon is inflated at the site of the stenosis. The proximal and distal end of the balloon are indicated by arrows. *D,* The site of stenosis is seen after balloon angioplasty. In this case a high-grade stenosis prevented a pacing lead from reaching the first lateral wall target vein. After the CS stenosis was dilated, an 8-F RDC1 guide was advanced into the lateral wall target vein and the lead was delivered.

## Angioplasty of Small or Stenotic Target Veins

The size of the vessel distal to the area of stenosis varies. It is usually easier to perform angioplasty on a large vein with a discrete stenosis because the directional guide fits securely in the OS of the vein. With a stable directional guide the angioplasty wire can be advanced distally against the resistance of the stenosis and the venous structures beyond without buckling. If needed a stiff angioplasty wire that generates more resistance as it advances can be used. As is true for over-the-wire pacing lead placement, it is important to have the angioplasty wire out beyond the stenosis as far as possible before attempting to advance the balloon. This insures that the balloon is advanced over the firm segment of the wire not the tip. Further, as the balloon is advanced it is important to keep the wire straight by gentle traction on the wire. If the wire is placed distally into small vessels or collaterals there is more friction between the veins and the wire operating over a longer length, holding it in place. Thus more traction can be placed on the wire to keep it straight without the wire retracting. In addition, if the wire does retract somewhat as the balloon is advanced there is sufficient wire left within the target vein to advance the balloon over the firm section of the wire. Finally, if the tip of the directional guide is inside the OS of the target vein the fine points of guide wire manipulation are less critical because the balloon is supported by the guide as it is advanced from the shoulder and relies less on the wire.

In Figure 6–72 the large lateral wall target vein is seen to have a stenosis near the origin. Neither the Medtronic ATTAIN 4193 nor the Guidant EASYTRAK leads would advance into the target vein. A 3.5-mm by 23.0-mm PowerSail balloon was advanced and inflated. The discrete nature of the stenosis preventing the lead from advancing is appreciated by the indentation (bone) in the balloon. Once the stenosis was relieved, the bone appearance disappeared and the pacing lead advanced. The resistance to dilation can be quite remarkable.

What happens if excess pressure is applied to a balloon in an attempt to relieve a stenosis? Figure 6–73 demonstrates a case in which a prior attempt at LV lead placement was unsuccessful. Because of prior OHS, surgical placement of an LV lead was denied. Using a telescoping system with a stable CS platform the only target vein is identified and selectively cannulated with an 8-F 55-cm Cordis Vistabritetip directional guide catheter. Initial attempts to place a lead were again unsuccessful. A 3.5-mm by 23-mm PowerSail balloon was placed in the target vein and inflated to 20 atm (see Figure 6–73*B*) without relief of the stenosis (*arrow*). The inflation pressure was taken to 24 atm, at which point the balloon burst. As seen in Figure 6–73*C,* the contrast in the balloon (*arrows*) is extravasated into the pericardial space. A 3.5-mm by 12-mm NC Monorail balloon was then advanced and inflated to 25 atm. With this the final inflation, tip of the guide (*G*) advanced further into the target vein. The ATTAIN 4193 lead was placed but did not pace at less than 3 V. The 4193 lead was replaced with an ATTAIN 2187 lead. The directional guide and stiffer lead provided sufficient support to advance the lead to the lead further onto the epicardial surface where it paced at less than 1 V. There were no acute or chronic complications related to the contrast extravasation.

## Angioplasty of Venous Collaterals

In some cases there are extremely limited options for LV lead placement. The target veins to the lateral wall may be extremely small or totally occluded but fill by collaterals.

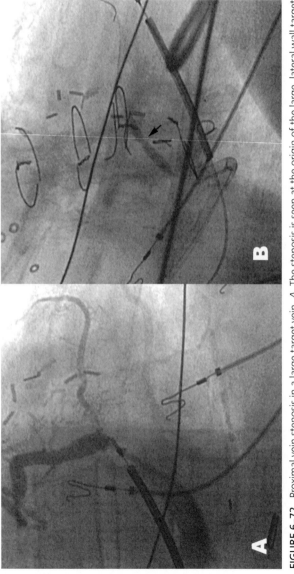

**FIGURE 6–72.** Proximal vein stenosis in a large target vein. *A,* The stenosis is seen at the origin of the large, lateral wall target vein. *B,* An indentation in the balloon persists despite inflation to 18 atm.

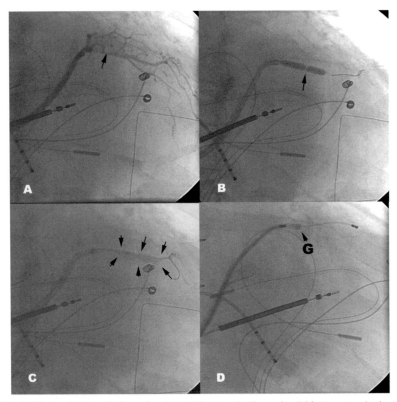

**FIGURE 6–73.** Angioplasty balloon bursts at 24 atm. *A,* The only viable target vein (*arrow*) is identified and selectively cannulated with an 8-F 55-cm Cordis Vistabritetip directional guide catheter. Neither a 4193 nor a 2187 lead advanced into the target vein. *B,* A 3.5-mm by 18-mm PowerSail balloon (noncompliant) is inflated to 24 atm without relief of the stenosis (*arrow*). *C,* The balloon ruptures from overinflation. Contrast (*arrows*) is seen in the pericardial space limited by adhesions from prior open heart surgery. *D,* After inflation of a noncompliant monorail balloon to 25 atm, the tip of the guide (*G*) advances further into the target vein. After the ATTAIN 4193 lead is removed because of high thresholds, an Attain 2187 lead is advanced.

In the course of placing angioplasty wires for pacing lead delivery or venous angioplasty it is not uncommon to see a wire pass from one vein to another through a collateral and re-enter the CS through the second vein (Figure 6–74). In patients with previous OHS where there is no direct access to the lateral wall the collateral network can be used to reach the target area. Figure 6–74 demonstrates the dilation of the venous collateral between the posterior lateral and lateral coronary veins. The patient had previous attempts to place an LV lead on the lateral wall fail due to limited access and phrenic pacing. In Figure 6–74*A,* selective injection of the posterior vein reveals a collateral connection (*arrows*) to the lateral wall target vein that could not be entered from the CS. Prior to proceeding with angioplasty of the collateral for lead placement, a test pacing system was created from a Luge angioplasty wire and a Cordis Transit infusion catheter, as follows. There is electrical continuity between the proximal and distal 3 cm of the tip of the Luge angioplasty wire (there is no electrical insulation on the distal 3 cm or on the proximal end of the wire). The Transit is a plastic 2.5-F infusion catheter

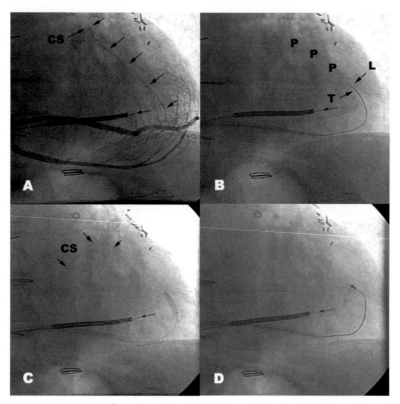

**FIGURE 6–74.** Angioplasty of venous collateral for left ventricular lead placement. *A,* A collateral venous structure connects the posterior lateral coronary vein to the lateral vein (*arrows*). Contrast injected into the posterior lateral vein is seen entering the coronary sinus through the lateral vein as a blush at the superior arrow. *B,* The Luge (*L*) angioplasty wire covered with Transit (*T*) is directed into the collateral to confirm pacing without phrenic stimulation before balloon dilation. Areas of phrenic pacing are indicated with a *P. C,* A 3.5-mm by 15-mm noncompliant balloon (PowerSail) is advanced into the collateral and inflated to 18 atm to create a channel for the pacing lead. *D,* A Medtronic ATTAIN 4193 OTW left ventricular pacing lead is advanced into position. The lead captured at 0.5 V without phrenic pacing at 10.0 V.

with .021 ID that is used to cover and insulate the Luge leaving the terminal 3–5 mm of the conducting tip of the Luge exposed. In Figure 6–74*B*, an arrow from the letter *T* indicates the distal marker of the Transit. The exposed electrically active segment of the Luge is indicated by the arrow from the letter *L*. Pacing of the distal 3–5 mm of the Luge is accomplished by attaching the negative clip to the proximal end of the Luge and the positive clip to the distal coil of the defibrillator lead or other suitable ground. In this way we were able to establish that there was viable myocardium along the collateral and also establish where phrenic pacing was a problem (indicated by the letter *P* in Figure 6–74*B*). The Transit infusion catheter was then removed, leaving the angioplasty wire left in place. In Figure 6–74*C*, the Luge enters the posterior cardiac vein within the guide and re-enters the CS through the lateral cardiac vein (*arrows*). A 3.5-mm by 18.0-mm PowerSail balloon is inflated in the collateral to 18 atm to provide a channel for the pacing lead. The Luge/Transit test pacing system detected phrenic pacing at sites further along the collateral (letter *P* in Figure 6–74*B*); thus balloon dilation was not carried out further along the collateral. The ATTAIN 4193 was easily advanced over the wire to the lateral wall of the left ventricle (Figure 6–74*D*) after percutaneous venous angioplasty (PCVA). Based on these observations the lateral wall of the left ventricle can be reached indirectly through dilated venous collaterals when the circumstances dictate.

### Angioplasty with Stent Placement

Tortuous vein segments are usually overcome with a directional guide or the buddy wire technique. However, in some cases the coronary vein to the lateral wall may be folded back on itself from prior surgery, particularly mitral valve ring, repair or replacement. In these cases a stent may be required to straighten the vein long enough to allow the pacing lead to pass. In Figure 6–75 a case is demonstrated in which the target cardiac vein (*T* in Figure 6–75*A*) is folded back on itself.

# Choosing the Appropriate Pacing Lead

Prior to the availability of multiple LV leads, inability to enter the target vein, high pacing thresholds, phrenic pacing, and/or an unstable lead position frequently resulted in the use of a less desirable target vein or implantation failure. Today, simply replacing the lead with a more appropriate size and shape solves the problem. This section introduces the LV leads available for implantation and will help you to match the lead to the target vein. Considerations for lead choice include the following:

1. Size
2. Location of the pacing electrode (tip vs. ring)
3. Presence or absence on tines
4. Preformed lead shape (straight or curved)
5. Over-the-wire or stylet driven
6. Steroid eluting

### Lead Size

Matching the size of the lead to the target vein is the most important first step. It is obvious that if the LV lead is too large for the target vein, it will not advance into the vein. However, a small lead in a large target vein will be unstable and have high thresholds. The Medtronic 2188 Bipolar Coronary Sinus Lead is the largest lead. It will pass through a 9-F ID sheath (remember the ID of a 9-F sheath is the same as the ID of an 11-F guide). The Medtronic ATTAIN OTW 4193 LV pacing lead is the smallest lead. It will pass through a 5-F sheath (or a 7-F guide).

### Electrode Location

LV pacing leads with the pacing electrode at the tip will behave differently from those with the ring set back from the tip. The Guidant EASYTRAK LV pacing lead is the only LV pacing lead with a ring pacing electrode set back from the tip. In order for the electrode on the EASYTRAK lead to make contact with the myocardium the lead must be wedged into the target vein. By comparison, when the pacing electrode is at the tip, the electrode may contact the myocardium without being wedged, depending on its shape.

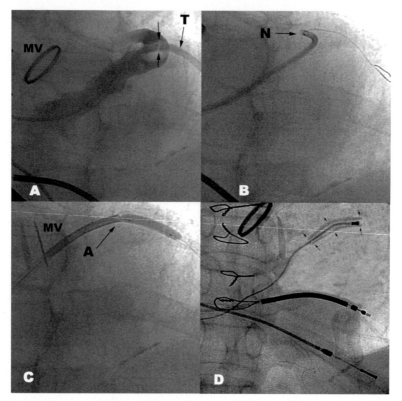

**FIGURE 6–75.** Stent to straighten folded cardiac vein. *A,* The ring of the mitral valve is indicated with the letters *MV.* The target vein (*T*) is seen folded back on itself (*arrow*). *B,* An 8-F Cardima Naviport deflectable tip guiding catheter (*N*) is in place at the ostium of the lateral wall target vein. An angioplasty wire is in place in the vein. *C,* The Naviport is replaced with the Medtronic ATTAIN Guide (*A*). A 3.5-mm by 18-mm PowerSail balloon is shown inflated in the target vein. Note there is no indentation in the balloon. *D,* The Medtronic ATTAIN 4193 pacing lead is in place just inside the two 3.5-mm Boston Scientific MultiLink Zeta stents (*arrows*).

## Presence or Absence of Tines

Tines are added to the tip of the pacing lead to help ensure the stability. In the right atrium and right ventricle the tines catch in the trabeculae. The mechanism by which tines promote stability in a venous branch of the CS is less clear. The intent is that the tines wedge in the vein as it is advanced distally. The Guidant EASYTRAK LV pacing lead is the only lead specifically designed for LV pacing that has tines. When the Medtronic CapSureSP 4023 lead is adapted for LV pacing, two or more of the four tines are usually removed.

## Preformed Lead Shape

The Medtronic ATTAIN LV 2187 and ATTAIN OTW 4193 LV pacing leads have preformed shapes of the lead body intended to promote stability and orient the tip electrode toward the myocardium. While the body of the lead is straight, the tip of the

Medtronic 2188 Bipolar Coronary Sinus Lead is canted. When the Medtronic CapSureSP 4023 lead is adapted for LV pacing, the tip of the lead may be canted by hand to resemble the 2188 lead. Although intended to promote stability, the preformed shape of the lead body of the 2187 and 4193 leads may actually induce lead dislodgement or less desirable pacing thresholds in some cases. Once the stylet or wire is removed, the lead attempts to assume it's preformed shape within the confines of the coronary vein. The tip may migrate forward or back (usually back) a few millimeters to a stable position. On occasion the physical characteristics of the CS vein and the preformed lead shape results in the lead "walking back" to a very proximal location or out of the vein entirely.

### Over-the-Wire or Stylet-Driven Leads

LV leads come in two basic types based on the method of delivery: (1) traditional stylet driven and (2) new over-the-wire approach. The Guidant EASYTRAK LV pacing lead and the Medtronic ATTAIN OTW 4193 LV pacing lead are over-the-wire leads. The 4193 lead may also be used with the included stylets. Stylet-driven leads, as a rule, are more difficult to advance to the lateral wall than the over-the-wire leads, particularly without a directional guide of a telescoping delivery system. However, when a telescoping delivery system is used and the tip of a directional guide is placed in the target vein, stylet-driven leads are easily placed and frequently work in the same target vein that failed with an over-the-wire lead. Over-the-wire leads are inserted by first advancing a conventional angioplasty wire into the target vein then advancing the pacing lead over the wire. The characteristics of the angioplasty wire (floppy, standard, and extra support) influence not only the ability of the wire to advance into the target vein but also the ability to of the pacing lead to be advanced over the wire. Stiff angioplasty wires (Platinum Plus, Choice PT Extra Support) are more difficult to advance into the target vein but tend to provide more support for the lead once in place. Conversely, softer wires may pass easily into the target vein but not provide enough support for the lead. Generally, a middle weight angioplasty wire (Luge or equivalent) is the best choice. More details on the selection of angioplasty wires is contained in the venoplasty portion of this section (Figure 6–76).

### Review of Left Ventricular Lead Type, Size and Personality

#### Medtronic ATTAIN LV 2187 Pacing Lead

The ATTAIN LV 2187 transvenous, unipolar, LV, cardiac vein pacing lead is a stylet-driven lead with the electrode at the tip. The electrode is not steroid-eluting. The lead can be difficult to deliver without a telescoping system. However, once in place the 2187 ATTAIN provides the best position on the lateral LV free-wall with the lowest thresholds, particularly in a large target vein. Once in place with the stylet and guide/sheath removed, the 2187 ATTAIN lead will not advance further into a target vein. Unless excess slack is added the 2187 rarely works its way back out of the target vein toward the CS. Even with the stylet and guide removed, the 2187 has enough body to be displaced from the target vein if excess slack is added. The 2187 ATTAIN can be inserted directly through any interventional guide with an internal diameter of greater than 0.088 inch (2.2 mm). Some 8-F guides and all 9-F or greater guides have an internal diameter of 0.088 inch or greater. The Cordis Vistabrite tip guide is an example of

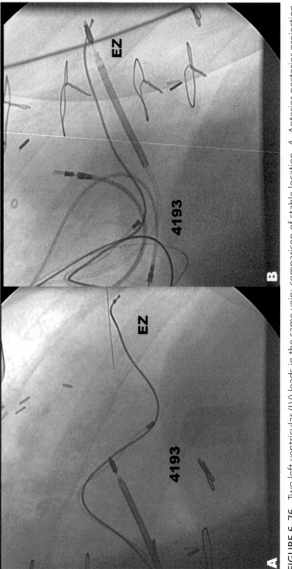

**FIGURE 6–76.** Two left ventricular (LV) leads in the same vein: comparison of stable location. A, Anterior-posterior projection. B, Right anterior oblique projection. The ATTAIN 4193 OTW LV pacing lead (4193) and the EASYTRAK lead (EZ) are in stable positions based on their individual physical characteristics.

an 8-F guide with an internal diameter of 0.088 inch, whereas the Boston Scientific Guider Softtip Guide must be 9-F to have sufficient internal diameter for direct lead delivery. The 2187 ATTAIN will pass through any 7-F sheath (Figure 6–77).

The ATTAIN OTW 4193 is a steroid eluting, transvenous, unipolar, LV over-the-wire, cardiac vein pacing lead with the electrode at the tip (Figure 6–78*A*). It has a preformed shape that it assumes when the stylet or wire is removed. The box shape is designed to direct the tip toward the myocardium and stabilize the lead in the target vein. It is delivered over a .014 angioplasty wire or using a stylet. Because the 4193 ATTAIN is smaller and can be delivered over an angioplasty wire, it is easier to place than the 2187 ATTAIN. Like the 2187 it does not tend to migrate more distally in the target vein. However, it will migrate proximally if the target vein is large or the proximal bend (*white arrow*) is not within the target vein. As a result, the tendency at the time of implantation is to advance the 4193 more distally than is desirable for optimal resynchronization. Distal locations are also more prone to phrenic stimulation. In situations where the 4193 lead has high-pacing thresholds (large target vein) or diaphragmatic/phrenic stimulation, replacing it with the 2187 frequently solves the problem. The 4193 lead can be delivered through any *directional guide* with an internal diameter of 0.076 inch (1.93 mm) or greater. The internal diameter of most 7-F guides is greater than 0.076 inch. The 4193 ATTAIN will pass through any 5-F introducer/sheath.

## Guidant EASYTRAK Left Ventricular Pacing Lead

The Guidant EASYTRAK LV pacing lead (Figure 6–79) is a steroid-eluting single electrode pace/sense lead. The model numbers 4510/4511/4512/4513 designate the available lengths of the lead (65, 72, 80, 90 cm). The EASYTRAK lead has a unique connector (LV-1) that is smaller than the standard IS-1 connector (Figure 6–79*C*). Oscor manufactures an adapter to convert an LV-1 connector to IS-1 connector, if needed. The pacing electrode is a ring that is located 2 mm from the tip (Figure 6–79*B, white arrow*). The EASYTRAK lead is delivered over a .014 angioplasty wire. Once in the target vein, the tendency is for the lead to migrate either proximal or distal unless it is wedged in a small branch of the target. Also, because the pacing electrode of the EASYTRAK lead is not at the tip, it must be wedged in a small branch to achieve satisfactory thresholds. It is often difficult or impossible to find a suitable location in a large target vein due diaphragmatic/phrenic stimulation distally with high-pacing thresholds and lead instability proximally.

Review of our experience with 38 sequential single site cases where the EASY-TRAK lead was placed in the target vein revealed that 11 were unsuccessful due to high pacing thresholds or diaphragmatic/phrenic stimulation. The EASYTRAK lead was successfully replaced with an ATTAIN 2187 or 4193 in the same target vein. Worse, our experience is that if the lead is placed distally, it may result in failure of resynchronization. We have five patients who failed to respond clinically to resynchronization with a distally placed EASYTRAK lead. They went on to a dramatic clinical improvement when the lead was replaced in the same target vein with a proximally placed 2187 or 4193 ATTAIN lead (Figure 6–80).

## Medtronic 2188 Bipolar Coronary Sinus Lead

The Medtronic 2188 Bipolar Coronary Sinus Lead (Figure 6–81*A*) is a bipolar lead originally designed to pace the atrium from the CS OS. In an occasional case it

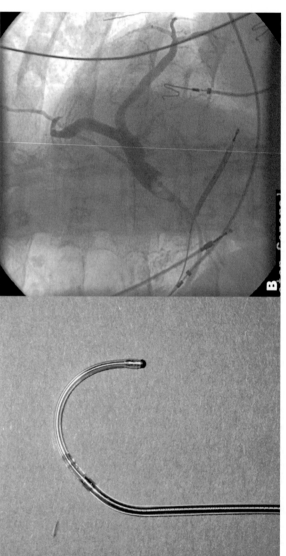

**FIGURE 6–77.** Medtronic ATTAIN LV 2187 pacing lead and suitable target vein. *A,* The 2187 lead shown with the stylet removed. *B,* A target vein suitable for a 2187 lead. If an ATTAIN 4193 lead is placed in this vein, the thresholds are likely to be high and the lead unstable unless the tip is wedged into a distal branch, which is more likely to result in phrenic pacing. In addition, patients with leads placed distally may not respond as well.

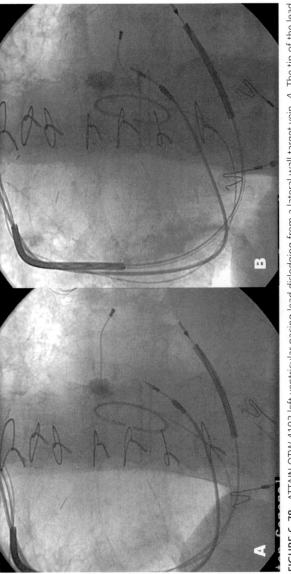

**FIGURE 6–78.** ATTAIN OTW 4193 left ventricular pacing lead dislodging from a lateral wall target vein. *A,* The tip of the lead is in the target vein but the proximal curve is in the coronary sinus. *B,* The 4193 works it way back into the coronary sinus. Unless the proximal curve is in the target vein, the lead tends to work its way out.

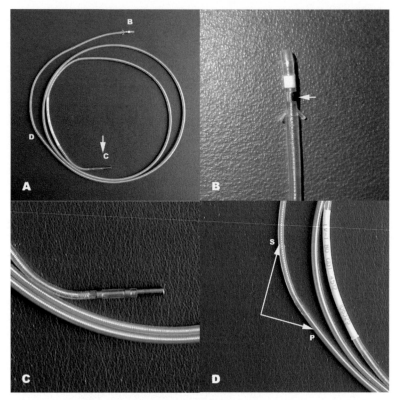

**FIGURE 6–79.** Guidant EASYTRAK left ventricular pacing lead. *A,* The entire lead. The tip of the lead (*B*), connector (*C*), and transition from polyurethane to silicone (*D*) are demonstrated in detail in *B-D. B,* Close-up of the lead tip. Note there are two tines at 180 degrees proximal to the pacing ring electrode. The white band is the steroid eluting collar. The ring pacing electrode (*white arrow*) is 2 mm proximal to the tip of the electrode. Unless the lead is wedged in a small target vein (or a branch of a large target vein), the ring electrode does not make good contact with the myocardium, and pacing thresholds are high. *C,* Close-up of the LV1 connector. It does not fit in a standard IS1 connector. *D,* Transition from polyurethane sheath over silicone (*P*) to silicone alone (*S*). The lead is insulated with silicone but also has an abrasion-resistant polyurethane coating that extends from the connector to a point 5 cm from the tip of the lead. The polyurethane coating increases the stiffness of the lead. Unless the lead is deep enough in the target vein that the polyurethane coated body is within the target vein, the lead tends to dislodge.

may be placed in an extremely large target vein. The 2188 lead has a canted tip which may provide lead stability not possible with other leads. The 2188 lead fits through the 9-F sheath or 11-F guide.

## Medtronic CapSureSP 4023

The Medtronic CapSureSP 4023 is a steroid-eluting unipolar implantable, tined ventricular transvenous lead. It is insulated with polyurethane and is available in 65- and 85-cm lengths. The 4023 is not specifically designed for LV pacing use but is essential for an occasional case. Other unipolar or bipolar leads could be used but

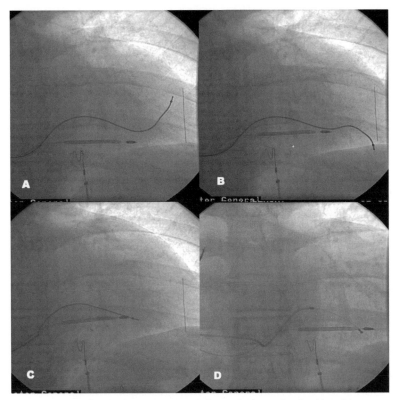

**FIGURE 6–80.** Failure of a Guidant EASYTRAK left ventricular pacing lead in a large target vein. *A* and *B*, The distal location of the lead resulted in phrenic pacing. *C,* The proximal location of the lead resulted in pacing thresholds over 5 V. *D,* An ATTAIN 2187 lead paced at 0.7 V. Without the option of an alternative lead, the target vein would have to be abandoned. This figure demonstrates the problem of placing an EASYTRAK lead in a large target vein.

are not available off the shelf in lengths over 58 cm. A 58-cm lead is usually not long enough to reach a lateral wall target vein in a patient with heart failure and a dilated heart. The recommended introducer/sheath size is 7-F. The 4023 lead fits through most 8-F or larger guides. The 4023 lead is usually modified for LV pacing. Two tines at 180 degrees are removed. The tip of the lead may be bent 30 degrees to improve contact and allow the lead tip to negotiate tight curves. Figure 6–82 is a case with a single lateral wall target vessel where both the ATTAIN 2187 and 4193 caused phrenic pacing. However, the 4023 lead delivered to the same vessel was placed in a different position that did not cause phrenic pacing.

## Avoiding Complications

Judicious use of contrast in the properly prepared (hydrated and premedicated) patient improves the efficiency and safety of resynchronization. It is essential to an understanding of the individual patient's venous anatomy and, because the implanter

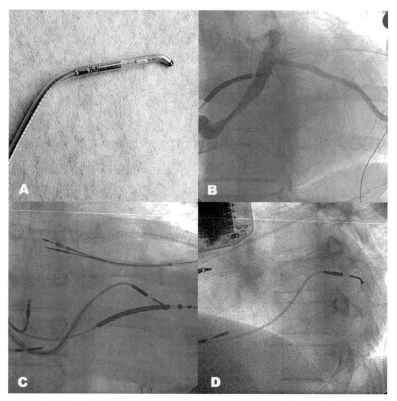

**FIGURE 6–81.** Medtronic ATTAIN CS 2188 lead. *A,* Lead tip. Note the canted tip. *B,* Venogram demonstrating the vein into which the 2188 lead was placed. *C,* Lead in place in the anterior-posterior projection. *D,* Lead in place in the left anterior oblique projection.

is aware of the catheter location at all times, to limiting unintentional trauma inflicted by EP catheters. When open-lumen catheters and contrast are used, missteps are quickly identified by staining. The same misstep with an EP catheter frequently goes unrecognized until announced by pain or hypotension. Thus the potential for staining with contrast is what makes it safe.

Contrast staining can occur at the time of CS venography but is not of hemodynamic significance. Staining can result from one of three mechanisms:

1. Unmasking of CS trauma inflicted by the EP catheter used to cannulate the CS. EP physicians frequently use a deflectable EP catheter to cannulate the CS and to serve as a guide wire over which to advance a guide. The EP catheter is not designed to prevent vascular trauma. It does not have a soft tip (like an open lumen catheter) nor does it have a J-tip (like a guide wire) to prevent vascular trauma. Thus unrecognized trauma to the CS is likely and will be made apparent when contrast is injected under pressure in the CS. In this case occlusive CS venography does not cause the staining but unmasks the unrecognized trauma inflicted by the sharp stiff EP catheter.

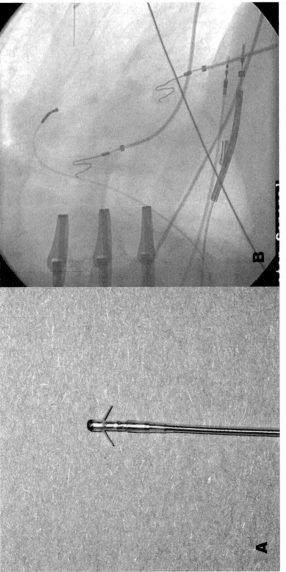

**FIGURE 6–82.** Medtronic CapSure SP 4023 lead. *A,* Lead with two tines removed. *B,* The 4023 lead in place on the lateral wall of the left ventricle in a location where both the 2187 and 4193 ATTAIN leads caused phrenic pacing. No other suitable target veins were available. The tip of the lead was bent to allow the lead to turn the corner into the vein. Bending the tip also seems to improve contact and lower pacing thresholds.

2. Local contrast extravasation at the tip of the balloon. If the tip of the balloon is or becomes lodged in a small venous branch during contrast injection the vein is disrupted and contrast is extravasated into the interstitial space, causing a stain.
3. Balloon-induced trauma due to overinflation of a non compliant balloon. Balloon trauma is limited by careful inflation of the balloon in the CS under fluoroscopy while contrast is being injected. Inflation is stopped when the balloon occludes the CS, preventing reflux of contrast. When overinflation occurs, a noncompliant balloon is more likely to inflict CS trauma than a compliant balloon. When a noncompliant balloon is overinflated for the size of the CS, it distorts and conforms to the CS. When a noncompliant (nondeformable) balloon is overinflated it enlarges without conforming to the CS, resulting in local trauma (Figure 6–83).

## Manipulation of Open-Lumen Catheters in and Around the Coronary Sinus

EP physicians are often not comfortable (due to a lack of experience) with the manipulation of open-lumen catheters in the heart, yet they feel safe with fixed curve or deflectable EP catheters. However, if one objectively compares a soft tip open-lumen catheter to an EP catheter, the EP catheter is much stiffer and prone to inflict vascular trauma. Further, there is concern that manipulation of catheters in and around the coronary venous structures is intrinsically more "dangerous" than the arteries because they are thin-walled structures. Nothing is further from the truth. Consider the three possible effects trauma to the coronary veins and compare the same event in a coronary artery.

### Dissection

The effect of an intimal disruption in a coronary artery versus a coronary vein are dramatically different. In an artery the blood is under high pressure and thus will get under the flap and extend the dissection. In a vein the blood is flowing in the opposite direction from the flap and is under low pressure; thus the dissection is not extended (Figure 6–84).

### Occlusion

If catheter trauma results in coronary artery closure, the consequences are abrupt and profound, leading to an acute myocardial infarction. However, the effect of catheter-induced trauma resulting in closure of a venous structure is of no acute or long-term significance other than the lack of venous access. Figure 6–85 demonstrates occlusion of a lateral wall target vein.

### Perforation

Catheter-induced trauma that results in coronary artery perforation presents a difficult situation, because the pressure gradient forces blood into the pericardial space, rapidly resulting in cardiac tamponade. However, perforation of a coronary vein does not have a similar effect, because the pressure gradient is in the opposite direction. Following a venous perforation, blood within the vein follows the pressure gradient into the CS and to the right atrium (Figure 6–86).

*Text continued on page 227*

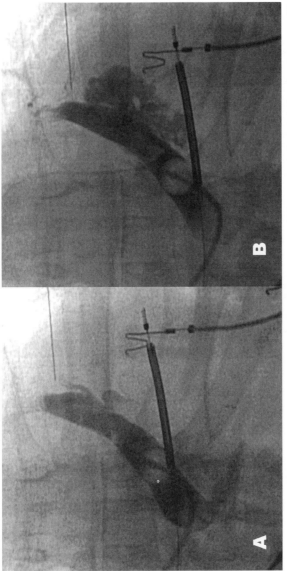

**FIGURE 6–83.** Contrast stain at the time of occlusive coronary sinus venography. *A*, The balloon is inflated and contrast fills the coronary sinus retrograde. *B*, The tip of the balloon catheter engages a small venous branch and contrast is extravasated into the interstitial tissue. Despite their ominous appearance, contrast stains do not result in hemodynamic complications. At their worst they obscure the venous anatomy.

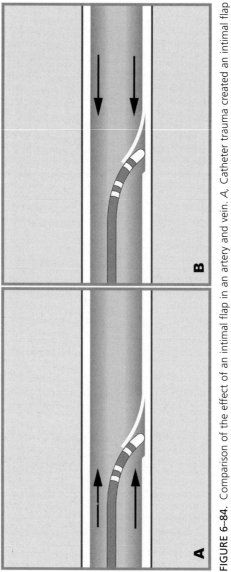

FIGURE 6-84. Comparison of the effect of an intimal flap in an artery and vein. A, Catheter trauma created an intimal flap in an artery. High pressure and the direction of blood flow in the artery will lift the flap and extend the dissection. B, Catheter trauma created an intimal flap in a vein. The direction of blood flow in the vein will close and seal the flap.

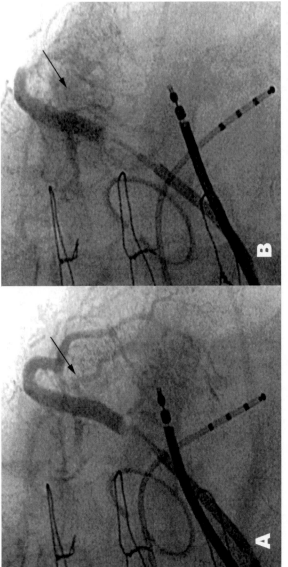

**FIGURE 6–85.** Occlusion of a lateral wall target vein. *A,* A small lateral wall target vein *(arrow)* is seen during the initial occlusive coronary sinus venography. *B,* The target vein is no longer seen when repeat venography is performed after an unsuccessful venoplasty. The patient suffered no ill effects. An alternative lateral wall target vein was used for left ventricular lead placement.

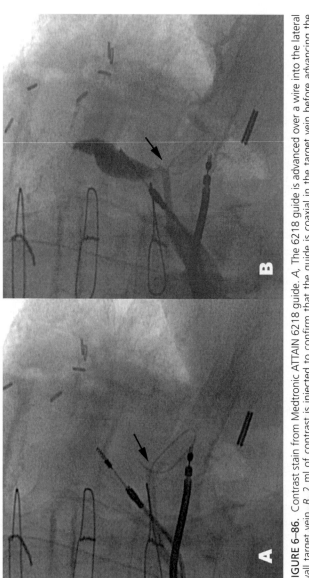

**FIGURE 6–86.** Contrast stain from Medtronic ATTAIN 6218 guide. *A,* The 6218 guide is advanced over a wire into the lateral wall target vein. *B,* 2 ml of contrast is injected to confirm that the guide is coaxial in the target vein before advancing the ATTAIN 2187 left ventricular pacing lead. The tip of the guide is not coaxial with the lumen of the vein and 1 ml of contrast is extravasated into the tissues around the vein. The position of the guide was adjusted and the lead advanced without incident. Vein perforation is likely if the pacing lead was advanced without contrast injection.

## Lead Perforation

In our experience, it is far more common for stylet-driven pacing leads to perforate the coronary veins than catheters, guides, or sheaths. Stylet-driven pacing leads, like EP catheters, have a solid metal tip with a wire reinforced shaft. A considerable amount of tip force can be delivered as evidenced by their ability to perforate the right ventricle. However, unlike RV perforation, coronary venous perforation rarely if ever cause tamponade. The explanation for the difference is explained by the fact that the pressure in the right ventricle is much higher than the pericardial space. Thus a pressure gradient favoring tamponade exists between the right ventricle and pericardial space. The pressure in a vein is much lower than the right ventricle. Further, a pressure gradient exists from distal to proximal in the vein. Thus the pressure gradient favors the flow of blood into the more proximal vein rather than out into the pericardial space. Figure 6–87 demonstrates the truth of this contention.

The complications particularly associated with LV lead implantation include CS dissection, vein perforation, LV lead dislodgement, and device-associated complications resulting from integration of additional leads placed in cardiac chambers not previously sensed or paced.[7] Although CS/venous trauma has emerged as a new procedural complication associated with LV lead implantation, most perforations produce little if any clinical consequence.[8] One should recognize when a catheter tip enters the subintimal space and thus avoid injecting large amounts of contrast to create a stain. Venous perforation usually does not produce hemodynamic instability, since the CS blood circulates at low pressure and the pericardium contains the perforation. When hypotension occurs in the setting of suspected perforation, immediate echocardiography can define the need for intervention with administration of fluids, vasopressors, or pericardial drainage. In the absence of hemodynamic instability, large contrast stains that prevent proper visualization of cardiac venous anatomy, or occlusion of the CS, repositioning the guiding catheter or pacing lead into the proper position usually permits the continuation of the implantation procedure. Should injection of contrast stain create a large stain, or should a dissection occlude the CS, the implantation procedure should be aborted, and another attempt considered after a delay of at least two weeks to allow the injury or stain to resolve.

## Patient Preparation When Using Contrast

The use of contrast agents in patients with CHF often causes concern among noninterventional cardiologists. However, interventional cardiologists routinely perform procedures on patients with CHF that require contrast. What is the real risk of contrast induced nephrotoxicity? In an unselected patient population of 220 patients who received $122 \pm 90$ ml of contrast material (75% received high-osmolarity contrast) Parfrey et al. found, "There is little risk of clinically important nephrotoxicity attributable to contrast material for patients with diabetes and normal renal function or for nondiabetic patients with preexisting renal insufficiency. The risk for those with both diabetes and preexisting renal insufficiency is about 9 percent, which is lower than previously reported."[9] None of the patients required dialysis. Despite these data, noninterventional physicians contend that patients with CHF who need cardiac resynchronization are unique and at higher risk than other patients. However, Meisel et al.

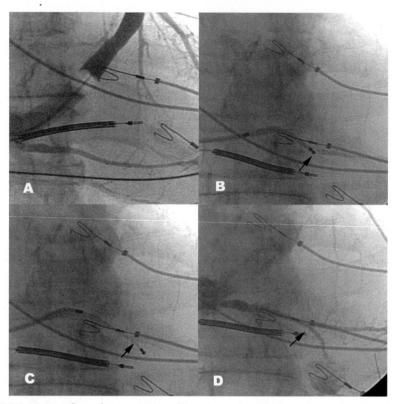

**FIGURE 6–87.** Free flow of contrast injected into the pericardial space after perforation of a vein with an ATTAIN 2187 left ventricular (LV) pacing lead. *A,* The posterior lateral target vein is demonstrated with occlusive coronary sinus venography. *B,* The ATTAIN 2187 LV pacing lead (*arrow*) is advanced into the vein. *C,* The tip of the 2187 lead (*arrow*) advances beyond the limits of the vein. *D,* The 2187 lead is removed and contrast is injected into the posterior lateral vein. Contrast under pressure from the injection (3 ml) exits the vein into the pericardial space. Despite the ominous appearance of *D,* there was no pericardial effusion on echo or hemodynamic consequences. The lead was successfully placed in an anterior lateral vein during the same procedures.

reported using 169 ± 105 ml of contrast in 129 patients with ventricular tachycardia and CHF to locate and investigate the CS anatomy. "Transient renal failure occurred... in 1 of 129 patients. Several unsuccessful attempts to enter the CS... resulted in the use of 420 ml of contrast agent. Serum creatinine level increased from 1.5 mg/100 ml before the procedure to 2.64 mg/100 ml after the procedure.... The patient recovered completely (without dialysis)."[10] Thus the objective data do not support the fear of using contrast in patients with CHF. However, proper respect must be paid to the potential for nephrotoxicity in patients with CHF because of the day-to-day variability in serum creatinine.

Patients who receive contrast, particularly those with renal insufficiency, should be prepared properly to minimize contrast nephropathy. Because the serum creatinine in patients with class III-IV CHF varies significantly from day to day, we regard all patients who undergo resynchronization therapy as having renal insufficiency.

## Hydration

The most important step in reducing contrast nephrotoxicity in patients with renal insufficiency is hydration. Patients should be pretreated with 0.45% saline 1ml/kg per hour for 12 hours before and 12 hours after the procedure.[11] The volume infused is intended to compensate for insensible loss while the patient is fasting and rarely results in an exacerbation of CHF.

## Mucomyst

In addition to hydration, "Prophylactic oral administration of the antioxidant acetylcysteine (Mucomyst) along with hydration, prevents the reduction in renal function induced by…contrast agent, in patients with chronic renal insufficiency." [12,13]

## Nonionic Contrast

Earlier data suggested there was no difference in the incidence of nephrotoxicity of ionic contrast or nonionic contrast when evaluated prospectively.[9] However, a recent article compared iodixanol (iso-osmolar, nonionic, dimeric contrast medium) to iohexol (low-osmolar, nonionic, monomeric contrast medium) and concluded that nephropathy induced by contrast medium may be less likely to develop in high-risk patients when iodixanol was used.[14] Thus the iso-osmolar nonionic contrast medium iodixanol seems to be the preferred agent at this time.

In summary, since the serum creatinine of patients with class III-IV CHF varies from day to day we regard all patients undergoing resynchronization therapy as having renal insufficiency and pretreat with acetylcysteine and hydration. Specifically, we hydrate all patients with 0.45% saline 1 ml per kg per hour starting 12 hours before the procedure, during the procedure (while the patient is NPO), and for 12 hours following the procedure. When questioned about throwing patients with chronic CHF into acute CHF via hydration, it is important to remember that the patients are NPO and continue to receive diuretics. In addition, we pretreat all patients with the antioxidant acetylcysteine (600 mg every 12 hours the day before the procedure, as well as the day of and the day after the procedure). Acetylcysteine (Mucomyst) is inexpensive and non-toxic. We do use nonionic contrast because of the attenuated hemodynamic effects. You can not count on nonionic contrast to eliminate the risk of renal insufficiency, however, based on the recent data noted previously the iso-osmolar nonionic contrast medium iodixanol is the preferred agent at this time. Remember not all nonionic contrast agents are the same. It is important to specify iodixanol.

## *Dislodgment*

Dislodgement of the LV lead after successful implantation eliminates the beneficial response to CRT. A review of data from the CRT trials shows lead dislodgement rate approach up to 10%.[7] When encountering a patient with recurrent symptoms of CHF after a CRT device implant, evaluating capture thresholds may reveal loss of capture as the cause. Chest radiographs may confirm movement of the LV lead from its original site. However, microdislodgement of the lead may produce loss of capture without the appearance of obvious changes in the chest X-ray. Successful reposition of dislodged LV leads usually requires reinsertion of the guiding catheter to provide enough support for advancement of either stylet-directed or over-the-wire leads. One may attempt to advance the lead over a guide wire or by inserting a stylet without the use of a guiding catheter. Failure to move the lead to a desired position quickly calls for the insertion of a new guiding catheter. Inserting a heavyweight (0.014–0.018) guide wire into the lumen of a dislodged over-the-wire lead will create vascular access over which to place subclavian introducers, and even a new guiding catheter. If removal of the chronically implanted lead does not dislodge the guide wire from the CS, careful insertion of the guiding catheter-introducer combination over the guide wire may allow tracking of the guide catheter directly into the CS. Removal of the introducer then allows "back loading" of the new LV pacing lead. If one cannot preserve the guide wire position within the CS, then insertion of the heavy guide wire into the lumen of the dislodged lead at least provides central venous access without the need to repeat the subclavian puncture. The implanter should consider what factors contributed to the dislodgement of the original lead when choosing a site for the new lead. Avoiding a mismatch in lead-vein size, proximal lead positions, excessive slack in the lead, and prolonged observation to detect early lead instability in the new position may decrease the probability of repeat dislodgement.

## Conclusion

Successful delivery of CRT requires a technique that safely implants pacing leads into an LV free-wall vein for biventricular stimulation. Understanding the anatomy of the failing heart allows the implanter to overcome most of the hurdles complicating CS catheterization. The technologic improvements in delivery system and LV pacing lead design provide tools to advance pacing leads to desired positions along the LV free-wall. Early recognition of potential complications increases the safety of the implantation procedure and allows the implanter to take remedial action to correct problems that may decrease the efficacy of CRT.

### REFERENCES

1. Ciocon JO, Galindo-Cocon D: Arm edema, subclavian thrombosis, and pacemakers. *Angiology*1998;49(4):315-319.
2. Roberts WC, Ferrans VJ: Pathologic anatomy of the cardiomyopathies. *Hum Pathol* 1975;6:287-342.
3. Curnis A, Neri R, Mascioli G, Cesario AS: Left ventricular pacing lead choice based on coronary sinus venous anatomy. *Eur Heart J Suppl* 2000;2:J31-J35.
4. Lattouf O, Leon A, DeLurgio D, et al: Minimally invasive surgical CRT, an alternative to transvenous lead placement. PACE 2003;26(2)II:S36.
5. DeRose JJ, Ashton RC, Belsley S, et al: Robotically assisted left ventricular epicardial lead implantation for biventricular pacing. *J Am Coll Cardiol* 2003;41(8)414-419.
6. Butter C, Auricchio A., Stellbrink C., et al: Effects of resynchronization therapy stimulation site on the systolic function of heart failure patients. *Circulation* 2001;104(25):3026-3029.
7. Greenberg JM, Mera FV, DeLurgio DB, et al: Safety of implantation of cardiac resynchronization devices: A review of major biventricular pacing trials. *PACE* 2003;26(4):952.
8. Hill PE: Complications of permanent transvenous cardiac pacing: A 14-year review of all transvenous pacemakers inserted at one community hospital. *Pacing Clin Electrophysiol* 1987;10:564-570.
9. Parfrey PS, Griffiths SM, Barrett BJ, et al: Contrast material-induced renal failure in patients with diabetes mellitus, renal insufficiency, or both: A prospective controlled study. *N Engl J Med* 1989;320(3);43-49.

10. Meisel E, Pfeiffer D, Engelmann L, et al: Investigation of coronary venous anatomy by retrograde venography in patients with malignant ventricular tachycardia. *Circulation* 2001;104(4)42-47.

11. Solomon R, Werner C, Mann D, et al: Effects of saline, mannitol, and furosemide to prevent acute decreases in renal function induced by radiocontrast. *N Engl J Med* 1994;331(21):416-420.

12. Shyu KG, Cheng JJ, Kuan P: Acetylcysteine protects against acute renal damage in patients with abnormal renal function undergoing a coronary procedure. *J Am Coll Cardiol* 2002;40:8383-8388.

13. Tepel M, van der Giet M, Schwarzfeld C, et al: Prevention of radiographic-contrast-agent-induced reductions in renal function by acetylcysteine. *N Engl J Med* 2000;343:380-384.

14. Aspelin P, Aubry P, Fransson SG, et al: Nephrotoxicity in High-Risk Patients Study of Iso-Osmolar and Low-Osmolar Non-Ionic Contrast Media Study Investigators. Nephrotoxic effects in high-risk patients undergoing angiography. *N Engl J Med* 2003;348(6):91-99.

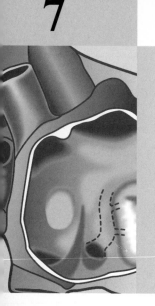

# 7

# Troubleshooting and Programming of Cardiac Resynchronization Therapy

G. Neal Kay

Although randomized clinical trials have demonstrated that most patients who have standard indications for cardiac resynchronization therapy (CRT) will experience improvement in both subjective and objective measures of cardiac function, a significant minority seem not to benefit.[1-4] There are a variety of potential explanations for the apparent failure of CRT, such as improper patient selection, limitations on placement of the cardiac venous lead, improper programming, and intrinsic limitations of the CRT device. When faced with a patient whose congestive heart failure (CHF) has not improved after implantation of a CRT device, the clinician must determine whether the device has been optimally programmed, whether the leads have been properly positioned, and whether a device with different features would be more appropriate. Troubleshooting and programming of CRT devices can be quite complex and involves both biologic and engineering considerations. Despite this complexity, the process of troubleshooting a CRT device involves asking oneself a series of rather basic clinical questions.

Several questions should be addressed for all patients who have received a CRT device. First, has the physiology of CRT been optimized for this patient? Has diastolic timing been optimally adjusted? Has systolic resynchronization been fully enhanced? Indeed, the answers to these questions are often interrelated, so that optimization of diastolic function will improve systolic function (and vice versa). Second, is CRT being consistently delivered? Simply implanting a CRT device will not benefit the patient if the ventricles are not being consistently paced at all physiologic heart rates. Is there appropriate upper-rate behavior? In order to answer these basic questions, the clinician must convince himself or herself that there is consistent capture of the left ventricle. Is the left ventricular (LV) stimulus consistently suprathreshold? Is there consistent atrial and ventricular sensing? Answering these questions requires an understanding of how to use diagnostics from the CRT device; how timing cycles interact with the intracardiac electrograms of patients with interventricular conduction delay; and the effects of such features as automatic mode switching, rate-adaptive atrioventricular (AV) delay, and rate smoothing. Finally, the function of implantable cardioverter-defibrillator (ICD) tachyarrhythmia therapy can be dramatically impacted by factors unique to sensing from both ventricles. The limitations of ICD timing cycles that are inherent to sensing of multiple tachyarrhythmia rate zones may limit the ability to deliver CRT at all pacing rates.

This chapter will review the factors that must be considered when patients with a CRT device present for follow-up, whether they are feeling well or not. The intent is to present an approach to troubleshooting the CRT device that is practical and clinically relevant.

# Troubleshooting the Physiology of CRT

## Optimization of the Atrioventricular Delay

It must be recognized that CRT not only resynchronizes intraventricular and, perhaps, interventricular systolic contraction, but it also may greatly improve diastolic filling of the left and right ventricles.[5-7] Indeed, improvement in diastolic function may have equal or more importance than enhancement of systolic performance for some patients with CHF who receive a CRT device. When assessing diastolic function, the clinician must keep a few important principles in mind[6,7]: the optimal AV delay will allow the onset of LV systole to occur at the peak of the left atrial (LA) systolic pressure wave (Figure 7–1); the optimal AV delay will maximize the time available for passive LV filling without limiting active filling related to LA contraction; and the optimal AV delay for the left ventricle may be different than that for the right ventricle.

Figure 7–1 illustrates the effects that the AV delay may have on LA and LV pressure waveforms, flow across the mitral valve, and cardiac output. Note that when there is a prolonged AV delay with atrial pacing (left panel), the peak of the LA pressure wave related to atrial contraction occurs in mid-diastole, far earlier than the onset of LV systolic pressure rise. As a result, the LA pressure falls during late diastole so that the LV end-diastolic pressure (LVEDP) exceeds the LA pressure. When LA pressure is less than LV pressure, flow across the mitral valve stops, as noted in the transmitral Doppler flow tracing. Also note that the total duration available for diastolic filling is only 220 msec with superimposition of the transmitral E (passive) and A (active) filling waves. With an excessive AV delay the LV end-diastolic pressure (the distending pressure in the left ventricle at the onset of systole) is low. Because the Frank-Starling mechanism is directly related to LVEDP and volume, the peak LV + dP/dt is reduced.

When the AV delay is excessively shortened to 60 msec (center panel), the LA systolic peak pressure occurs after the onset of LV systole. As a result, the LA contraction is not able to open the mitral valve because LV pressure greatly exceeds the LA peak systolic pressure. Thus although the time available for passive filling of the left ventricle might in theory be increased, the duration of the E wave is actually shortened to 200 msec, because the LV pressure is equal to or exceeds the LA pressure during late diastole. In addition, there is no active filling wave (absence of the transmitral Doppler A wave). Also note that the LVEDP is very low, reducing the contractility of the left ventricle and the LV + dP/dt by the Frank-Starling mechanism. The hemodynamic condition is further worsened by a marked increase in the mean LA pressure (averaged over the entire cardiac cycle). As a result of this improper timing of LA and LV contraction, the cardiac output is markedly reduced,

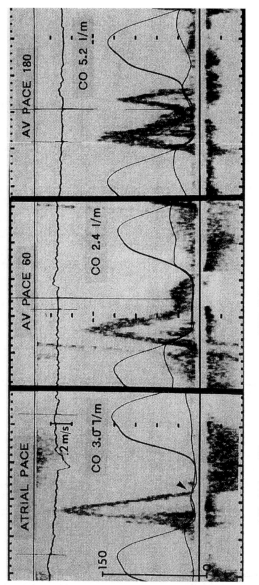

**FIGURE 7-1.** High-fidelity hemodynamic pressure tracings from the left atrium and left ventricle recorded simultaneously with pulse Doppler mitral inflow recordings in a patient with dilated cardiomyopathy and prolonged PR interval. *Left panel*, Atrial pacing with a long PR interval. Note that the peak of the atrial pressure wave occurs during mid-diastole (*arrowhead*). The mitral inflow tracing shows fusion of the E and A flow waves with a shortened duration of diastolic filling. During late diastole there is virtually no forward flow across the mitral valve. *Center panel*, Pacing recorded during atrioventricular (AV) pacing with an AV interval of 60 msec. Note that the left atrial pressure wave occurs during ventricular systole. The mitral E wave is preserved. There is absence of the A wave because atrial contraction occurs during ventricular systole. *Right panel*, Pacing recorded during AV pacing with an AV interval of 180 msec. Note that the mitral Doppler tracing demonstrates normal E and A waves with the onset of rise in LV pressure occurring simultaneously with the end of the A wave. (*Reproduced from Nishimura RA, Hayes DL, Holmes DR, et al: Mechanisms of hemodynamic improvement by dual chamber pacing for severe left ventricular dysfunction: an acute Doppler and catheterization study.* J Am Coll Cardiol *1995;25:281-288, with permission from The American College of Cardiology Foundation.*)

the mean LA pressure is increased, and the patient is likely to experience symptoms of both low cardiac output and pulmonary congestion.

In contrast to an AV delay that is either too long or too short, a properly timed AV delay (right panel of Figure 7–1) allows the peak of the LA systolic pressure wave to occur just prior to the onset of LV systole. This results in a markedly increased LV end-diastolic pressure, improvement in LV contractility (+dP/dt), and a greater cardiac output. Note that the increased LV end-diastolic pressure is associated with a low LA mean pressure. Also note that optimal LA-LV timing increases the total duration of transmitral flow to 320 msec and allows both passive (E) and active (A) filling waves to be recorded on the transmitral Doppler flow tracing. The transmitral flow due to atrial contraction is not truncated such that mitral valve closure occurs simultaneously with the end of LA systole. Thus an optimally timed AV delay allows the LA pressure to exceed the LV pressure throughout diastole. Figure 7–1 further illustrates how optimization of diastolic function improves systolic function.

Figure 7–2 illustrates the phenomenon of diastolic mitral regurgitation, which may occur in patients with CHF when the AV delay is excessive. In the presence of a long AV delay *(left panel)*, the LA pressure may fall below LV pressure during late diastole. This is illustrated by the Doppler flow signal by sampling from the left atrium, which demonstrates regurgitant flow into the left atrium prior to LV contraction. This reversal of diastolic flow reduces LV end-diastolic pressure and compromises LV contractility by failure to optimize the Frank-Starling mechanism. In contrast, when the LA-LV timing is optimal *(right panel)*, diastolic mitral regurgitation is eliminated because the LA pressure exceeds LV pressure throughout diastole and cardiac output is increased. In the PATH-CHF study,[7] patients were classified as "responders" and "nonresponders" on the basis of whether the aortic pulse pressure increased by at least 5% with biventricular pacing. For responders to biventricular pacing, the peak improvement in aortic pulse pressure occurred at an AV delay equal to 43% of the intrinsic PR interval. This was also the shortest AV delay that did not decrease the LVEDP. At AV delays less than 40% of the intrinsic PR interval, there was a decline in both LVEDP and aortic pulse pressure (Figure 7–3). In contrast to responders, the nonresponder group showed a progressive decrease in pulse pressure as the paced AV delay was progressively decreased from the intrinsic PR interval. Thus although preload and the Frank-Starling mechanism are important in biventricular pacing, the improvement in LV systolic function cannot be explained by this mechanism alone. It is also important to recognize whether a patient is a "responder" or a "nonresponder," because responders will require an AV delay that ensures biventricular pacing and nonresponders should have an AV delay programmed to minimize ventricular pacing. Indeed, recognition that a patient is a "nonresponder" allows the physician the opportunity to consider repositioning of the LV lead.

Because it is impractical to measure hemodynamics invasively during implantation and follow-up of the patient with a CRT device, the transmitral Doppler flow recording is used to guide programming of the AV delay. Figure 7–4 illustrates the effects of AV delay on Doppler transmitral flow. If the AV delay is appropriately programmed, there are distinct E and A waves without limitation of the active filling component. When programmed optimally, the mitral valve closes immediately after completion of the A wave. In contrast, if the AV delay is too long, the time available for transmitral flow is reduced, with fusion of the E and A waves and a reduction in the total duration of diastolic transmitral flow. Because the LV pressure can exceed the LA pressure during late diastole, diastolic mitral regurgitation may be recorded,

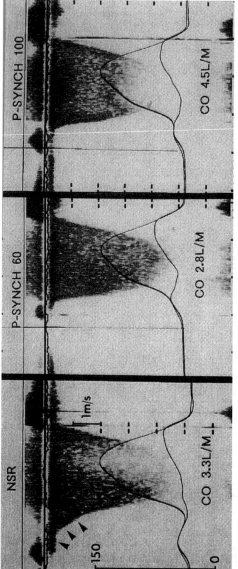

**FIGURE 7–2.** Simultaneous left atrium (LA) and left ventricle (LV) pressure tracings in a patient with a long PR interval. Pulse Doppler sampling from above the mitral valve demonstrate late diastolic mitral regurgitation (*left panel*) during sinus rhythm with a prolonged PR interval (*arrowheads*). Note that during late diastole the LV pressure exceeds the LA pressure. During atrioventricular (AV) pacing with an AV delay of 60 msec (*center panel*) there is elimination of diastolic mitral regurgitation. With an appropriately timed AV delay of 100 msec (*right panel*), there is marked improvement in the cardiac output with elimination of diastolic mitral regurgitation and an increase in the LV end-diastolic pressure. (*Reproduced from Nishimura RA, Hayes DL, Holmes DR, et al: Mechanisms of hemodynamic improvement by dual chamber pacing for severe left ventricular dysfunction: an acute Doppler and catheterization study. J Am Coll Cardiol 1995;25:281-288, with permission from The American College of Cardiology Foundation.*)

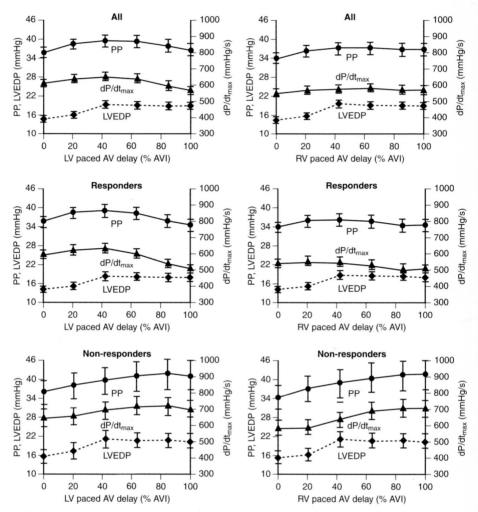

**FIGURE 7–3.** Aortic pulse pressure (PP) and left ventricular (LV) end-diastolic pressure (LVEDP), and maximum rate of increase in LV pressure rise (+dP/dt$_{max}$) during LV *(left panels)* and right ventricular (RV) *(right panels)* pacing at various atrioventricular (AV) delays normalized to the intrinsic PR interval (100%). All patients in the study are shown in the *upper panels;* patients who responded to LV pacing by an increase in PP and +dP/dt$_{max}$ are shown in the *middle panels;* and nonresponders are shown in the *lower panels.* Note that responders had peak improvement in PP and +dP/dt$_{max}$ with an AV delay that was approximately 40% of the intrinsic PR interval, whereas nonresponders showed progressive deterioration as the AV delay was shortened. *(Reproduced from Auricchio A, Ding J, Spinelli JC, et al: Cardiac resynchronization therapy restores optimal atrioventricular mechanical timing in heart failure patients with ventricular conduction delay. J Am Coll Cardiol 2002;39:1163-1169, with permission from The American College of Cardiology Foundation.)*

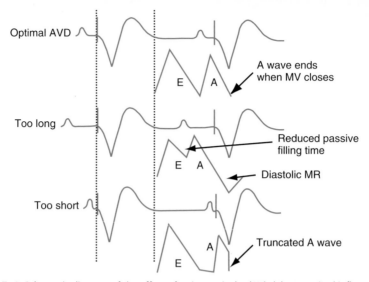

**FIGURE 7–4.** Schematic diagram of the effect of atrioventricular (AV) delay on mitral inflow tracings. Note that when the AV delay is optimal, the mitral valve closes at the end of the mitral A wave. If the AV delay is too long, the E and A waves become fused and the duration of diastolic filling is reduced. Late diastolic mitral regurgitation may occur. If the AV delay is too short, the A wave is truncated as the mitral valve closes before active filling from atrial contraction has completed.

further reducing LVEDP and volume. If the AV delay is too short, active filling cannot complete before the onset of LV contraction and the A wave is either absent or is truncated by abrupt closure of the mitral valve during the rise in LV systolic pressure. Although several formulas have been proposed to guide optimization of the AV delay,[8] the important concept is to program the shortest AV delay that does not compromise the transmitral Doppler A wave (closure of the mitral valve should occur immediately after the end of the A wave). Figure 7–5 illustrates the basic concept of AV delay optimization.[9] Note that if the interval from the end of the mitral A wave to closure of the mitral valve (S1) is too long, there is the potential for late diastolic mitral regurgitation. The optimal AV delay should place the first heart sound simultaneous with the end of the A wave.[9,10]

Figure 7–6 illustrates the practical application of Doppler echocardiography to optimization of the AV delay. Note that when the AV delay is programmed to 200 msec (see Figure 7–6A), there is fusion of the E and A waves. Closure of the mitral valve occurs well after the end of the A wave, with no transmitral flow during late diastole and a reduced total duration of LV filling. When the AV delay is programmed to 100 msec (see Figure 7–6B), the E and A waves are no longer fused and there is an increase in the total duration of LV filling. However, the A wave is truncated by LV contraction as the mitral valve closes before LA systole completes. When the AV delay is increased to 120 msec (see Figure 7–6C), the mitral valve closes simultaneously with the end of the A wave and LV diastolic filling is maximized. Thus programming of the AV delay need not be complicated when this simple method is utilized.

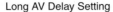

Long AV Delay Setting

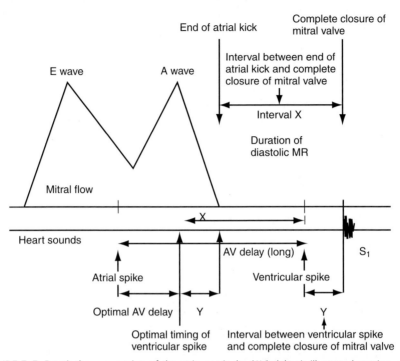

FIGURE 7–5. Practical programming of the atrioventricular (AV) delay is illustrated starting with a long AV delay that allows completion of the A wave from the pulse Doppler mitral inflow tracing. The optimal AV delay (point *X*) is one in which the first heart sound ($S_1$) is timed to occur at point *Y* simultaneous with the end of the A wave. *(Reproduced from Ishikawa T, Sumita S, Kimura K, et al: Prediction of optimal atrioventricular delay in patients with implanted DDD pacemakers. PACE 1999;22:1365-1371, with permission from Blackwell Publishing Ltd.)*

Because the AV nodal conduction interval normally shortens with exercise, careful attention must be paid to programming of the rate-adaptive AV delay in patients with a CRT device, if resynchronization is to be maintained throughout the range of metabolic need. If the rate-adaptive delay shortens excessively in comparison to normal AV nodal physiology with an increasing sinus rate during exercise, the LA-LV timing may become suboptimal, thereby forcing LV contraction before active LA contraction. This is especially likely to occur in the Medtronic 8040 CRT pacemaker if mode switching is programmed "on," which automatically adjusts the minimum sensed AV delay to 30 msec. In contrast, if the rate-adaptive AV delay is programmed "off," shortening of the intrinsic AV nodal conduction time with exercise may lead to loss of ventricular tracking and loss of ventricular resynchronization. Thus the rate-adaptive AV delay should be programmed "on," with a minimum AV delay that shortens in proportion to the intrinsic AV nodal conduction interval. In practical terms, the rate-adaptive AV delay is programmed by first optimizing the resting AV delay by the transmitral Doppler flow pattern and then asking the patient to exercise while recording the surface electrocardiogram to ensure that ventricular tracking is

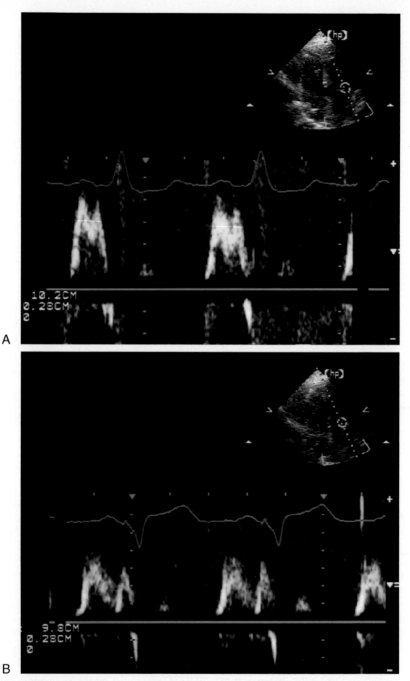

A

B

**FIGURE 7–6.** Pulsed Doppler mitral inflow tracings during atrioventricular (AV) optimization for a patient with left bundle branch block and a biventricular pacemaker. Note that when the AV delay is programmed to 200 msec (*A*), there is intrinsic conduction with fusion of E and A waves. With a programmed AV delay of 100 msec (*B*),

*Continued*

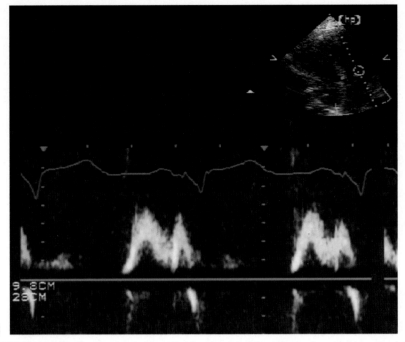

C

**FIGURE 7–6, cont'd.** The A wave is truncated by closure of the mitral valve. At the optimal AV delay of 120 msec (C), the mitral valve closes simultaneous with the end of the A wave.

maintained at all rates. The difference between maximal and minimal sensed AV delay is usually between 20 and 40 msec for most patients, although there can be some dramatic exceptions (see Interatrial Conduction Delay). However, care must be taken to note the heart rate during AV delay optimization at rest so that the range of AV delays from the lower to the maximal tracking rate can be adjusted appropriately. Because all CRT devices offer the DDDR pacing mode, care should also be taken not to allow an inappropriately aggressive increase in atrial rate in response to the rate-adaptive sensor. If the rate-adaptive sensor is too aggressive, the paced AV delay will shorten inappropriately, forcing the left ventricle to be paced before LA contraction. It is often prudent to limit the maximum sensor rate to 120 bpm while allowing the maximum tracking rate to be age-adjusted (220 – Age).

## Interatrial Conduction Delay

A potential reason for failure of patients receiving a CRT device to experience improvement in CHF is prolongation of the interatrial conduction interval. In some patients with advanced heart disease the interval from right atrial (RA) to LA activation may be quite prolonged. Figure 7–7 illustrates surface electrogram leads and coronary sinus electrograms at the time of biventricular ICD implantation. Note that whereas the P wave has a notched morphology with an apparent duration of 186 msec, the interval from the onset of the P wave to coronary sinus activation is markedly prolonged (368 msec). Biventricular pacing with an RA pacing lead and an AV delay of 200 msec would result in LV stimulation 180 msec earlier than

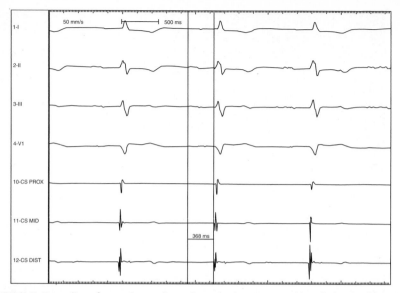

**FIGURE 7–7.** Recordings from a hexapolar catheter in the coronary sinus during implantation of a cardiac resynchronization therapy device. Note that the interval from the onset of the surface P wave to coronary sinus activation measures 368 msec, indicating marked interatrial conduction delay.

LA activation. As a result, the left atrium would contract after the left ventricle. Thus the only solution to this problem is to resynchronize atrial contraction by pacing the left atrium from the coronary sinus (Figure 7–8). In this situation a pacing lead was placed in the proximal coronary sinus so that the interval between LA and LV contraction could be precisely controlled. Thus the status of interatrial conduction is a potentially important consideration during implantation of a CRT device and failure to appreciate this problem may result in failure of CRT to improve CHF. It is our practice to routinely measure the interval from the RA pacing stimulus to the coronary sinus electrogram at the time of coronary sinus cannulation so that this problem can be avoided.

Another critical feature of CRT is to recognize that the sensed and paced interatrial conduction intervals may differ dramatically in some patients. Kinderman and colleagues[10] studied the effect of atrial sensing and atrial pacing on the timing of right and LA contraction. Using echocardiographic analysis of atrial contraction, these investigators demonstrated that atrial pacing may dramatically increase the interval between RA contraction and LA contraction. As a result, optimization of the AV delay during atrial sensing (VDD mode) may not provide optimal timing of LA and LV contraction during atrial pacing (DDD mode). It is also important to recognize that the major clinical trials of CRT (MUSTIC, MIRACLE, InSynch ICD, Contak CD, and Companion) all used the VDD pacing mode. Thus it may not be reasonable to extrapolate the benefits of CRT in these clinical trials to the routine use of the DDD or DDDR pacing modes. Because most patients receiving a CRT device do not have a standard pacing indication, it may be prudent to use the VDD mode whenever possible.

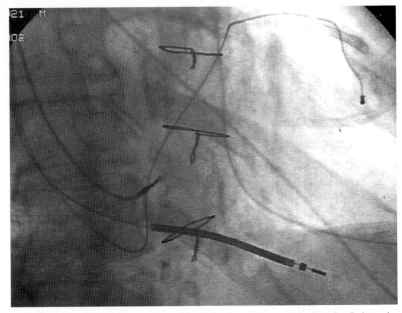

**FIGURE 7–8.** Right anterior oblique view of leads in the right ventricle (ICD lead), lateral cardiac vein, and active fixation lead in the coronary sinus.

## Optimization of Systolic Function

A prolonged QRS duration usually results in both interventricular (right ventricle to left ventricle) and intraventricular (LV septum to LV lateral wall) dyssynchrony. Reduction in the amount of LV dyssynchrony has been the goal of CRT.[11-35] Using Fourier phase analysis of the radionuclide angioscintigram, Fauchier and colleagues[11] demonstrated that intraventricular dyssynchrony was the more important cause of hemodynamic deterioration in dilated cardiomyopathy (Figure 7–9). Patients with the greatest degree of intraventricular dyssynchrony in the left ventricle were more likely to have a lower LV ejection fraction and cardiac index. In contrast, dyssynchrony between the right ventricle and left ventricle was not associated with hemodynamic deterioration. Intraventricular dyssynchrony in either the right ventricle or the left ventricle was predictive of adverse clinical events, such as need for cardiac transplantation or death. Delay between contraction of the right ventricle and left ventricle was not predictive of adverse clinical events.

Briethardt et al.[13] used two dimensional echocardiography to predict which patients receiving a CRT device in the PATH-CHF study would respond to this therapy. These investigators analyzed the timing of peak systolic septal and lateral wall motion as an indicator of intraventricular dyssynchrony.(Figure 7–10). The difference in phase angle of displacement of the lateral and septal LV walls was used as the measure of intraventricular synchrony. During sinus rhythm without pacing, the mean difference in lateral to septal phase angle was $104 \pm 41$ degrees and improved to $71 \pm 50$ degrees with LV pacing and to $66 \pm 42$ degrees with biventricular pacing ($P = 0.001$). Three distinct patterns of lateral to septal phase angles were identified (Figure 7–11). Type 1 patients (n = 4) were similar to normal controls with nearly simultaneous contraction

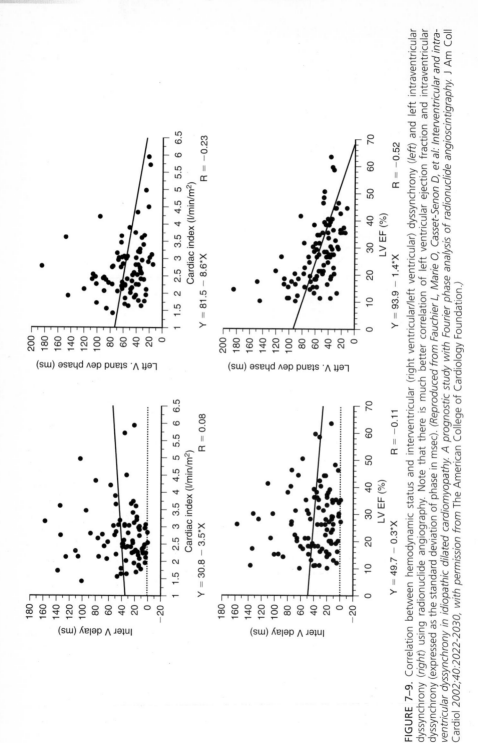

**FIGURE 7-9.** Correlation between hemodynamic status and interventricular (right ventricular/left ventricular) dyssynchrony (*left*) and left intraventricular dyssynchrony (*right*) using radionuclide angiography. Note that there is much better correlation of left ventricular ejection fraction and interventricular dyssynchrony (expressed as the standard deviation of phase in msec). (Reproduced from Fauchier L, Marie O, Casset-Senon D, et al: Interventricular and intraventricular dyssynchrony in idiopathic dilated cardiomyopathy. A prognostic study with Fourier phase analysis of radionuclide angioscintigraphy. J Am Coll Cardiol 2002;40:2022-2030, with permission from The American College of Cardiology Foundation.)

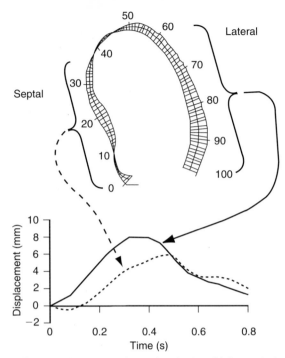

**FIGURE 7–10.** Apical four-chamber echocardiographic display of left ventricular septal and lateral walls with peak displacement for 100 endocardial segments. Note that the septal and lateral walls contracted out of phase (*graph*) when displacement is plotted over time. *(Reproduced from Breithardt OA, Stellbrink C, Kramer AP, et al. for the PATH-CHF Study Group: Echocardiographic quantification of left ventricular asynchrony predicts an acute hemodynamic benefit of cardiac resynchronization therapy.* J Am Coll Cardiol *2002;40:536-545, with permission from* The American College of Cardiology Foundation.*)*

of the lateral and septal walls. A type 2 pattern was identified in 17 patients and was characterized by septal contraction before lateral contraction with a difference in phase angle >25 degrees and was associated with the greatest improvement with biventricular pacing. A type 3 pattern (n = 3) was characterized by nearly opposite phases of contraction in the septal and lateral walls with a late component of septal contraction and a mean difference in phase angle of −115 ± 33 degrees. Based on their hemodynamic response to biventricular pacing (+LV dP/dt) (Figure 7–12), no patient with a type 1 pattern improved, whereas significant improvement was noted for 16 of 17 patients with a type 2 pattern and 10 of 13 patients with a type 3 pattern.

Pitzalis et al.[14] used the short axis M-mode echocardiogram to calculate the delay between peak motion of the LV posterior and septal walls (SPWMD = septal to posterior wall motion delay) in 25 patients with CHF and interventricular conduction delay (IVCD) undergoing CRT device implantation (Figure 7–13). The baseline QRS duration correlated significantly with the SPWMD (r = 0.62; $P < 0.01$). Patients who responded to CRT with a reduction of LV end systolic volume index >15% had a greater SPWMD (246 ± 68 msec) than did nonresponders (110 ± 55 msec; $P < 0.0001$). All responders to CRT had a baseline SPWMD >130 msec, a QRS duration >150 msec, and a PQ interval >180 msec. However, there was no difference in baseline QRS

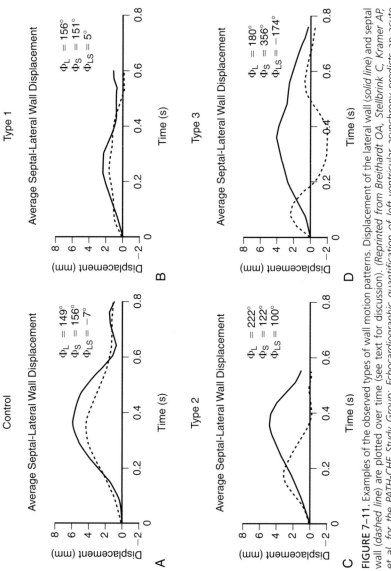

**FIGURE 7-11.** Examples of the observed types of wall motion patterns. Displacement of the lateral wall (*solid line*) and septal wall (*dashed line*) are plotted over time (see text for discussion). (*Reprinted from Breithardt OA, Stellbrink C, Kramer AP, et al. for the PATH-CHF Study Group: Echocardiographic quantification of left ventricular asynchrony predicts an acute hemodynamic benefit of cardiac resynchronization therapy. J Am Coll Cardiol 2002;40:536-545, with permission from The American College of Cardiology Foundation.*)

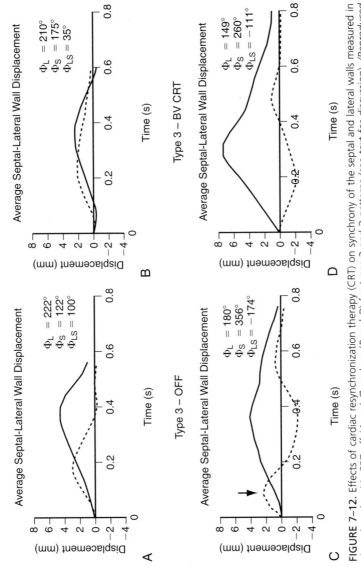

**FIGURE 7–12.** Effects of cardiac resynchronization therapy (CRT) on synchrony of the septal and lateral walls measured in phased angle with CRT off (A and C) and on (B and D) for types 2 and 3 patterns (see text for discussion). *(Reproduced from Breithardt OA, Stellbrink C, Kramer AP, et al: for the PATH-CHF Study Group. Echocardiographic quantification of left ventricular asynchrony predicts an acute hemodynamic benefit of cardiac resynchronization therapy. J Am Coll Cardiol 2002;40:536-545, with permission from The American College of Cardiology Foundation.)*

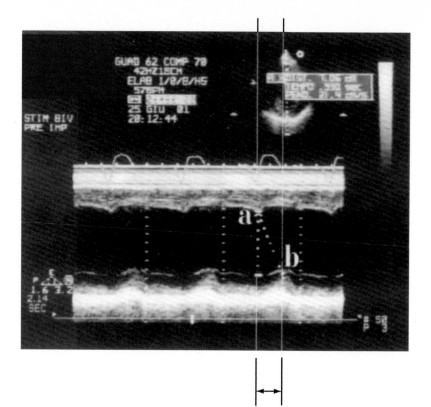

SPWMD = 330 ms.

**FIGURE 7–13.** M-mode echocardiographic illustration of the septal to posterior wall motion delay (SPWMD) as measured from the maximum displacement of the septal (*a*) and posterior (*b*) walls. *(Reproduced from Pitzalis MV, Iacoveillo M, Romito R, et al: Cardiac resynchronization therapy tailored by echocardiographic evaluation of ventricular asynchrony. J Am Coll Cardiol 2002;40:1615-1622, with permission from The American College of Cardiology Foundation.)*

duration between responders and nonresponders ($173 \pm 18$ vs. $164 \pm 12$ msec). Thus echocardiographic or nuclear angioscintigraphic measures of intraventricular dyssynchrony may be better predictors of response to CRT than the baseline electrocardiogram. Tissue Doppler imaging is a newer technique that has been used to quantitate the degree of intraventricular dyssynchrony in patients receiving CRT devices.[15-22] Using color tissue Doppler imaging, Yu and colleagues[15] noted that peak regional contraction was earliest in the basal anteroseptal region and latest in the basal lateral region in patients with a QRS duration >140 msec and CHF. After biventricular pacing with simultaneous right ventricular (RV) and LV stimulation, there was marked improvement in the synchrony of the septal and lateral walls (Figure 7–14). Sogaard, et al.[16] demonstrated that tissue Doppler imaging, when used to calculate changes in the percentage of the LV base with delayed longitudinal contraction with biventricular pacing, was highly predictive of changes in LV ejection fraction (Figure 7–15). Color Doppler imaging has also been used to quantitate myocardial strain in patients receiving

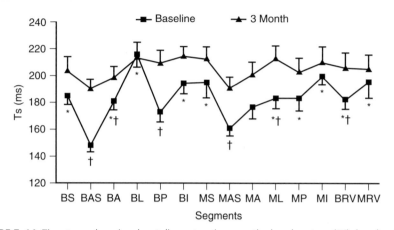

**FIGURE 7–14.** Time to peak regional systolic contraction over the basal septum (*BS*), basal anterior (*BA*), basal lateral (*BL*), basal posterior (*BP*), basal inferior (*BI*), midseptum (*MS*), basal RV (*BRV*) and mid-RV (*MRV*) walls. Before pacing (*squares*) there was marked variability in the time to peak systolic contraction (*Ts*). BAS = Basal anteroseptal; MA = Midanterior; MAS = Midanterior septum; MI = Midinferior; ML = Midlateral; MP = Midposterior. After pacing (*triangles*), there is homogeneous prolongation of the time to peak systolic contraction. (*Reproduced with permission from Yu CM, Chau E, Sanderson JE, et al: Tissue Doppler echocardiographic evidence of reverse remodeling and improved synchronicity by simultaneously delaying regional contraction after biventricular pacing therapy in heart failure. Circulation 2002;105:438-445.*)

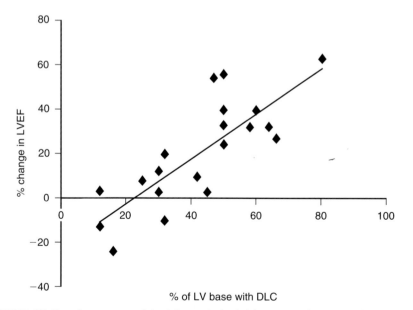

**FIGURE 7–15.** Plot of percentage of the left ventricular (*LV*) base circumference exhibiting delayed longitudinal contraction (DLC) versus the percentage change in left ventricular ejection fraction (*LVEF*) that occurs after onset of biventricular pacing using tissue Doppler imaging.

CRT devices.[18] Biventricular pacing improved overall regional LV strain and decreased the coefficient of variation of strain throughout the LV significantly as compared with baseline (Figures 7–16 and 7–17). It is important to point out that both of these studies used CRT devices that simultaneously stimulated the right and left ventricles.

Despite the benefits of the first generation of CRT devices that stimulate both ventricles in parallel, there is considerable reason to believe that intraventricular synchrony can be better optimized by individualization of the timing of RV and LV pacing.[15,17,23] Because the location of cardiac venous lead placement differs between individual patients, as does the pattern of intraventricular dyssynchrony, adjustment of RV and LV timing provides a way to optimize the function of the CRT device for each individual. The effect of the RV to LV interval on QRS duration in patients undergoing biventricular pacemaker implantation has been investigated by O'Cochlain and colleagues,[23] who noted that the most narrow-paced QRS was produced by an LV-RV delay ranging from −50 msec to +50 msec (Figure 7–18). In more than 80% of patients the most narrow QRS was produced by an RV-LV interval other than 0 msec. Despite this finding, it is unlikely that the QRS duration alone will provide the most physiologic information regarding resynchronization. The velocity time integral of LV ejection measured by continuous wave Doppler from the suprasternal notch may also be used as a method for optimizing the RV-LV timing interval (Figure 7–19). To optimize the RV-LV interval, the AV delay is first optimized from the mitral Doppler inflow tracing. Once the best RA-LV interval has been determined, an apical 5-chamber echocardiographic view with sampling from the aortic root is used to determine the best RV-LV timing (defined as the maximal aortic Doppler time velocity integral). In the Medtronic InSync III pacemaker

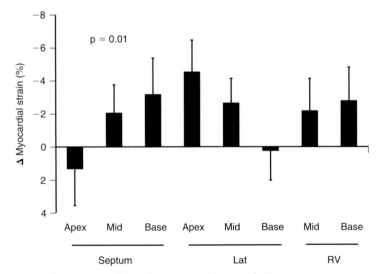

FIGURE 7–16. Regional myocardial strain change with biventricular pacing. Note that regional strain improved with CRT for all regions except the apical septum and the basal lateral walls.

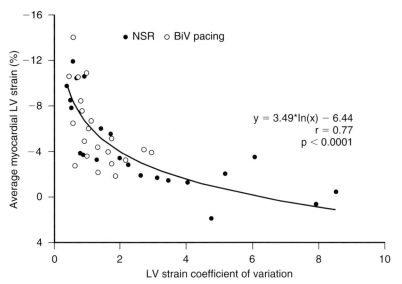

FIGURE 7–17. Correlation between the average myocardial left ventricular (LV) strain and the coefficient of variation of LV strain during normal sinus rhythm (*closed circles*) and during biventricular pacing (*open circles*).

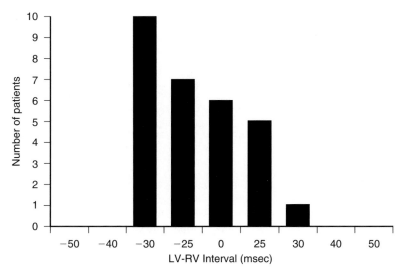

FIGURE 7–18. Distribution of left ventricular/right ventricular pacing interval that produced the shortest paced QRS duration (see text for discussion).

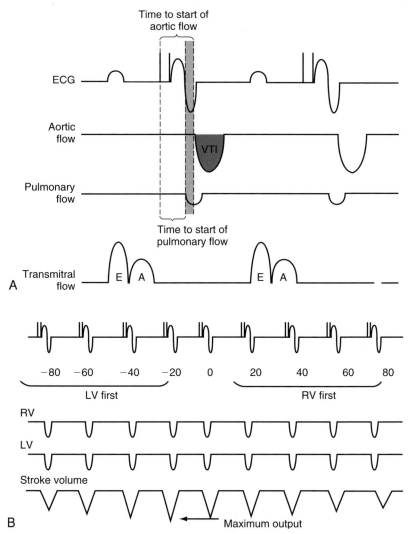

**FIGURE 7–19.** *A,* The use of the aortic velocity time integral as a method of estimating relative stroke volume from the left ventricle. *B,* The right ventricular/left ventricular interval is varied to produce the greatest aortic velocity time integral. *(Courtesy Medtronic, Inc.)*

(Figure 7–20), the AV delay (RA-LV) that is optimal is referred to as the "AV$_{opt}$." The RV-LV delay is referred to as the "V-V pace delay." Which of the two ventricles is stimulated first is then programmed (left ventricle first or right ventricle first). Programming the AV delay to the AV$_{opt}$ value, left ventricle first, and a V-V pace delay to 20 msec results in LV stimulation 20 msec before RV stimulation. In contrast, programming the AV delay to (AV$_{opt}$ – 20 msec), the right ventricle first, and the V-V pace delay to 20 msec results in RV stimulation 20 msec before LV stimulation. Thus the optimal AV delay remains constant, whereas the V-V pace delay

A

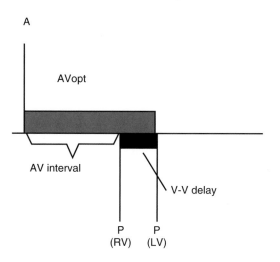

AV interval = AVopt-$\lfloor$V-V delay$\rfloor$

**FIGURE 7–20.** Optimization of the atrioventricular (AV) interval. The optimal right atrial/left ventricular interval is first determined by the mitral inflow Doppler tracing. The AV interval is equal to the AV optimal interval minus the right ventricular/left ventricular delay. *(Courtesy Medtronic, Inc.)*

is varied (AV interval = $AV_{opt}$ – V-V delay). It is important to remember that when pacing is programmed $LV_{tip}$ to $RV_{ring}$, anodal stimulation in the right ventricle is possible. Thus the clinician must be certain that RV anodal capture does not occur if the intention is to pace the left ventricle before the right ventricle. On the other hand, if the intention is to pace the right ventricle before the left ventricle, anodal stimulation in the right ventricle is not likely to be a problem because the right ventricle will be refractory to pacing during the LV stimulation pulse.

Tissue Doppler imaging of the left ventricle has been reported as a more sophisticated means for optimizing the RV-LV timing of CRT devices offering independent RV and LV stimulation.[15,17] Using tissue Doppler imaging to determine the extent of delayed longitudinal contraction (DLC) in 20 patients with left bundle branch block (LBBB) and CHF, Sogaard and colleagues[17] demonstrated that simultaneous stimulation of the right ventricle and left ventricle (RV-LV interval = 0 msec) reduced the proportion of the left ventricle with DLC from 49 ± 16% to 23 ± 13%; $P < 0.01$). However, by evaluation of a range of RV to LV stimulation intervals (–80 to +80 msec), an optimum interval could be individualized that further reduced the amount of DLC from 23 ± 13% to 11 ± 7%; $P < 0.01$ (Figure 7–21). Optimal resynchronization was achieved by pre-exciting the left ventricle in 9 patients and the right ventricle in 11 patients (range, –12 to +20 msec). These authors further demonstrated that the site of delayed contraction may differ between patients with idiopathic dilated cardiomyopathy (the lateral and posterior LV walls) and those with ischemic heart disease (the septum and inferior wall). As a result, the patients with idiopathic dilated cardiomyopathy were more likely to require LV pre-excitation, whereas those with ischemic heart disease usually required RV pre-excitation. The correct timing in the patient with CHF with

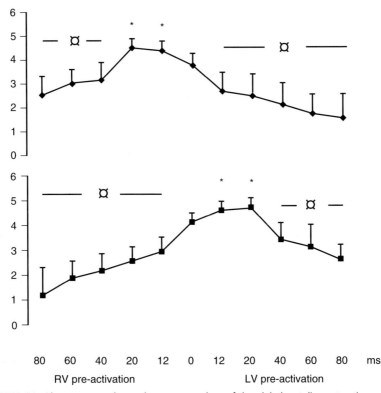

**FIGURE 7–21.** The top curve shows the average values of the global systolic contraction amplitude calculated from the average shortening amplitude of 16 LV segments by tissue Doppler imaging for 11 patients with optimal resynchronization by pacing the RV before the LV. The bottom tracing shows the average global systolic contraction amplitude for 9 patients with optimal synchrony by pacing the LV before the RV.

large regions of akinesia or dyskinesia from prior myocardial infarction has not been adequately defined. It is quite likely that the optimal RV-LV timing may be dependent on the site of infarction (anterior or inferior) as well as the location of the LV lead. Thus when a patient appears not to respond to CRT, imaging techniques should be considered to determine that the site of pacing and the timing of RV and LV stimulation have been optimized.

### Ensuring Biventricular Capture

For CRT to improve hemodynamics, the left ventricle must be continuously paced. An important aspect of CRT is an appreciation of the differences between endocardial and cardiac venous pacing. In contrast to endocardial pacing, in which the stimulating electrode is in direct contact with the endocardium, a pacing electrode in the cardiac venous system may be considerably farther from excitable myocardium. For example, the cardiac venous electrode may be separated from the myocardium by the venous wall, by epicardial fat, and by fibrosis in a region of prior myocardial infarction. In addition, the conduction velocity away from the site of stimulation may be slower with cardiac venous pacing due to a greater distance from the Purkinje network. As a result of these differences, cardiac venous pacing thresholds are considerably higher than endocardial RV pacing thresholds. The greater distance of the stimulating electrode from excitable myocardium often results in a rightward and upward shift of the strength-duration curve (Figure 7–22). Thus chronaxie is often longer for cardiac venous pacing than for endocardial pacing. The practical application of this finding is that the LV voltage threshold can be dramatically lowered by extending the pulse duration from a customary value of 0.4 msec (typical of endocardial pacing) to as long as 2.0 msec. The strength-duration curve may be shifted downward and to the left by placing the coronary venous lead more distally in the targeted cardiac vein.

### Effect of Pacing Configuration on Left Ventricular Stimulation Threshold and Impedance

Only unipolar leads have been commercially released in the United States for CRT. There are several potential ways in which a unipolar lead in a cardiac vein, and either a unipolar or bipolar lead in the right ventricle, can be configured for biventricular stimulation.[36,37] The first CRT devices used the tip electrodes of the cardiac venous lead and the RV lead as a split cathode. The anode was usually configured as the ring electrode of a bipolar RV lead (termed the *bipolar split cathodal configuration*)

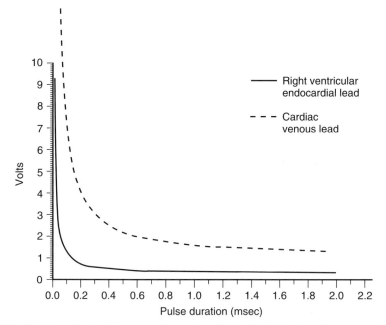

**FIGURE 7–22.** Strength duration curves for endocardial (*solid line*) and cardiac venous (*dashed line*) pacing electrodes. Note that the cardiac venous pacing lead has both higher rheobase voltage and longer chronaxie msec.

(Figures 7–23*A* and 7–24*A*). Alternatively, when the CRT pulse generator is programmed to the unipolar pacing configuration, the pulse generator casing becomes the anode (termed the *unipolar split cathodal configuration*) (Figures 7–23*B* and 7–24*B*). Both of these split cathodal configurations stimulate the right and left ventricles in parallel, such that the pulse from the output capacitor is applied to both the LV

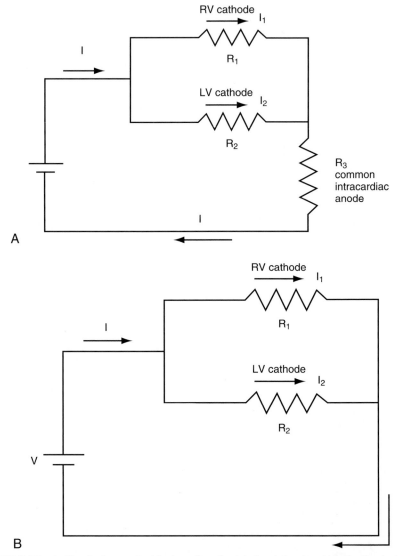

**FIGURE 7–23.** *A,* Circuit diagram for bipolar split cathodal stimulation in which the tip electrodes of the right ventricular (RV) and the left ventricular (LV) leads are in parallel with a common anode at the pulse generator housing. *B,* Circuit diagram for unipolar split cathodal stimulation with the RV and LV tip electrodes in parallel and a common anode at the RV ring electrode. *(Reproduced with permission from Barold SS, Levine PA. Significance of stimulation impedance in biventricular pacing. J Intervent Cardiac Electrophysiol 2002;6:67-70.)*

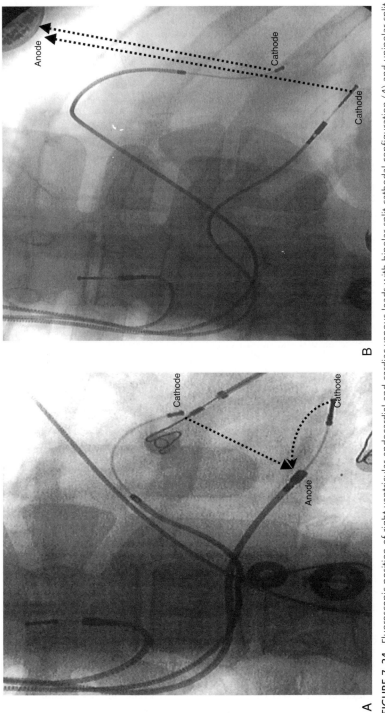

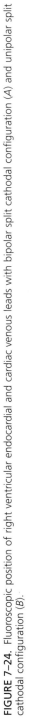

**FIGURE 7-24.** Fluoroscopic position of right ventricular endocardial and cardiac venous leads with bipolar split cathodal configuration (*A*) and unipolar split cathodal configuration (*B*).

and the RV electrodes. As a result, current simultaneously flows to both the LV and the RV tip electrodes. Because the LV and RV circuits are stimulated in parallel, the total impedance of the circuit is less than when either the LV or the RV tip electrodes are stimulated alone. However, there are several alternative configurations that have been used to achieve CRT, especially when pre-existing leads or pulse generators are used. One possible configuration uses the tip electrode of the cardiac venous lead as the cathode (or anode) and the tip electrode in the right ventricle as the anode (or cathode) (Figure 7–25A). Such a configuration has been employed when a pre-existing unipolar RV pacing lead has been employed for CRT. This widely split bipolar configuration utilizes two unipolar leads, each having electrodes with small surface areas, thereby increasing the overall impedance of the circuit. Alternatively, a Y-adapter can be placed to combine the tip electrodes of two unipolar leads as a split cathode and the pulse generator casing as the anode for unipolar split cathodal stimulation (Figure 7–25B). More recent generations of FDA-approved CRT devices utilize separate output circuits for both the cardiac venous and the RV leads that allow independent programming of stimulation amplitude, pulse duration, and polarity. Ultimately, bipolar leads will be used for both the right ventricle and the left ventricle, each with its own output circuit. Each of these configurations has different electrical characteristics and inherently different advantages and disadvantages.

A limitation of the split cathodal configuration is that assessment of the electrical integrity of either the LV or the RV lead may be difficult. A complete fracture of the LV lead conductor or the RV tip conductor would have only a small effect on impedance. A fracture of the RV ring conductor would create a dramatic rise in impedance only if the output circuit is programmed bipolar. In addition, a low impedance of one of the leads due to an insulation failure may be difficult to detect because of the already low impedance of the parallel circuit.

### Off-label Upgrading of Implantable Cardioverter-Defibrillators to Provide Biventricular Pacing

There are several potential ways in which standard dual chamber ICDs can be upgraded to provide biventricular pacing after implantation of a cardiac venous lead (Figure 7–26A-D). However, one must be very careful with such off-label use and understand how different adapters will configure pacing, sensing, and the high-voltage circuits. Because most coronary venous leads that have been used so far have been unipolar, an adapter is required. However, it must be remembered that ICDs often utilize the distal high-voltage coil as the anode for pacing. Thus an adapter that is placed only on the pace/sense connector pin of an ICD lead that is connected to such an ICD pulse generator will not necessarily provide the anticipated result. For example, when a unipolar cardiac venous lead is connected to a St. Jude Medical ICD, a bipolar-to-bipolar Y-adapter should be used (such as the Medtronic 2872). When the RV defibrillation lead is a dedicated bipolar design (Figure 7–26A), pacing will be biventricular split cathodal and sensing is bipolar with a composite RV plus LV cathode. Similarly, if an integrated bipolar RV defibrillation lead is used, this adapter will provide biventricular pacing and sensing (Figure 7–26B). When a bipolar LV lead is used in conjunction with a dedicated bipolar RV defibrillation lead, a bipolar-to-bipolar adapter must be used to prevent the LV ring electrode from being incorporated into the high-voltage circuit (Figure 7–26C). When a unipolar-to-bipolar connector is used with a unipolar LV lead placed in the cathodal port of the Y-adapter (Medtronic 5866-38m), only the left

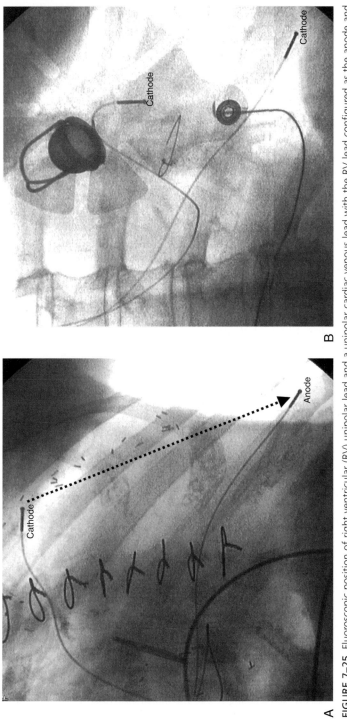

**FIGURE 7-25.** Fluoroscopic position of right ventricular (RV) unipolar lead and a unipolar cardiac venous lead with the RV lead configured as the anode and the cardiac venous lead as the cathode (*A*). Alternatively, both the RV and cardiac venous leads can be configured with a Y-adapter in parallel as a split cathodal configuration with the pulse generator case as the common anode (*B*).

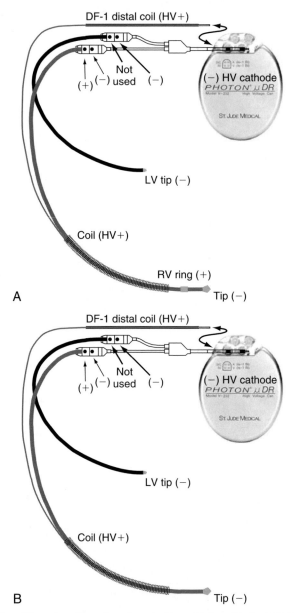

**FIGURE 7–26.** Five different configurations for adapting a St. Jude Medical ICD that uses the right ventricular (*RV*) distal defibrillation coil as the anode for pacing to achieve biventricular pacing. When a unipolar left ventricular (*LV*) lead is used in combination with a dedicated bipolar defibrillation lead (*A*), it is important to use a bipolar-to-bipolar adapter as shown. This configuration provides biventricular pacing and sensing. When using an integrated bipolar defibrillation lead and a unipolar LV lead (*B*), a bipolar-to-bipolar adapter also provides biventricular pacing and sensing.

*Continued*

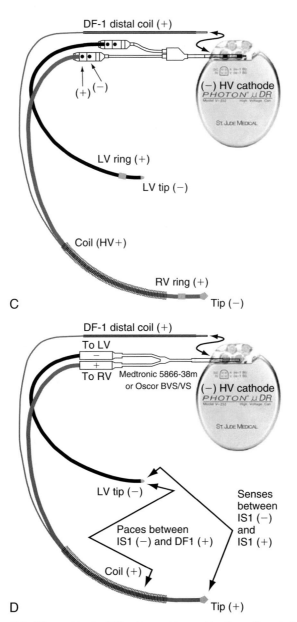

DF-1 distal coil (+)

(+) (−)

(−) HV cathode
*PHOTON μ DR*

St. Jude Medical

LV ring (+)

LV tip (−)

Coil (HV+)

RV ring (+)

**C**    Tip (−)

DF-1 distal coil (+)

To LV

−
+

To RV    Medtronic 5866-38m
or Oscor BVS/VS

(−) HV cathode
*PHOTON μ DR*

St. Jude Medical

LV tip (−)

Paces between
IS1 (−) and DF1 (+)

Senses
between
IS1 (−)
and
IS1 (+)

Coil (+)

**D**    Tip (+)

**FIGURE 7–26, cont'd.** When a bipolar LV lead is used in combination with a dedicated bipolar RV defibrillation lead (*C*), a bipolar-to-bipolar adapter must be used to prevent the LV ring electrode from being incorporated into the high-voltage circuit. When a bipolar LV lead is used with a unipolar to bipolar adapter (*D*), pacing will only occur in the left ventricle, whereas sensing will be biventricular.

*Continued*

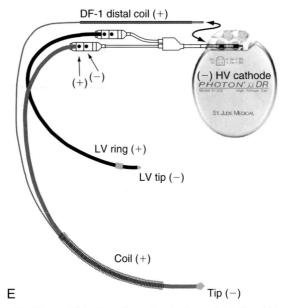

DF-1 distal coil (+)

(+) (−)

(−) HV cathode
*PHOTON' μDR*

LV ring (+)

LV tip (−)

Coil (+)

E                                    Tip (−)

FIGURE 7–26, cont'd. The prohibited configuration is shown in *E*, in which a bipolar LV lead is used with an integrated bipolar RV defibrillation lead, as this configuration includes the LV ring electrode in the high-voltage circuit.

ventricle will be used for pacing, whereas sensing will be biventricular (Figure 7–26*D*). It is important never to use a bipolar LV lead with an integrated bipolar RV defibrillation lead because this configuration will incorporate the LV ring electrode into the high-voltage circuit (Figure 7–26*E*).

## Implantation Stimulation Thresholds with Cardiac Venous Leads

The implant stimulation threshold measurements of cardiac venous leads in 19 patients undergoing CRT are shown in Table 7–1. The LV unipolar stimulation threshold (0.7 + 0.5 V) was significantly lower than the bipolar threshold with use of the endocardial RV ring electrode as the anode ($1.0 \pm 0.7$ V; $P = 0.01$). Combining the tip electrodes as a split cathode results in a marked increase in the apparent LV threshold for both the bipolar and unipolar shared-cathodal configurations. The apparent LV threshold increased by 30%, from $1.0 \pm 0.7$ V in the bipolar left ventricle–alone configuration to $1.3 \pm 0.9$ V in the bipolar split-cathodal configuration ($P < 0.001$). Similarly, the apparent RV bipolar threshold increased by 67%, from $0.3 \pm 0.2$ V to $0.5 \pm 0.2$ V in the bipolar split-cathodal configuration ($P = 0.005$). The apparent LV threshold also increased from $0.7 \pm 0.5$ V in the unipolar left ventricle–alone configuration to $1.0 \pm 0.8$ V in the unipolar split-cathodal configuration (43% increase; $P = 0.01$).

## Long-Term Stimulation Thresholds

The 1-year LV and RV stimulation thresholds measured with the pulse generator in the shared-cathodal configurations are shown in Table 7–2. The long-term

**Table 7–1.** Pacing Thresholds (Volts) at Implantation

| | | | | (Pulse Duration 0.5 msec) | | | |
|---|---|---|---|---|---|---|---|
| Patient No. | RV Bipolar | LV Unipolar | LV Bipolar | LV Bipolar Split Cathode | RV Bipolar Split Cathode | LV Unipolar Split Cathode | RV Unipolar Split Cathode |
| 1 | 0.2 | 0.3 | 0.4 | 0.4 | 0.4 | 0.4 | 0.3 |
| 2 | 0.4 | 0.5 | 0.6 | 0.8 | 0.5 | 0.6 | 0.4 |
| 3 | 0.5 | 0.1 | 0.3 | 0.6 | 0.3 | 0.3 | 0.3 |
| 4 | 1.0 | 0.9 | 1.0 | 1.5 | 1.0 | 1.0 | 1.0 |
| 5 | 0.3 | 0.2 | 0.3 | 0.8 | 0.4 | 0.5 | 0.2 |
| 6 | 0.3 | 0.5 | 0.8 | 1.3 | 0.5 | 0.6 | 0.2 |
| 7 | 0.3 | 0.3 | 0.5 | 0.7 | 0.4 | 0.6 | 0.2 |
| 8 | 0.4 | 0.7 | 1.9 | 2.0 | 0.6 | 2.2 | 0.4 |
| 9 | 0.3 | 1.3 | 2.1 | 2.6 | 0.4 | 1.9 | 0.3 |
| 10 | 0.3 | 1.5 | 1.5 | 1.9 | 0.4 | 1.4 | 0.2 |
| 11 | 0.3 | 0.3 | 0.5 | 0.5 | 0.4 | 0.3 | 0.2 |
| 12 | 0.2 | 1.9 | 2.3 | 2.5 | NA | 2.5 | 0.3 |
| 13 | 0.3 | 1.0 | 0.6 | 0.6 | 0.5 | 0.5 | 0.3 |
| 14 | 0.3 | 0.3 | 0.6 | 0.8 | 0.3 | 0.5 | 0.1 |
| 15 | 0.2 | 0.3 | 0.7 | 0.7 | 0.2 | 1.1 | 0.4 |
| 16 | 0.1 | 0.7 | 0.7 | 1.3 | 0.3 | 0.9 | 0.2 |
| 17 | 0.1 | 0.5 | 0.5 | 0.7 | 0.6 | 0.6 | 0.5 |
| 18 | 0.2 | 1.7 | 2.3 | 3.6 | 1.1 | 3.0 | 0.6 |
| 19 | 0.4 | 1.2 | 1.0 | 1.6 | 0.8 | 1.0 | 0.4 |
| Mean | 0.3 | 0.7 | 1.0 | 1.3 | 0.5 | 1.0 | 0.3 |
| Standard Deviation | 0.2 | 0.5 | 0.7 | 0.9 | 0.2 | 0.8 | 0.2 |

Source: Reproduced with permission from Mayhew M, Bubein RS, Slabaugh J, et al. Effect of a split cathodal configuration on pacing threshold and impedance. *PACE* 2003: in press.
LV = Left ventricular; RV = right ventricular.

apparent bipolar split-cathodal LV and RV thresholds were $2.4 \pm 1.6$ V and $0.8 \pm 0.3$ V, respectively ($P < 0.001$). In the unipolar split-cathodal configuration, the 1-year follow-up apparent LV and RV thresholds were $1.8 \pm 1.6$ V and $0.7 \pm 0.3$ V, respectively ($P = 0.004$). As compared with the unipolar split-cathodal configuration, the bipolar split-cathodal configuration increased the apparent LV threshold by 33% ($P = 0.003$) and the RV threshold by 14% ($P = 0.02$). Thus programming a CRT device that combines the RV and cardiac venous tip electrodes as a split cathode to the bipolar configuration significantly increases the threshold. Although programming to the unipolar split-cathodal configuration improves the LV threshold, there is a significant risk for pectoral muscle stimulation. The advantage of bipolar split-cathodal stimulation is the elimination of the potential for pectoral muscle stimulation.

## Impedance Measurements

The impedance measurements at CRT lead implantation as a function of stimulation configuration are shown in Table 7–3. The average impedance of the LV lead in a bipolar configuration was $874 \pm 299$ ohms and the average impedance of the RV lead in a bipolar configuration was $705 \pm 152$ ohms. The measured

Table 7–2. Pacing Thresholds (Volts) at 1 Year

| | (Pulse Duration 0.5 msec) | | | |
|---|---|---|---|---|
| Patient No. | LV Bipolar Split Cathode | RV Bipolar Split Cathode | LV Unipolar Split Cathode | RV Unipolar Split Cathode |
| 1 | NA | NA | NA | NA |
| 2 | 3.5 | 1.0 | 2.0 | 1.0 |
| 3 | 1.5 | 1.0 | 1.0 | 0.5 |
| 4 | 7.5 | 1.0 | 7.5 | 1.0 |
| 5 | 2.5 | 1.0 | 3.0 | 0.5 |
| 6 | 2.5 | 0.5 | 1.5 | 0.5 |
| 7 | 1.0 | 0.5 | 1.0 | 0.5 |
| 8 | 3.5 | 1.0 | 1.0 | 0.5 |
| 9 | 1.0 | 0.5 | 1.0 | 0.5 |
| 10 | 1.5 | 1.0 | 1.0 | 0.5 |
| 11 | 1.5 | 0.5 | 1.0 | 0.5 |
| 12 | 2.5 | 1.5 | 2.0 | 1.5 |
| 13 | 3.5 | 1.0 | 3.0 | 1.0 |
| 14 | 3.5 | 1.0 | 1.5 | 0.5 |
| 15 | 1.5 | 0.5 | 1.5 | 0.5 |
| 16 | 2.0 | 1.0 | 1.5 | 1.0 |
| 17 | 1.0 | 0.5 | 0.5 | 0.5 |
| 18 | 2.0 | 0.5 | 1.5 | 0.5 |
| 19 | 1.5 | 0.5 | 1.0 | 0.5 |
| Mean | 2.4 | 0.8 | 1.8 | 0.7 |
| Standard Deviation | 1.6 | 0.3 | 1.6 | 0.3 |

Source: Reproduced with permission from Mayhew M, Bubein RS, Slabaugh J, et al. Effect of a split cathodal configuration on pacing threshold and impedance. *PACE* 2003: in press.
LV = Left ventricular; RV = right ventricular.

impedance in the bipolar split-cathodal configuration was $516 \pm 64$ ohms. Assuming a parallel circuit that follows ohm's Law, the predicted impedance in the bipolar split-cathodal configuration would equal 390 ohms. This finding highlights the fact that impedance is a complex parameter that depends on several factors, such as capacitance at the electrode-tissue interface, polarization, and resistance of the lead conductors. The impedance measurements at 1 year are shown in Table 7–4. At 1 year, the average impedance in the bipolar split-cathodal configuration was $526 \pm 68$ ohms and the average impedance in the unipolar split-cathodal configuration was $339 \pm 72$ ohms ($P < 0.001$).

## Ventricular Electrogram Amplitudes with Different Sensing Configurations

The measured ventricular electrogram amplitudes at lead implantation are shown in Table 7–5. On average, the R wave in the RV bipolar configuration measured $16.9 \pm 7.4$ mV. This value was significantly greater than the R waves measured in the unipolar and bipolar split-cathodal configurations ($10.2 \pm 5.3$ mV and $11.9 \pm 5.4$ mV, respectively; $P < 0.001$). The R waves in the unipolar split-cathodal configuration measured $12.0 + 4.0$ mV and $15.0 \pm 5.0$ mV in the bipolar split-cathodal configuration ($P = 0.01$).

TABLE 7–3. Impedance Measurements (Ohms) at Implantation

| Patient No. | RV Bipolar | LV Unipolar | LV Bipolar | Bipolar Split Cathode | Unipolar Split Cathode |
|---|---|---|---|---|---|
| 1 | 899 | 771 | 899 | 599 | 442 |
| 2 | 744 | 732 | 861 | 497 | 441 |
| 3 | 992 | 664 | 664 | 530 | 493 |
| 4 | 528 | 648 | 759 | 460 | 343 |
| 5 | 639 | 511 | NA | 491 | 395 |
| 6 | 667 | 569 | 597 | 442 | 546 |
| 7 | 869 | 978 | 1092 | 568 | 514 |
| 8 | 802 | 645 | 805 | 522 | 440 |
| 9 | 664 | 1052 | 1086 | 505 | 395 |
| 10 | 687 | 564 | 707 | 446 | 357 |
| 11 | 789 | 792 | 771 | 487 | 379 |
| 12 | 519 | 546 | 628 | 425 | 347 |
| 13 | 585 | 752 | 707 | 471 | 334 |
| 14 | 1012 | 603 | 704 | 504 | 452 |
| 15 | 642 | 546 | 732 | 640 | 432 |
| 16 | 582 | 1854 | 1915 | 633 | 503 |
| 17 | 533 | 395 | 776 | NA | 643 |
| 18 | 674 | 741 | 1025 | 583 | 583 |
| 19 | 560 | 596 | 891 | 488 | 364 |
| Mean | 705 | 735 | 874 | 516 | 442 |
| Standard Deviation | 152 | 313 | 299 | 64 | 87 |

Source: Reproduced with permission from Mayhew M, Bubein RS, Slabaugh J, et al. Effect of a split cathodal configuration on pacing threshold and impedance. *PACE* 2003: in press.
LV = Left ventricular; RV = right ventricular.

## *Practical Guidelines for Programming of CRT Stimulation*

The preceding discussion allows us to propose several practical guidelines for programming the stimulation pulse of CRT devices. First, when possible, separate output circuits are desirable, both in terms of minimizing the LV pacing threshold and for optimization of intraventricular synchrony. This allows independent programming of RV and LV stimulus amplitude, pulse duration, timing, and polarity so that each chamber can be individually optimized. Second, when a split-cathodal CRT device is used, the LV stimulation threshold will be lower in the unipolar than in the bipolar configuration. If the LV stimulation threshold is low, programming to the unipolar configuration is unlikely to result in pectoral muscle stimulation. On the other hand, if the LV threshold is high, the chances of pectoral muscle stimulation increase and unipolar pacing may not be tolerated. Third, it must be remembered that the LV voltage threshold may be significantly reduced by programming a longer pulse duration. Thus the LV threshold may decrease from 5.0 V at 0.4 msec to as low as 2.5 V at 1.9 msec. The net result on stimulus energy (E) is a factor of the square of the stimulus voltage (V) but is directly related to the pulse duration (t) as given by the equation $E = V^2 t/R$ (R being resistance). Thus if the voltage is doubled from 2.5 V to 5.0 V, the energy of the pulse increases by a factor of 4. If the pulse duration is increased from 0.4 msec to 1.9 msec, the energy is increased by 4.75 times. Although it may be more energy-efficient to increase the stimulus voltage in some cases, in others it may be more efficient to increase the pulse duration. However, it must also

TABLE 7–4. **Impedance Measurements (Ohms) at 1 Year**

| Patient No. | Split Bipolar | Split Unipolar |
|---|---|---|
| 1 | 539 | 335 |
| 2 | 439 | 267 |
| 3 | 515 | 313 |
| 4 | 492 | 293 |
| 5 | 525 | 376 |
| 6 | 387 | 219 |
| 7 | 642 | 406 |
| 8 | 652 | 546 |
| 9 | 577 | 407 |
| 10 | 504 | 294 |
| 11 | 519 | 344 |
| 12 | 558 | 358 |
| 13 | 424 | 246 |
| 14 | 474 | 276 |
| 15 | 584 | 377 |
| 16 | 548 | 332 |
| 17 | 492 | 329 |
| 18 | 575 | 368 |
| 19 | 540 | 349 |
| Mean | 526 | 339 |
| Standard Deviation | 68 | 72 |

Source: Reproduced with permission from Mayhew M, Bubein RS, Slabaugh J, et al. Effect of a split cathodal configuration on pacing threshold and impedance. *PACE* 2003: in press.
LV = Left ventricular; RV = right ventricular

be remembered that the primary goal of CRT is to achieve optimal cardiac resynchronization, whereas battery longevity is of lower priority. Fourth, a lower margin of safety may be appropriate for the LV stimulus of CRT devices than when programming a standard pacemaker or ICD in a patient who is dependent on pacing. For example, the CRT device will usually have a very high margin of safety for the RV lead, such that failure of LV capture is unlikely to result in severe symptoms. In addition, many patients implanted with a CRT device do not have a standard pacing indication. Both of these factors may allow a lower margin of safety for LV stimulation. Finally, when the stimulation polarity is programmed to bipolar with use of the RV ring electrode as the anode, anodal stimulation of the right ventricle is possible, even when the intention is to pace the left ventricle (LV tip to RV ring configuration).

## Timing Cycles of Cardiac Resynchronization Devices

The first CRT device approved for commercial sale in the United States (Medtronic Model 8040) was based on the Thera family of dual chamber pacemakers. This device utilizes a split-cathodal pacing and sensing configuration in which the tip electrodes of the LV and RV leads are stimulated in parallel. The sensed ventricular electrogram is a composite of the tip electrograms of the two chambers. The polarity of pacing and sensing can be programmed either unipolar (with the pulse generator casing as the anode) or bipolar (with the ring electrode of the RV lead as the anode). Because both ventricular leads are stimulated in parallel, there is no flexibility for independent

**TABLE 7–5. R waves (mV) at Implantation**

| Patient No. | RV Bipolar | LV Unipolar | LV Bipolar | Bipolar Split Cathode | Unipolar Split Cathode |
|---|---|---|---|---|---|
| 1 | 16.8 | 18.3 | 15.9 | 5.6 | 9.9 |
| 2 | 11.5 | 12.2 | 19.8 | 8.0 | 8.2 |
| 3 | 30.0 | 30.0 | 30.0 | 23.0 | 11.8 |
| 4 | 16.1 | 18.2 | 2.5 | 9.9 | 9.9 |
| 5 | 20.8 | NA | 29.8 | 11.5 | 11.5 |
| 6 | 11.6 | 3.3 | 3.0 | 10.9 | 3.0 |
| 7 | 7.0 | 4.0 | 4.4 | 4.0 | 3.0 |
| 8 | 28.5 | 14.5 | 13.5 | 5.7 | 23.1 |
| 9 | 16.0 | 17.4 | 17.5 | 13.3 | 5.5 |
| 10 | 13.9 | 8.4 | 8.9 | 8.2 | 7.2 |
| 11 | 4.2 | 3.5 | 7.6 | 6.2 | 6.2 |
| 12 | 26.1 | 10.4 | 10.5 | 13.0 | 12.9 |
| 13 | 13.5 | 23.7 | 30.0 | 16.7 | 15.6 |
| 14 | 28.3 | 20.9 | 12.3 | 17.4 | 16.5 |
| 15 | 19.8 | 7.8 | 28.7 | 10.4 | 2.9 |
| 16 | 12.1 | 8.5 | 11.6 | 16.8 | 9.9 |
| 17 | 12.5 | 8.4 | 3.2 | NA | NA |
| 18 | 10.9 | 18.9 | 10.9 | 13.4 | 13.4 |
| 19 | 21.7 | 4.9 | 4.8 | 20.6 | 12.8 |
| Mean | 16.9 | 13.0 | 13.9 | 11.9 | 10.2 |
| Standard Deviation | 7.4 | 7.7 | 9.6 | 5.4 | 5.3 |

Source: Reproduced with permission from Mayhew M, Bubein RS, Slabaugh J, et al. Effect of a split cathodal configuration on pacing threshold and impedance. *PACE* 2003: in press.
LV = Left ventricular; RV = right ventricular.

timing of LV and RV stimulation, and the same amplitude and duration of the ventricular output waveform is applied to both chambers. Although this device provides biventricular pacing without the requirement for a specialized lead adapter, the timing cycles are the same as for a standard dual-chamber pacemaker. Timing of the Medtronic 8040 pacemaker is atrial based (A-A) when programmed to a mode with atrial pacing (DDD, DDDR, DDIR, AAI, AAIR), with separately programmable sensed (SAV) and paced (PAV) AV delays. The AV delay can be programmed to be rate-adaptive with flexibility for the maximum and minimum values, as well as the lowest and highest rates for which these AV delays apply. The postventricular atrial refractory period (PVARP) is programmable and occurs after paced, sensed, and refractory sensed ventricular events. In the event of a device-defined premature ventricular complex (PVC), the PVARP is extended to 400 msec (a programmable on/off feature). The PVARP is automatically adjusted by the rate-adaptive sensor to allow tracking of higher atrial rates. The ventricular refractory period (VRP) is also programmable in duration and serves to prevent oversensing of T waves. It is initiated with ventricular-paced, ventricular-sensed, or refractory-sensed ventricular events. The atrium is blanked after ventricular paced or sensed events (PVAB) and is programmable. Atrial sensing is also blanked during the first 50–100 msec of the AV delay, depending on the programmed atrial amplitude and pulse duration. Ventricular blanking occurs after a sensed, paced, or refractory-sensed ventricular event and is a nonprogrammable value of 50–100 msec, depending on the amplitude of the ventricular stimulus.

The first generation of biventricular ICDs also utilized standard timing cycles. However, there are significant differences between sensing with the Medtronic InSync ICD and the Guidant Contak CD. Both of these ICDs stimulate the right ventricle and the left ventricle simultaneously with a parallel, split-cathodal configuration, without an option for independent timing of the LV and RV pulse. The major difference between these ICDs is in the sensing configuration. The Medtronic InSync ICD utilizes only the RV channel for sensing. As such, the sensing function is the same as for standard dual chamber ICDs. In contrast, the Guidant Contak CD and Contak CD II devices use a composite electrogram from both the left ventricle and right ventricle for sensing (similar to the Medtronic 8040 pacemaker). As a result of this composite electrogram, there is an increased risk of double counting of the electrogram during intrinsic conduction or loss of capture in either ventricle (Figure 7–27). This may lead to an increased risk of inappropriate shocks[38] and may require reprogramming of ventricular sensitivity (to a less sensitive value). In addition, careful analysis of the intracardiac electrogram and marker channels is required at the time of implantation device testing to reduce this occurrence. In cases in which this cannot be resolved by reprogramming, repositioning of the LV lead or change of the pulse generator to a device that senses only in the right ventricle to define the cardiac cycle may be required.

### Upper Rate Behavior in Cardiac Resynchronization Therapy Devices

There are many reasons why biventricular pacing may not occur despite a programmed ventricular output amplitude that exceeds threshold in both ventricles (Table 7–6). The most common causes of failure to deliver consistent biventricular pacing relate to sensing near the maximal tracking rate. Upper rate behavior of the Medtronic 8040 CRT pacemaker may be Wenckebach or 2:1, as determined by the programmed upper tracking rate and the total atrial refractory period. If every other atrial event falls within PVARP, 2:1 block occurs. If the atrial rate exceeds the upper tracking rate but is less than the 2:1 rate, the ventricular rate is limited and pacemaker Wenckebach pacing occurs. The upper tracking limit is determined by the total atrial refractory period (TARP), the combination of the AV delay and the PVARP. Thus if the TARP is equal to 450 msec (an AV delay of 150 msec and a PVARP of 300 msec), 2:1 block will occur when the atrial rate exceeds 133 bpm, regardless of the programmed upper tracking rate.

An especially important aspect of CRT devices that sense with a composite electrogram from both the left ventricle and right ventricle is the difference between the TARP during biventricular pacing (pTARP) and the TARP during intrinsic (nonpaced) rhythm (iTARP). Figure 7–28 illustrates this distinction. In the presence of a prolonged QRS duration and IVCD, a CRT device that senses in both the left ventricle and right ventricle often double counts the intrinsic ventricular electrogram (Figure 7–29). As a result, the ventricular refractory period and the PVARP are reset by the electrogram component from the chamber with latest activation. For example, in a patient with LBBB the composite ventricular electrogram includes an early RV component and a late LV component, with the interval between the LV and RV electrogram components reflecting the interventricular conduction delay (see Figure 7–29). Thus if there is double counting of the ventricular electrogram during a sensed intrinsic ventricular rhythm, the PVARP is reset by the last sensed component of the composite ventricular

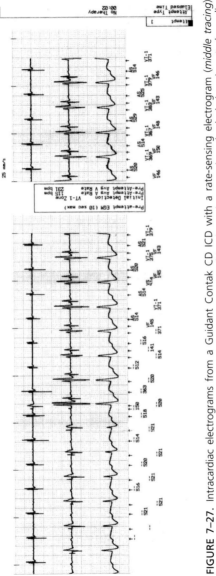
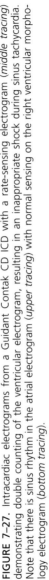

**FIGURE 7–27.** Intracardiac electrograms from a Guidant Contak CD ICD with a rate-sensing electrogram (*middle tracing*) demonstrating double counting of the ventricular electrogram, resulting in an inappropriate shock during sinus tachycardia. Note that there is sinus rhythm in the atrial electrogram (*upper tracing*) with normal sensing on the right ventricular morphology electrogram (*bottom tracing*).

TABLE 7–6. **Differential Diagnosis of Causes for Loss of Biventricular Pacing without Loss of Left Ventricular Capture**

| PROGRAMMING CONSIDERATIONS |
| --- |
| Long AV Delay |
| Failure to program sensed AV delay offset |
| Failure to optimize rate adaptive AV delay |
| Prolonged PVARP |
| Low maximal tracking rate |
| Post PVC extension of PVARP |
| AV Search Hysteresis |
| Rate smoothing up |
| Rate smoothing down |
| DDI or DDIR pacing mode |

| ELECTROGRAM CONSIDERATIONS |
| --- |
| Atrial undersensing |
| Ventricular double counting |
| Far-field atrial potentials in the ventricular electrogram |
| T wave oversensing |
| Myopotentials |
| Atrial fibrillation with mode switching |
| Blanked atrial flutter search |
| Diaphragmatic oversensing |
| Ventricular crosstalk |
| Prolonged intrinsic PR interval |
| Junctional rhythm |

electrogram and the iTARP will be equal to the AV delay plus the IVCD plus the PVARP (iTARP = AVD + IVCD + PVARP). As an example, if there is normal biventricular pacing (with single counting of the ventricular electrogram) with an AV delay of 120 msec and a PVARP of 300 msec, the pTARP will equal 420 msec and atrial tracking will occur at rates up to 142 bpm. However, if there is an intrinsic ventricular rhythm with a ventricular double counting and an IVCD of 150 msec, the iTARP will equal 570 msec and 2:1 block will occur at rates greater than 105 bpm. Because of double counting of the ventricular electrogram, the iTARP exceeds the pTARP by an interval equal to the IVCD.

The practical importance of the iTARP concept is that patients may demonstrate lack of ventricular pacing at slower heart rates than would be predicted by addition of the AV delay to the PVARP. Of course, without ventricular pacing the CRT device will not provide the hemodynamic benefits of cardiac resynchronization. This phenomenon is especially likely to occur in the presence of PVCs with automatic extension of the PVARP to 400 msec. Following a PVC, the next atrial event may fall within PVARP and the next ventricular stimulus will be inhibited (Figure 7–30). The intrinsic QRS complex will then be double counted and the subsequent PVARP delayed by an interval equal to the IVCD. Thus intrinsic conduction begets intrinsic conduction by continuous resetting of the PVARP by an interval equal to the IVCD. This leads to at least three potential upper-rate behavior zones. At rates above the upper tracking rate and below the 2:1 rate, pacemaker Wenckebach conduction may occur. If a higher upper tracking rate is programmed, the conditional upper tracking limit will be equal

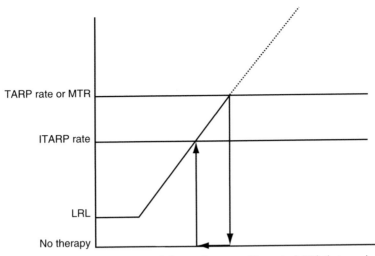

**FIGURE 7–28.** Graphical presentation of the maximum tracking rate (MTR) that can be achieved during consistent biventricular pacing (total atrial refractory period [TARP] rate), which is determined by adding the atrioventricular (AV) delay + postventricular atrial refractory period (PVARP). However, during a sensed ventricular rhythm using a composite ventricular electrogram from both the right ventricle and left ventricle, the intrinsic TARP (iTARP) is equal to AV delay + intraventricular conduction delay (IVCD) + PVARP. Thus the atrial rate that will be tracked is equal to the TARP rate during biventricular pacing but the iTARP rate during double sensing of the composite ventricular electrogram. The difference between TARP and iTARP is equal to the IVCD in the ventricular electrogram. *(Reproduced from Wang P, Kramer A, Estes M, Hayes DL. Timing cycles for biventricular pacing. PACE 2002;25:62-75, with permission from Blackwell Publishing Ltd.)*

to that consistent with the pTARP. However, if ventricular pacing is inhibited for any reason, the upper tracking limit will decrease to that consistent with the iTARP. The width of this conditional tracking zone is equal to the IVCD. Thus the wider the intra-cardiac electrogram, the more marked this effect. Another potential cause of double counting of the ventricular electrogram, despite continued ventricular pacing, is that associated with loss of LV capture (Figure 7–31). If the pacing stimulus fails to capture the left ventricle, RV pacing may result in a prolonged interventricular conduction interval and double counting. Thus the PVARP is extended by an interval equal to the IVCD and 2:1 block may occur at relatively slow ventricular rates. In order to minimize double counting and anomalous upper rate tracking behavior, the post PVC extension of the PVARP should be programmed "off" and the ventricular pacing stimulus must be of sufficient amplitude and duration to ensure consistent biventricular capture. Careful analysis of pacemaker diagnostics will provide a clue to this phenomenon by demonstrating a significant proportion of ventricular sensed rather than paced events (Figure 7–32).

Another way of considering this difference between the pTARP and the iTARP intervals is that they add a zone of hysteresis to the atrial tracking of CRT devices. As the atrial rate increases, atrial tracking is maintained until the maximum tracking rate (MTR) is reached, unless an intrinsic QRS is sensed. However, once the MTR has been exceeded and tracking has been interrupted by pacemaker Wenckebach or 2:1 upper rate behavior, the atrial rate must fall significantly below the MTR in order

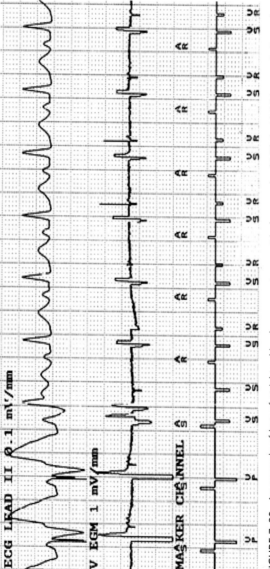

**FIGURE 7-29.** An example of loss of atrial tracking by a premature ventricular complex (PVC) that inhibits ventricular pacing for one beat, followed by a double counting of the intrinsically conducted ventricular electrogram. Because of a long intraventricular conduction delay, double counting resets the ventricular refractory period and the postventricular atrial refractory period (PVARP) such that the next atrial electrogram occurs during PVARP. As a result, there is perpetuation of intrinsic conduction and failure to maintain consistent cardiac resynchronization therapy. (*Courtesy Medtronic, Inc.*)

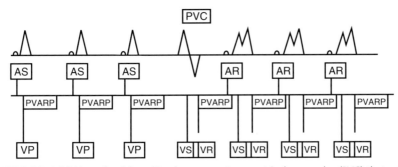

**FIGURE 7–30.** Inhibition of atrial tracking by a premature ventricular complex (PVC) that extends the postventricular atrial refractory period (PVARP) to 400 msec. As a result of post-PVC PVARP extension, the subsequent atrial electrogram falls within the PVARP, inhibiting tracking and leading to persistent double counting of the ventricular electrograms during left bundle branch block intrinsic conduction. *(Courtesy Medtronic, Inc.)*

for atrial tracking to be reestablished. The disadvantage of this phenomenon is that the patient would lose the hemodynamic benefits of cardiac resynchronization at rates that the clinician had expected pacing to be maintained. A specific feature of newer generations of CRT devices is to shorten the PVARP at high rates to maintain tracking even in the iTARP zone (a feature known as Tracking Preference in the Guidant Renewal CRT device; Figure 7–33). Tracking Preference allows retraction of the PVARP when an atrial sensed event occurs after a ventricular sensed event for two consecutive cycles and the atrial rate is below the MTR. The PVARP remains

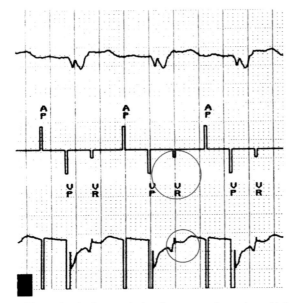

**FIGURE 7–31.** Double sensing in the ventricular electrogram due to loss of left ventricular capture. The pacing stimulus captures the right ventricle but not the left ventricle. The prolonged conduction time from the right ventricle to the left ventricle results in double counting of the ventricular rate. *(Courtesy Medtronic, Inc.)*

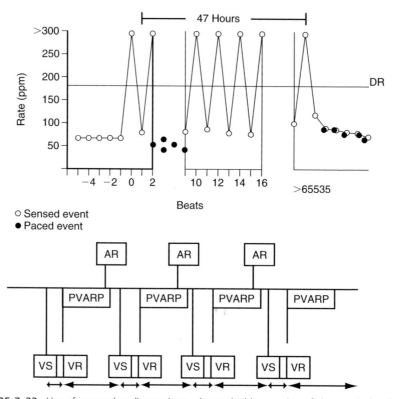

FIGURE 7–32. Use of pacemaker diagnostics to detect double counting of the ventricular electrogram. Note that double counting in the ventricular electrogram (*open circles*) occurs and lasts for 47 hours. During this period no effective cardiac resynchronization therapy is delivered.

retracted until a ventricular paced event occurs at the programmed AV delay. Thus the iTARP is made to equal the pTARP by this feature, allowing more physiologic MTRs to be achieved (Figure 7–34). The potential disadvantage of this feature is the possibility of promoting pacemaker-mediated tachycardia.

## Timing Cycles of Cardiac Resynchronization Therapy Devices with Independent Left Ventricular and Right Ventricular Output Circuits

Because optimal management of intraventricular synchrony in the left ventricle requires flexibility in the timing of RV and LV stimulation, the present generation of CRT devices offer independent programmability of the RV and LV output circuits. Although this added flexibility allows greater chances to achieve optimal hemodynamic function, it also greatly increases the complexity of follow-up and troubleshooting.[39] True biventricular pacing and sensing offer several possibilities for control of the ventricular rate. For example, after a ventricular sensed event, the VA interval could be timed to either the RV or the LV electrogram, depending on the site of earliest ventricular sensing (Figure 7–35). However, timing could also be based on either the right ventricle or left ventricle alone, resulting in timing that is either RV-based or LV-based

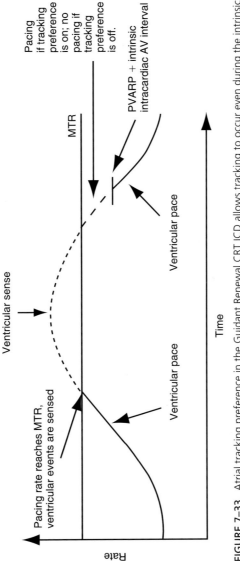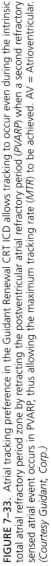

**FIGURE 7–33.** Atrial tracking preference in the Guidant Renewal CRT ICD allows tracking to occur even during the intrinsic total atrial refractory period zone by retracting the postventricular atrial refractory period (*PVARP*) when a second refractory sensed atrial event occurs in PVARP, thus allowing the maximum tracking rate (*MTR*) to be achieved. AV = Atrioventricular. (*Courtesy Guidant, Corp.*)

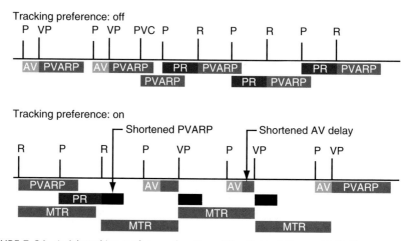

**FIGURE 7–34.** Atrial tracking preference function of the Guidant Renewal ICD. If two successive cycles occur in which a sensed right ventricular event is preceded by an atrial event that occurs in postventricular atrial refractory period (*PVARP*), the PVARP shortens until normal atrial tracking is restored. The atrial electrogram is tracked at rates up to the maximum tracking rate (*MTR*). At rates above MRT, atrial tracking preference is disabled. *(Courtesy Guidant Corporation.)*

(Figure 7–36). By allowing the left ventricle to be stimulated either before or after the right ventricle (either a negative or positive RV-LV interval, respectively), the AV delay (RA-LV) will vary directly with the RV-LV interval (Figure 7–37). At the lower pacing rate, the atrium will be paced while various combinations of RV and LV sensing or pacing or both may occur. For example, an atrial pacing stimulus could be followed by an RV-sensed event and an LV-sensed event (RVs and LVs), an LV-sensed event and an RV-paced event (when a negative RV-LV interval is programmed), an RV-sensed and an LV-paced event (when a positive RV-LV interval is programmed) or an RV-paced event and an LV-paced event. Because of these multiple combinations, Wang et al.[39] have proposed a three-letter code to specify these features of pacing and sensing (Figure 7–38).

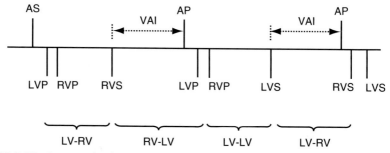

**FIGURE 7–35.** An example of a potential scheme for biventricular sensing in which a sensed or paced event in either the left ventricle or right ventricle could reset the ventriculoatrial interval (*VAI*) with a delay between the left ventricular pacing stimulus and the right ventricular pacing stimulus. This could lead to an irregular ventricular rhythm because the intervals could vary from one ventricle to the other. AP = Atrial paced; AS = atrial sensed; LVP = left-ventricular paced; LVS = left-ventricular sensed; RVP = right-ventricular paced; RVS = right-ventricular sensed. *(Reproduced from Wang P, Kramer A, Estes M, Hayes DL. Timing cycles for biventricular pacing. PACE 2002;25:62-75, with permission from Blackwell Publishing Ltd.)*

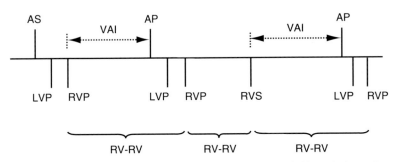

**FIGURE 7–36.** An example of right ventricular (*RV*)-based timing with biventricular pacing with a left ventricular (*LV*)-RV delay. RV sensed or paced events are used to reset the ventriculoatrial (VA) interval. This configuration is used in the Guidant Renewal III and the Medtronic InSync III cardiac resynchronization therapy devices. AP = Atrial paced; AS = atrial sensed; LVP = left-ventricular paced; LVS = left-ventricular sensed; RVP = right-ventricular paced; RVS = right-ventricular sensed; VAI = VA interval. *(Reproduced from Wang P, Kramer A, Estes M, Hayes DL. Timing cycles for biventricular pacing. PACE 2002;25:62-75, with permission from Blackwell Publishing Ltd.)*

The first letter in the code would indicate which of the ventricular chambers are paced (R = right, L = left, B = both). The second letter would indicate the ventricular chambers used for sensing (R, L, or B). The third letter would specify which ventricular chamber is used to reset the cardiac timing cycle (R, L, B, or T, where T = biventricular triggered mode). The triggered mode (a feature of the St. Jude Medical Model 5508 and Medtronic InSync III CRT pacemakers) can be programmed such that a simultaneous pacing stimulus is delivered to both the right ventricle and left ventricle when a sensed R wave is generated from either the right ventricle or the left ventricle (see the following discussion).

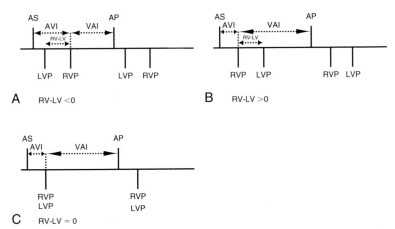

**FIGURE 7–37.** Examples of negative right ventricular (*RV*)-left ventricular (*LV*) delay (*A*), positive RV-LV delay (*B*), and simultaneous RV-LV stimulation with RV-based timing. All of these options are available in the Guidant Renewal III and the Medtronic InSync III cardiac resynchronization therapy devices. AP = Atrial paced; AS = atrial sensed; LVP = left-ventricular paced; LVS = left-ventricular sensed; RVP = right-ventricular paced; RVS = right-ventricular sensed; VAI = Ventriculoatrial interval. *(Reproduced from Wang P, Kramer A, Estes M, Hayes DL. Timing cycles for biventricular pacing. PACE 2002;25:62-75, with permission from Blackwell Publishing Ltd.)*

Biventricular Pacing Code and Lower Rate Limit Timing Events

| Biventricular Pacing Code | | | LRL Timing Events | | | |
|---|---|---|---|---|---|---|
| Ventricles Paced | Ventricles Sensed | Ventricular Timing | RVP | LVP | RVS | LVS |
| B | B | R | X |  | X |  |
| B | B | L |  | X |  | X |
| B | B | B | X | X | X | X |
| B | R | R* | X |  | X |  |
| B | R | B* | X | X | X |  |
| B | L | R* | X |  |  |  |
| B | L | L |  | X |  | X |
| B | L | B | X | X |  | X |
| R | B | R | X |  | X |  |
| R | B | L |  |  |  | X |
| R | B | B | X |  | X | X |
| R | R | L+ |  |  |  |  |
| R | R | B+ | X |  | X |  |
| R | L | R* | X |  |  |  |
| R | L | L |  |  |  | X |
| R | L | B | X |  |  | X |
| L | B | L |  | X |  | X |
| L | B | B |  | X | X | X |
| L | R | R |  |  | X |  |
| L | R | L* |  | X |  |  |
| L | R | B |  | X | X |  |
| L | L | R+ |  |  |  |  |
| L | L | L |  | X |  | X |
| L | L | B+ |  | X |  | X |

*Indicates timing using a channel in which sensing is absent.
+Indicates timing using a channel in which pacing or sensing is absent. LRL = lower rate limit; RVP = right-ventricular paced; LVP = left-ventricular paced; RVS = right-ventricular sensed; LVS = left-ventricular sensed; B = both ventricular chambers; R = right ventricle; L = left ventricle.

FIGURE 7–38. A proposed code for indicating biventricular pacing, sensing, and timing. Although potentially useful, most newer generations of cardiac resynchronization therapy devices will pace both ventricles, sense in both ventricles, and have right ventricular-based timing. Nevertheless, various combinations of sensing and timing are in use at present. (Reproduced from Wang P, Kramer A, Estes M, Hayes DL. Timing cycles for biventricular pacing. PACE 2002;25:62-75, with permission from Blackwell Publishing Ltd.)

## Upper Rate Behavior of CRT Devices with Independent Ventricular Channels

To maintain optimal cardiac resynchronization over the range of physiologic heart rates, the MTR should be programmed to a value at least as high as the expected exercise sinus rate (generally 220 − Age). The use of a nominal value for the MTR of 120 bpm in all patients only ensures that most patients will not have effective resynchronization during exercise. Because a low MTR will result in pacemaker Wenckebach block, this will result in loss of ventricular pacing due to intrinsic AV conduction or a variable AV delay and loss of optimal diastolic filling (in the presence of AV block). In either case, a low MTR will adversely impact hemodynamic function.

## Sensing Issues with Separate Right Ventricular and Left Ventricular Pacing Stimuli

Simultaneous biventricular stimulation may be combined with sensing that is right ventricle only (such as the Medtronic 7272 ICD) or from both the right ventricle and the left ventricle (Medtronic 8040 and Guidant Contak CD). Sensing issues become much more complex when stimulation is independently applied with a delay between the right ventricle and the left ventricle (Medtronic InSync III and Guidant Renewal). In the case of RV-only or LV-only sensing with a delay between the RV-LV pacing stimuli, there is a risk that a pacing stimulus will be delivered asynchronously in the chamber that is not sensed (Figure 7–39). For example, in an RV-only sensing CRT device with a positive RV-LV interval, it is possible for an unsensed LV event to be followed by an RV-paced event and a later LV-paced event. This may be especially likely in the presence of a long LV to RV conduction interval (IVCD) and a long AV delay. It is possible that this could result in LV pacing within the vulnerable period of the left ventricle. The Medtronic InSync Marquis ICD uses A-A timing. Ventricular sensing is based on the RV electrogram. Although this device offers biventricular stimulation, sensing does not occur in the left ventricle, and the VA interval is based on either an RV-sensed or RV-paced event. Because the RV-LV interval can be programmed from +80 (left ventricle after right ventricle) to −80 msec (right ventricle after left ventricle), there is the potential for an LV-sensed

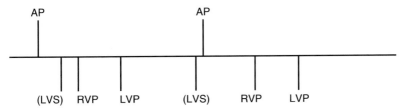

**FIGURE 7–39.** An example of right ventricular (*RV*) sensing with biventricular pacing having a delay between RV and left ventricular (*LV*) pacing stimuli. A premature ventricular complex (PVC) occurring in the LV that is not sensed (left-ventricular sensed [*LVS*]) will be followed by an RV pacing stimulus and then by an LV pacing stimulus. If the interval from the LV PVC to the RV pacing stimulus is long due to interventricular conduction delay, an LV pacing stimulus could potentially be delivered in the vulnerable period of the LV. AP = Atrial paced; LVP = left-ventricular paced; RVP = right-ventricular paced; RVS = right-ventricular sensed. *(Reproduced from Wang P, Kramer A, Estes M, Hayes DL. Timing cycles for biventricular pacing. PACE 2002;25:62-75, with permission from Blackwell Publishing Ltd.)*

to LV-paced interval to be as long as the IVCD plus 80 msec. For example, consider a patient with right bundle branch block with an RV to LV interval of 160 msec and a programmed RV- to LV-paced interval of 80 msec. If an unsensed event occurs in the left ventricle, it may not be sensed in the right ventricle for 160 msec and an RV-paced event could be delivered up to 160 msec after the unsensed LV event (LV-sensed to RV-paced). Because the LV stimulus is delivered 80 msec after the RV stimulus, the LV-sensed–to–LV-paced interval would be 240 msec, potentially in the LV vulnerable period. Although this example is extreme, such an occurrence is possible. Programming the RV-paced–to–LV-paced interval to a more realistic value of 20 msec or less would minimize the chance of LV capture in the vulnerable period. Therefore prevention of this theoretical possibility will require that the clinician appreciate this risk and limit the RV-LV interval that is programmed.

The Medtronic InSync III pacemaker allows clinicians to select the ventricular sensing configuration between RV bipolar (nominal), RV tip to LV tip, or left ventricle. RV bipolar sensing is certainly the easiest to understand and avoids double counting, whereas LV unipolar sensing is usually reserved for testing of the LV lead. This device also offers an interventricular refractory period (IVRP) that is active when sensing is RV tip to LV tip and should be programmed to the patient's IVCD + 30 msec (Figure 7–40). This programmable interval is designed to prevent double counting of ventricular events that are sensed in one ventricle, thereby avoiding reset of the VRP, PVAB, and PVARP. The Medtronic InSync III also offers a feature known as *Ventricular Sense Response* (Figure 7–41) that is designed for use when the sensing configuration is programmed LV tip to RV tip. The ventricular sense response is designed to deliver a pacing triggered stimulus to both the right ventricle and the left ventricle at the minimum V-V pace delay (4 msec) when a sensed ventricular event occurs in the AV interval. This feature is intended to prevent loss of CRT pacing during rapid atrial rates or in response to late-coupled PVCs.

Another sensing option for CRT devices is to sense in both the right ventricle and left ventricle and to use the first sensed event to change the VA interval. The challenge with this method of sensing is that it may be difficult to discriminate between IVCD and a PVC. The option that has been chosen for sensing in the most recent generation of Guidant CRT-ICD devices is to use RV sensing to define the cardiac cycle for tachycardia and bradycardia sensing but to use LV sensing to protect the LV from pacing within its vulnerable period. This option has the significant advantages of maintaining the proven record of tachycardia detection of previous generation of ICDs and simplifying the understanding of device behavior. Because the cardiac cycle interval is based on the right ventricle only, timing is not dependent on the programmed pacing chamber(s), and only one cardiac cycle interval is used for tachycardia and bradycardia sensing. Thus the ventricular interval is timed from one RV-paced or sensed event to the next RV event (whether paced or sensed). Why then is there a need for LV sensing? The answer lies in prevention of unsafe LV pacing into the vulnerable period. Thus LV-sensed events are used to initiate a LV protection period during which LV pacing stimuli are inhibited (Figure 7–42). The LV protection period is programmable between 300 and 500 msec after an LV sensed event. The potential for inappropriate sensing with a unipolar LV lead is illustrated in Figure 7–43.

Another potentially hazardous aspect of a prolonged IVCD is that an abrupt change from a sensed intrinsic QRS to a biventricular paced QRS may also result in

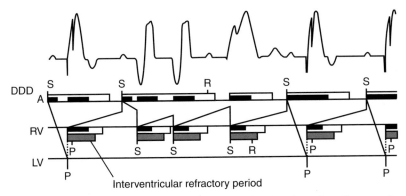

Interventricular refractory period

FIGURE 7–40. Interventricular refractory period of the Medtronic InSync III cardiac resynchronization therapy pacemaker. This device allows a right ventricular (*RV*)-left ventricular (*LV*) pacing delay
with options for RV bipolar sensing, RV-tip to LV-tip sensing, or LV unipolar sensing. When
programmed to RV-tip to LV-tip sensing, an interventricular refractory period is present in both chambers that should be programmed at least 30 msec longer than the intrinsic interventricular conduction
delay (IVCD). P = Paced event; R = refractory event; S = sensed event. *(Courtesy Medtronic, Inc.)*

LV pacing into the LV vulnerable period. This is most likely to occur when the atrial
rate falls from above to below the maximum tracking rate. For example, consider a
patient with LBBB with an IVCD of 150 msec during intrinsic conduction who has
a programmed maximum tracking rate of 150 bpm (400 msec). If the atrial rate
decreases from 151 to 150 bpm there will be an abrupt change from an intrinsically

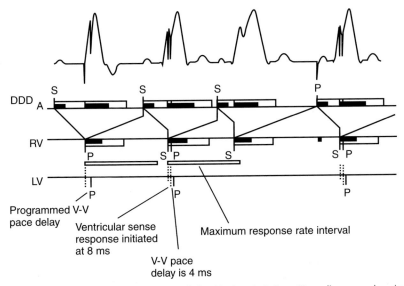

Programmed V-V
pace delay

Ventricular sense
response initiated
at 8 ms

V-V pace
delay is 4 ms

Maximum response rate interval

FIGURE 7–41. Ventricular sense response of the Medtronic InSync III cardiac resynchronization
therapy pacemaker. This function is designed to ensure biventricular pacing without inhibition in
the presence of ventricular sensing. When programmed to "pace" and a ventricular-sensed event
occurs in the atrioventricular interval, a biventricular stimulus is delivered at the minimum V-V delay
(4 msec). LV = Left ventricular; P = paced event; R = refractory event; RV = right ventricular;
S = sensed event. *(Courtesy Medtronic, Inc.)*

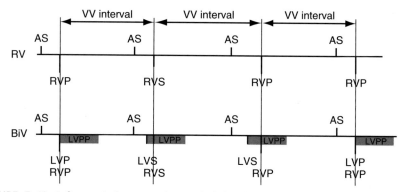

**FIGURE 7–42.** Left ventricular protection period (*LVPP*) of the Guidant Renewal ICD. This implantable cardioverter-defibrillator (ICD) has right ventricular (*RV*) timing and independent RV and left ventricular (*LV*) stimulation channels without a programmable RV-LV delay. The LVPP allows LV sensing to occur with inhibition of the LV stimulus for a period that is programmable to prevent pacing into the vulnerable period of the left ventricle. Thus this feature allows biventricular sensing but RV-based timing. AS = Atrial sensed; BiV = biventricular; LVP = left-ventricular paced; LVS = left-ventricular sensed; RVP = right-ventricular paced; RVS = right-ventricular sensed. *(Courtesy Guidant, Corp.)*

conducted LBBB QRS to biventricular pacing. In this case, the first cardiac cycle with resumption of normal tracking would result in an LV-sensed–to–LV-paced interval of 250 msec, a value that is potentially in the vulnerable period of the left ventricle. Thus the LV protection period is a potentially important feature for prevention of pacing-induced ventricular arrhythmias.

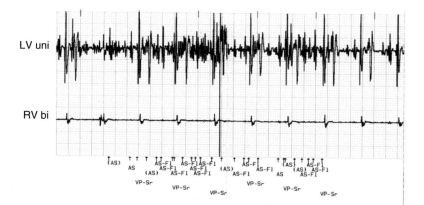

**FIGURE 7–43.** Example of unipolar left ventricular (*LV*) sensing and bipolar right ventricular (*RV*) sensing in a cardiac resynchronization therapy (CRT) device. In this patient with chronic atrial fibrillation and complete atrioventricular (AV) block, a unipolar cardiac venous lead, and a bipolar RV lead, the cardiac venous lead was connected to the atrial channel of a dual chamber pacemaker and the RV lead was connected to the ventricular channel. Biventricular pacing was accomplished by programming the pacemaker to the DDIR pacing mode with an AV delay of 10 msec. Thus the atrial channel records from the cardiac venous lead while the ventricular channel records from the RV lead. Note the marked myopotentials in the atrial but not the ventricular electrogram. This points out the potential hazards of unipolar LV sensing and explains why unipolar LV sensing is not used to time the cardiac cycle of implantable cardioverter-defibrillators offering CRT.

## Biventricular Sensing and Premature Ventricular Contractions

Standard dual chamber pacemakers or ICDs define a PVC as a ventricular-sensed event following either a ventricular paced or sensed event without an intervening atrial event (either paced or sensed). If there is biventricular sensing, two ventricular sensed events (RVs and LVs) will occur after an atrial event when there is intrinsic AV conduction, thereby potentially creating confusion that this was actually a PVC. A potential solution to this problem is to create a cross-chamber refractory period after sensing in the opposite ventricular chamber so that such double counting does not occur (Medtronic InSync III). An alternative approach to this problem is to use a triggered mode such that sensing in either chamber would result in an immediate pacing stimulus (St. Jude Medical Model 5508 or Medtronic InSync III). The triggered mode in the St. Jude Medical device is referred to as "DDT timing" and gives the user the option of triggering the pacing stimulus concurrently with the P wave, the R wave, or both the P wave and R wave (when DDT timing is set to "DDD"). When the DDT timing is set to "DDI" the pacing stimulus is triggered only by a sensed R wave. Figure 7–44 illustrates the function of a ventricular triggered event. In this example, a sensed event in the right ventricle may result in triggering of an early LV pacing stimulus to ensure resynchronization. Thus in a triggered mode, the RV-LV interval could be different for sensed than for paced events. In the triggered mode, it is important to sense in both the left ventricle and right ventricle so that both chambers are stimulated immediately without regard to the IVCD. This feature requires a limit on the maximum paced rate as well as the number of sequential triggered beats that will be delivered. The St. Jude Frontier CRT device also offers the option of an atrial-triggered mode in which an atrial sensed event in the atrial alert period generates a RA pacing stimulus. This feature is contraindicated for patients with chronic atrial tachyarrhythmias, and its utility to reduce paroxysmal atrial arrhythmias has yet to be demonstrated.

## Oversensing of Atrial Signals in the Ventricular Electrogram

Because the coronary sinus electrogram includes both LA and LV components, a cardiac venous lead that is positioned in a basal region may present a difficult oversensing problem. For example, the atrial component of the cardiac venous electrogram may inhibit delivery of the ventricular pacing stimulus. Figure 7–45A illustrates an example of triple sensing in the ventricular electrogram due to a cardiac venous lead that was placed in a basal region. As a result, the composite electrogram from the right ventricle and left ventricle includes an LA deflection, a LV deflection, and a RV deflection with a programmed ventricular sensitivity threshold of 2.8 mV. Reprogramming to a less sensitive ventricular value (5.6 mV) eliminated oversensing and allowed atrial tracking to be resumed (Figure 7–45B). The disadvantage of this strategy is that normal ventricular sensing may be lost, predisposing to ventricular arrhythmias. In such a case it is wise to reposition the cardiac venous lead to a new position.

## The Problem of a Long PR Interval

Standard dual chamber pacemakers have difficulty maintaining atrial tracking in the presence of a very prolonged PR interval. This may be especially troubling to

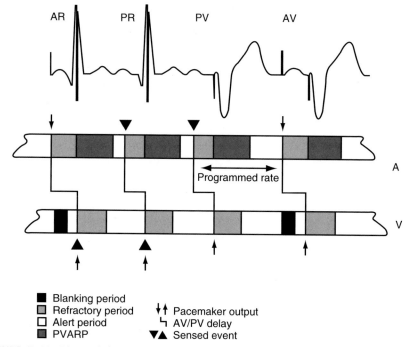

AR    PR    PV    AV

A

Programmed rate

V

■ Blanking period
□ Refractory period    ↓↑ Pacemaker output
□ Alert period          ↳ AV/PV delay
▨ PVARP                ▼▲ Sensed event

FIGURE 7–44. Triggered function of the St. Jude Medical Frontier cardiac resynchronization therapy device. This device can be programmed to deliver a synchronous pacing stimulus to the atrium or both ventricles in response to atrial or ventricular sensed events. AR = atrial paced, ventricular sensed; AV = atrial paced, ventricular paced; PR = atrial sensed, ventricular sensed; PV = atrial sensed, ventricular paced; PVARP = postventricular atrial refractory period. *(Courtesy St. Jude Medical.)*

some patients if the P wave occurs soon after the preceding R wave, because this may result in atrial contraction during ventricular systole. This may result in cannon A waves in the neck veins and pulmonary veins and pseudopacemaker syndrome. This same phenomenon may also occur in biventricular pacemakers, thereby inhibiting cardiac resynchronization. However, because of the IVCD and the iTARP mechanism discussed previously, biventricular pacing systems are even more likely to encounter this problem.[40] The use of downward rate smoothing may prevent this from occurring. In addition, the Guidant Renewal CRT device offers a feature to shorten the PVARP at rates between the iTARP and the MTR, which may help to minimize this problem. However, for patients with a very long PR interval that approaches the RR interval, the only solution may be catheter ablation of the AV node.

### Rate Smoothing

Rate smoothing is a potentially useful feature that prevents abrupt changes in the ventricular paced interval in response to an unstable sinus node, atrial arrhythmias, PACs, or PVCs. When programmed "on," rate smoothing uses the preceding R-R interval to determine a reference value, and the next paced ventricular event is not allowed to vary by more than a programmed percentage of this interval. The ventricular rate may be smoothed in the upward direction (preventing an abrupt increase in ventricular pacing rate) or in the downward direction (preventing an abrupt slowing

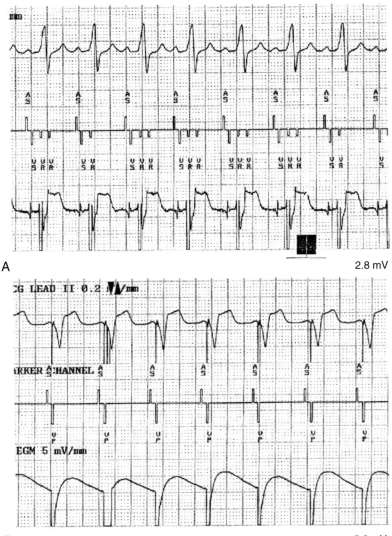

**FIGURE 7–45.** (*A*) Oversensing of the atrial component, right ventricular (RV) component, and left ventricular (LV) component of a composite ventricular electrogram from a lead located in the basal portion of the lateral cardiac vein. Persistent oversensing at a sensitivity setting of 2.8 mV prevented effective resynchronization. Programming to a less sensitive ventricular sensitivity setting of 5.6 mV (*B*) eliminated oversensing and restored cardiac resynchronization therapy.

in ventricular paced rate). Rate smoothing (down) has been demonstrated to prevent ventricular arrhythmias that are induced by a long-short sequence of ventricular intervals. In some cases rate smoothing (up) may prevent the induction of ventricular tachycardias by prevention of tracking PACs that would result in an S1S2 effect in the ventricle (Figure 7–46). However, rate smoothing (down) may prevent or delay detection of monomorphic ventricular tachycardia in some patients with ICDs.

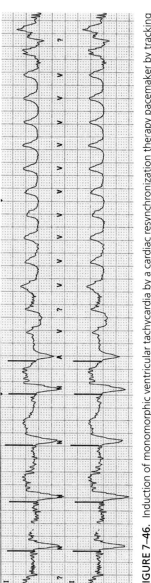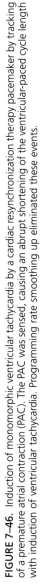

**FIGURE 7–46.** Induction of monomorphic ventricular tachycardia by a cardiac resynchronization therapy pacemaker by tracking of a premature atrial contraction (PAC). The PAC was sensed, causing an abrupt shortening of the ventricular-paced cycle length with induction of ventricular tachycardia. Programming rate smoothing up eliminated these events.

The mechanism for this interference with ventricular tachycardia (VT) detection is the induction of rapid pacing by rate smoothing during VT, which introduces ventricular blanking periods that follow paced events (Figure 7–47). For example, Glikson and colleagues[41] demonstrated that programming rate smoothing "down" delayed (two cases) or prevented (four cases) detection of 10 monomorphic ventricular tachycardias induced in 16 patients (cycle length ranging from 270 to 430 msec). In all cases, programming the AV delay to the dynamic mode eliminated nondetection. This adverse effect of rate smoothing was more significant when the percentage change allowed was 3% and decreased when greater percentage values were programmed. This effect was worse the higher the maximal pacing rate programmed. Rate smoothing down may also interfere with consistent delivery of resynchronization therapy, such that PVCs may lead to an increase in the ventricular-paced rate with VVI pacing and loss of AV synchrony (Figure 7–48). Rate smoothing in the upward direction may lead to prolongation of the AV interval and loss of optimal AV timing. If rate smoothing prevents tracking of an increase in atrial rate (Figure 7–49), intrinsic conduction may occur, leading to perpetuation of loss of tracking due to the iTARP mechanism discussed previously. As a result, it is usually best to program rate smoothing "off" in a CRT device.

In biventricular pacing, rate smoothing in the "up" direction may also limit consistent delivery of CRT, because prevention of change in the paced R-R interval may allow intrinsic AV conduction to occur. If intrinsic conduction is present, there may be double counting of the ventricular electrogram because of a long IVCD and perpetuation of ventricular pacing inhibition. This may be especially likely when the sinus node is unstable or when there are frequent PACs (thereby invoking rate smoothing in the upward direction). Because of this potential, it may be wise to turn off rate smoothing in a CRT device or to limit the aggressiveness of the programmed percentage value allowed.

## Mode Switching

Automatic mode-switching algorithms that prevent tracking of atrial tachyarrhythmias by conversion to a nontracking mode (VVIR or VDIR) have been

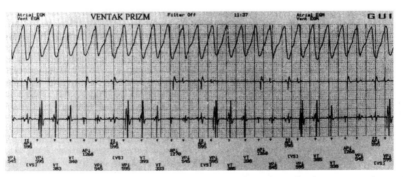

**FIGURE 7–47.** Example of sustained monomorphic ventricular tachycardia that was not detected by a dual chamber implantable cardioverter-defibrillator due to aggressive programming of rate smoothing down. Rate smoothing results in rapid ventricular pacing during ventricular tachycardia (VT), inhibiting detection of VT by introducing ventricular blanking periods at a rate similar to the tachycardia. *(Reproduced from Glikson M, Beeman AL, Luria DM, et al: Impaired detection of ventricular tachyarrhythmias by rate-smoothing algorithm in dual chamber implantable defibrillators: intradevice interaction.* J Cardiovasc Electrophysiol *2002;13:312-318, with permission from Blackwell Publishing Ltd.)*

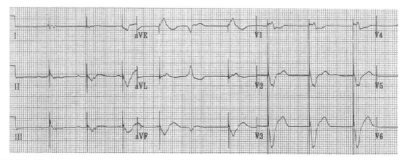

**FIGURE 7–48.** Rate switching down. In the left portion of the tracing, there is atrial tracking with a premature ventricular complex (fifth beat from left). Rate smoothing down results in an increase in the ventricular pacing rate with loss of atrioventricular synchrony for the subsequent beats as the ventricular rate gradually slows. Rate smoothing may prevent abrupt changes in ventricular pacing rate but may cause major disruption in consistent cardiac resynchronization therapy.

especially useful for patients with DDD pacemakers or ICDs. Despite their usefulness, some mode-switching algorithms may force the minimum sensed AV interval to a nonphysiologic value. In the Medtronic 8040 CRT pacemaker, programming mode switching "on" automatically assigns the minimum sensed AV delay a value of 30 msec. Because this sensed AV delay is not physiologic, biventricular pacing will occur before the left atrium has been activated. Thus at high atrial tracking rates the patient will lose the benefits of optimized LA-LV timing. Limiting the MTR to a relatively low value will only exacerbate this inappropriate shortening of the sensed AV delay. Thus mode switching should be programmed "on" only when there is a real indication to limit tracking of intermittent atrial arrhythmias. The aggressive use of antiarrhythmic medications such as amiodarone to prevent atrial fibrillation may be justified in patients who require CRT. Other CRT devices have overcome many of these limitations by more sophisticated mode-switching algorithms that do not place such limits on the rate-adaptive AV delay.

### Interactions between CRT and ICD Tachycardia Detection Zones

Antitachycardia therapy is based on heart rate zones. For ICDs offering CRT, the lowest VT detection rate that can be programmed is 5 bpm above the MTR (Figure 7–50). Because of this limitation, it may result in trade-offs between the rates for which CRT can be delivered and the slowest VT that can be detected. For example, a patient with a slow monomorphic VT at 130 bpm will usually require programming of the VT detection rate to 120 bpm. If this VT detection rate is programmed, then CRT will be limited to tracking of atrial rates <115 bpm. Alternative VT therapies such as antiarrhythmic drugs or catheter ablation may be required to control slow VT rates to provide effective CRT at all physiologic sinus rates.

### When Is It Time to Consider a Different Left Ventricular Pacing Site?

An important clinical question that the clinician must ask when evaluating patients who have not responded to CRT is whether or not they may improve with a different LV-pacing site. The first step is to be certain that the LV pacing lead

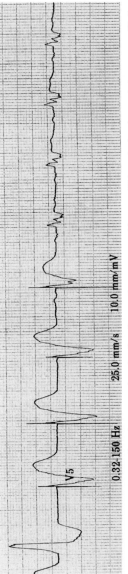

**FIGURE 7–49.** Inhibition of cardiac resynchronization therapy by rate smoothing up. Although the sinus rate increases with the fourth paced complex from the left, the ventricular paced cycle length is smoothed such that the atrioventricular delay of this beat is prolonged. Subsequent sinus beats are no longer tracked due to double counting in the ventricle, with the sinus electrogram falling into the postventricular atrial refractory period.

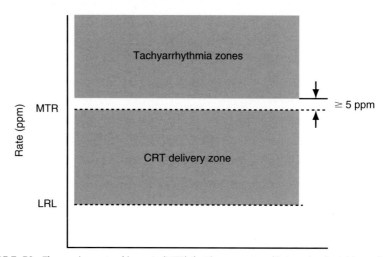

**FIGURE 7–50.** The maximum tracking rate (MTR) that is programmed into an implantable cardioverter-defibrillator (ICD) will limit the minimum ventricular tachycardia (VT) detection rate that is programmed. The slowest tachycardia detection zone must be at least 5 bpm faster than the *MTR*. This is most likely to be a problem when patients need both cardiac resynchronization therapy (*CRT*) and antitachycardia pacing for slow VT. In these instances it may be best to consider catheter ablation of VT, thereby allowing a faster MTR and more effective CRT. LRL = Lower rate limit. *(Courtesy Guidant, Corp.)*

captures the left ventricle. If LV capture is not consistent, one may consider upgrading to a device with separate ventricular output circuits as a way to decrease the pacing threshold (Figure 7–51). Second, assessment of the LA-LV timing is critically important and easily remedied by reprogramming. This should always be examined by Doppler echocardiography before considering an operative intervention. The most difficult

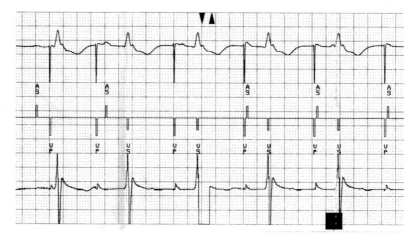

**FIGURE 7–51.** Dislodgement of the cardiac venous lead into the coronary sinus. During left ventricular lead threshold determination with a cardiac resynchronization therapy–implantable cardioverter-defibrillator (Medtronic 7272) capture of the distal coronary sinus is demonstrated. This lead required repositioning into a cardiac vein.

decision is whether the patient requires a different pacing site to achieve improvement in intraventricular synchrony. Before deciding on lead replacement, one should be certain that reprogramming of the RV-LV delay will not improve resynchronization. This requires an assessment of intraventricular synchrony, either with radionuclide angiography, M-mode echocardiographic assessment of septal and lateral wall synchrony or tissue Doppler imaging. If significant intraventricular dyssynchrony is present and cannot be improved by optimization of the RV-LV delay, one should at least consider repositioning of the LV lead. In many cases this will require epicardial lead placement. On the other hand, if the LV lead is located in the anterior interventricular vein, transvenous lead placement may remain feasible. Last, the risk-benefit ratio of reoperation to achieve more effective CRT must be weighed for each patient individually. Such consideration must include an assessment of the patient's ability to withstand reoperation, especially if an epicardial approach is needed.

# Conclusion

Cardiac resynchronization therapy is both very promising and very complex. Troubleshooting and programming can be a challenge, especially when a patient has not responded favorably to this therapy. The use of pulsed Doppler echocardiography to optimize the AV interval is an effective first step in tailoring CRT to the needs of each patient. However, careful attention to pacemaker diagnostics, pacing thresholds, and electrograms is critical in the follow-up of these patients to ensure that CRT is consistently delivered. Newer techniques such as tissue Doppler imaging hold promise for more effective optimization of intraventricular synchrony. In addition, programming of mode switching, rate smoothing, the rate-adaptive AV delay, post-PVC response, MTR, and VT detection zones are all important considerations that are special challenges with CRT devices.

## REFERENCES

1. Abraham WT, Fisher WG, Smith AL, et al: MIRACLE Study Group. Multicenter InSync Randomized Clinical Evaluation: Cardiac resynchronization in chronic heart failure. *N Engl J Med* 2002;346:1845-1853.
2. Auricchio A, Stellbrink C, Sack S, et al: Long-term clinical effect of hemodynamically optimized cardiac resynchronization therapy in patients with heart failure and ventricular conduction delay. *J Am Coll Cardiol* 2002;39:2026-2033.
3. Auricchio A, Stellbrink C, Block M, et al: Effect of pacing chamber and atrioventricular delay on acute systolic function of paced patients with congestive heart failure: The Pacing Therapies for Congestive Heart Failure Study Group and Guidant Congestive Heart Failure Research Group. *Circulation* 1999;99:2993-3001.
4. Cazeau S, Leclercq C, Lavergne T, et al: Effects of multisite biventricular pacing in patients with heart failure and intraventricular conduction delay. *N Engl J Med* 2001;344:873-880.
5. Morris-Thurgood JA, Turner MS, Nightingale AK, et al: Pacing in heart failure: Improved ventricular interaction in diastole rather than systolic re-synchronization. *Europace* 2000;2:271-275.
6. Nishimura RA, Hayes DL, Holmes DR, et al: Mechanisms of hemodynamic improvement by dual chamber pacing for severe left ventricular dysfunction: an acute Doppler and catheterization study. *J Am Coll Cardiol* 1995;25:281-288.
7. Auricchio A, Ding J, Spinelli JC, et al: Cardiac resynchronization therapy restores optimal atrioventricular mechanical timing in heart failure patients with ventricular conduction delay. *J Am Coll Cardiol* 2002;39:1163-1169.
8. Ritter P, Padeletti L, Gillio-Meina L, et al: Determination of the optimal atrioventricular delay in DDD pacing: comparison between echo and peak endocardial acceleration measurements. *Europace* 1999;1:126-130.

9. Ishikawa T, Sumita S, Kimura K, et al: Prediction of optimal atrioventricular delay in patients with implanted DDD pacemakers. *PACE* 1999;22:1365-1371.

10. Kinderman M, Frohlig G, Doerr T, et al: Optimizing the AV delay in DDD pacemaker patients with high degree AV block: mitral valve Doppler versus impedance cardiography. *Pacing Clin Electrophysiol* 1997;20:2453-2462.

11. Fauchier L, Marie O, Casset-Senon D, et al: Interventricular and intraventricular dyssynchrony in idiopathic dilated cardiomyopathy. A prognostic study with Fourier phase analysis of radionuclide angioscintigraphy. *J Am Coll Cardiol* 2002;40:2022-2030.

12. Le Rest C, Couturier O, Turzo A, et al: Use of left ventricular pacing in heart failure: evaluation by gated blood pool imaging. *J Nucl Cardiol* 1999;6:651-656.

13. Breithardt OA, Stellbrink C, Kramer AP, et al: for the PATH-CHF Study Group: Echocardiographic quantification of left ventricular asynchrony predicts an acute hemodynamic benefit of cardiac resynchronization therapy. *J Am Coll Cardiol* 2002;40:536-545.

14. Pitzalis MV, Iacoveillo M, Romito R, et al: Cardiac resynchronization therapy tailored by echocardiographic evaluation of ventricular asynchrony. *J Am Coll Cardiol* 2002;40:1615-1622.

15. Yu CM, Chau E, Sanderson JE, et al: Tissue Doppler echocardiographic evidence of reverse remodeling and improved synchronicity by simultaneously delaying regional contraction after biventricular pacing therapy in heart failure. *Circulation* 2002;105:438-445.

16. Sogaard P, Eneblad H, Kim WY, et al: Tissue Doppler imaging predicts improved systolic performance and reversed left ventricular remodeling during long-term cardiac resynchronization therapy. *J Am Coll Cardiol* 2002;40:723-730.

17. Sogaard P, Egeblad H, Persen AK, et al: Sequential versus simultaneous biventricular resynchronization for severe heart failure. Evaluation by tissue Doppler imaging. *Circulation* 2002;106:2078-2084.

18. Popovic ZB, Grimm RA, Perlic G, et al: Noninvasive assessment of cardiac resynchronization therapy for congestive heart failure using myocardial strain and left ventricular peak power as parameters of myocardial synchrony and function. *J Cardiovasc Electrophysiol* 2002;13:1203-1208.

19. Rodriquez L, Garcia M, Ares M, et al: Assessment of mitral annular dynamics during diastole by Doppler tissue imaging: Comparison with mitral Doppler inflow in subjects without heart disease and in patients with left ventricular hypertrophy. *Am Heart J* 1996;131:982-987.

20. Yu CM, Lin H, Zhang Q, Sanderson JE: High prevalence of left ventricular systolic and diastolic asynchrony in patients with congestive heart failure and normal QRS duration. *Heart* 2003;89:54-60.

21. Kawaguchi M, Murabayashi T, Fetics BJ, et al: Quantitation of basal dyssynchrony and acute resynchronization from left or biventricular pacing by novel echocontrast variability imaging. *J Am Coll Cardiol* 2002;39:2052-2058.

22. Eldadah ZA, Berger RD: The strain of resynchronizing the failing heart. *J Cardiovasc Electrophysiol* 2002;13:1209-1210.

23. O'Cochlain B, Delurgio D, Leon A, Langberg J: The effect of variation in the interval between right and left ventricular activation on paced QRS duration. *PACE* 2001;24:1780-1782.

24. Cazeau S, Leclercq C, Lavergne T, et al: Effects of multisite biventricular pacing in patients with heart failure and intraventricular conduction delay. *N Engl J Med* 2001;233:873-880.

25. Lupi G, Brignole M, Oddone D, Bolline R: Effects of left ventricular pacing on cardiac performance and on quality of life in patients with drug-refractory heart failure. *Am J Cardiol* 2000;86:1267-1270.

26. Kass DA, Chen CH, Curry C, et al: Improved left ventricular mechanisms from acute VDD pacing in patients with dilated cardiomyopathy and ventricular conduction delay. *Circulation* 1999;99:1567-1573.

27. Nelson GS, Berger RD, Fetics BJ, et al: Left ventricular or biventricular pacing improves cardiac function at diminished energy cost in patients with dilated cardiomyopathy and left bundle branch block. *Circulation* 2000;102:3053-3059.

28. Braunschweig F, Linde C, Gadler F, et al: Reduction of hospital days by biventricular pacing. *Eur J Heart Fail* 2000;2:399-406.

29. Etienne Y, Mansourati J, Touiza A, et al: Evaluation of left ventricular function and mitral regurgitation during left ventricular-based pacing in patients with heart failure. *Eur J Heart Fail* 2001;3:441-447.

30. Nelson GS, Curry CW, Wyman BT, et al: Predictors of systolic augmentation from left ventricular pre-excitation in patients with dilated cardiomyopathy and intraventricular conduction delay. *Circulation* 2000;101:2703-2709.

31. Gras D, Cebron J-P, Brunel P, et al: Optimal stimulation of the left ventricle. *J Cardiovasc Electrophysiol* 2002;13:S57-S62.

32. Lunati M, Paolucci M, Oliva F, et al: Patient selection for biventricular pacing. *J Cardiovasc Electrophysiol* 2002;13:S63-S67.

33. Stellbrink C, Breithardt O, Franke A, et al: Impact of cardiac resynchronization therapy using hemodynamically optimized pacing on left ventricular remodeling in patients with congestive heart failure and ventricular conduction disturbances. *J Am Coll Cardiol* 2001;38:1957-1965.

34. Rouleau F, Merheb M, Geffroy S, et al: Echocardiographic assessment of the interventricular delay of activation and correlation to the QRS width in dilated cardiomyopathy. *Pacing Clin Electrophysiol* 2001;24:1500-1506.

35. Butter C, Auricchio A, Stellbrink C, et al: Effect of resynchronization therapy stimulation site on the systolic function of heart failure patients. *Circulation* 2001;104:3026-3029.

36. Barold SS, Levine PA. Significance of stimulation impedance in biventricular pacing. *J Intervent Cardiac Electrophysiol* 2002;6:67-70.

37. Mayhew M, Bubien RS, Slabaugh J, et al: Effect of a split cathodal configuration on pacing threshold and impedance. *PACE* 2003: in press.

38. Schreieck J, Zrenner B, Kolb C, et al: Inappropriate shock delivery due to ventricular double detection with a biventricular pacing implantable cardioverter defibrillator. *PACE* 2001;24:1154-1157.

39. Wang P, Kramer A, Estes M, Hayes DL. Timing cycles for biventricular pacing. *PACE* 2002;25:62-75.

40. Glikson M, Beeman AL, Luria DM, et al: Impaired detection of ventricular tachyarrhythmias by rate-smoothing algorithm in dual chamber implantable defibrillators: intradevice interaction. *J Cardiovasc Electrophysiol* 2002;13:312-318.

41. Akiyama M, Kaneko Y, Taniguchi Y, Kurabayashi M. Pacemaker syndrome associated with a biventricular pacing system. *J Cardiovasc Electrophysiol* 2002;13:1061-1062.

# 8

# Programming Cardiac Resynchronization Therapy

Richard A. Grimm

Cardiac resynchronization therapy (CRT) has been found to improve New York Heart Association (NYHA) functional class, quality of life, and exercise capacity for patients with impaired left ventricular (LV) function, prolonged QRS duration, and functional class III/IV heart failure.[1,2] Subsequent data analysis also found evidence of LV reverse remodeling 6 months postimplantation, as demonstrated by reduction in LV volumes, increase in ejection fraction, attenuation in mitral regurgitation, increase in cardiac index, and a decrease in LV mass.[2,3] It is therefore believed that the symptomatic (NYHA class) and functional (6-minute hall walk) improvements experienced by patients may be mediated by reverse remodeling[4] as well as by coordination of ventricular contraction.[5] This effect of cardiac resynchronization therapy appears to be independent and additive to the positive benefit of beta-blockers. A recent meta-analysis of four randomized trials involving 1634 patients showed that CRT reduced death from progressive heart failure by 51% in comparison with the rate for controls, reduced heart failure hospitalization by 29%, and produced a trend toward reducing all-cause mortality.[6] These early yet powerful results not only have revolutionized heart failure therapy but also have caused a rethinking of more conventional pacemaker therapies and their resultant hemodynamic and clinical effects.[7]

Despite these astonishing results, investigators have only begun to understand the mechanisms responsible for improvement. Clinicians are struggling to identify those most and least likely to derive benefit from CRT and continue to perfect the technique. Furthermore, the establishment of appropriate protocols and methods for optimization of resynchronization therapy (i.e., lead position and timing of stimulation) and the characterization and monitoring of cardiac function before and after CRT have not been not well defined and are currently under investigation and development. The three primary aspects of programming or optimization of resynchronization therapy that have become salient to management have been the optimization of atrioventricular (AV) delay, mechanical synchrony, and interventricular timing. Although much of the attention to date has focused on optimization of the AV delay,

**294**

it has become evident that optimization of mechanical synchrony may be the most important parameter to target as an endpoint to ensure successful therapy. This chapter discusses this evolving field and current methods for assessing the impact of pacing therapy on cardiac function.

## Atrioventricular Delay Optimization

The optimal AV delay has been defined as that which allows completion of the end-diastolic filling flow prior to ventricular contraction, thereby providing the longest diastolic filling time.[8] In patients with high-grade AV block and paced in the DDD mode, the diastolic filling time (DFT) is abbreviated by premature mitral valve closure prior to the start of ventricular contraction if the AV delay is programmed too long. On the other hand, if the AV delay is programmed too short, the end-diastolic filling flow (mitral A-wave) is abruptly interrupted by the onset of ventricular contraction.

Several investigators have reported on the importance of optimal AV synchrony in paced patients with high-grade AV block. Whereas Carlton and colleagues[9] were the first to highlight the importance of AV synchrony in paced patients with high-grade AV block, Ronaszeki et al.[8] demonstrated the impact of optimal AV delay in minimizing LV filling pressures and mitral regurgitation. Rey et al.[10] noted that the longest ventricular filling time without interruption of the A-wave resulted in the highest cardiac outputs. Ritter[11] subsequently reported on a method taking advantage of the ability of Doppler echocardiography to assess electrical-mechanical intervals, whereby AV timing could be optimized with use of a relatively simple and clinically practical protocol.

### The Ritter Method for Optimizing the Atrioventricular Delay

This method as described by Ritter,[11, 12] requires programming the AV delay to a short interval and a long interval while testing each setting for its impact on end-diastolic filling with Doppler echocardiography (Figure 8–1). The interval is first set inappropriately short (e.g., 50 msec) so that mitral valve closure is postponed until end-diastolic filling is prematurely terminated by the onset of ventricular contraction (Figure 8–2B). This then provides the examiner with the longest time interval a in between the ventricular pacing artifact and mitral valve closure (Q-A interval) and hence the maximum diastolic filling time for any given heart rate. It should be emphasized that the measurement of this Q-A interval should be made from the onset of the V-pacing spike to the termination of the A wave. Identifying the termination of the A wave can be difficult because of suboptimal Doppler acquisition; however, careful extrapolation from the down slope of the Doppler profile to the baseline will minimize measurement error. The AV delay is then set inappropriately long (i.e., 200 or 250 msec, as dictated by underlying conduction disease), which usually shortens the time interval from the ventricular pacing artifact to mitral valve closure and may even generate a negative value for b (Figure 8–2C). The optimal AV delay is then determined by correcting the long AV delay by the time shift from letter a to letter b, $AV_{long} - (a-b)$. The goal is to allow for completion of end-diastolic filling precisely at the onset of ventricular contraction (Figure 8–2D).

Implementation of this protocol requires a knowledgeable and experienced staff, coordination between the echocardiography laboratory and the electrophysiology technical staff, and close attention to detail during acquisition of the Doppler data. Although the Ritter method is typically relatively quick and simple to perform,

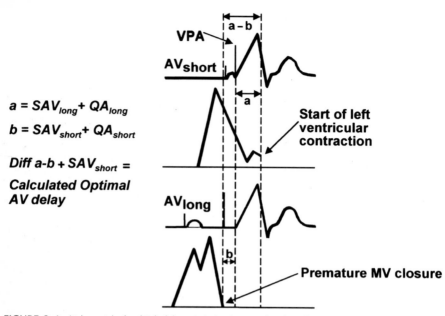

$a = SAV_{long} + QA_{long}$

$b = SAV_{short} + QA_{short}$

$Diff\ a\text{-}b + SAV_{short} =$

Calculated Optimal
AV delay

FIGURE 8–1. Atrioventricular (AV) delay optimization mechanics. The AV interval is set short (i.e., 50 msec) so that mitral valve closure is postponed until end-diastolic filling is prematurely terminated by the onset of ventricular contraction. The Q-A interval is then measured at this setting. The AV delay is thus set inappropriately long (i.e., 200–250 msec), which shortens the time interval from ventricular pacing to mitral valve closure and may even generate a negative value for b. Again the Q-A interval is measured. The optimal AV delay is then determined by correcting the long AV delay by the time shift from letter a to letter b, $AV_{short} + (a\text{–}b)$. (Adapted from Kindermann M, Frohlig G, Doerr T, Schieffer H: Optimizing the AV DELAY in DDD pacemaker patients with high degree av block: mitral valve Doppler versus impedance cardiography. PACE 1997;20:2453-2462, with permission from Blackwell Publishing Ltd.)

individual cases may be particularly involved, technically difficult, or complex and may require considerably more time and deliberation. It should be noted, however, that this method has not been validated or been proven to be superior to fixed (e.g., empiric) setting of the AV interval in the CRT population. Last, yet another index of myocardial performance that may prove useful when conducting an AV optimization procedure is the Tei index.[13] This method is relatively simple to perform yet provides reliable data on both systolic and diastolic function. This index is obtained from the sampling of mitral inflow as well as LV outflow by pulsed Doppler echocardiography. The ejection time is then subtracted from the interval between cessation and onset of the mitral inflow velocity to give the sum of the isovolumic contraction time and isovolumic relaxation time. Further study is required to assess its utility in this patient population.

## Limitations of the Ritter Method for Optimizing the Atrioventricular Delay

Limitations of the Ritter method are many and primarily are related to the lack of data in the CRT patient population, as well as technical issues related to the acquisition of Doppler information. This method was originally reported and previously validated

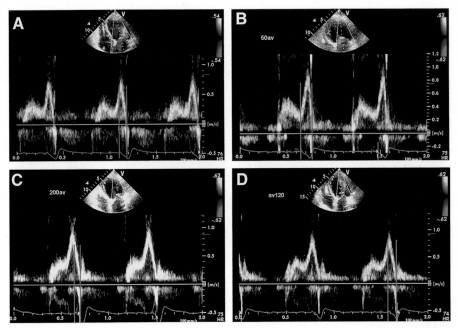

**FIGURE 8–2.** The atrioventricular (AV) delay optimization procedure as proposed by Ritter. *A,* Mitral inflow at the baseline setting upon presentation to cardiac function laboratory, AV delay of 100 msec. *B,* AV delay reset to a short interval of 50 msec. The Q-A interval was measured at 130 msec. *C,* The AV delay was then changed to a long interval of 200 msec and the Q-A interval was measured at 50 msec. *D,* The mitral inflow was resampled at the calculated optimal AV delay of 120 msec. *(Reprinted from Sogaard P, Egeblad H, Kim WY, et al: Tissue Doppler imaging predicts improved systolic performance and reversed left ventricular remodeling during long-term cardiac resynchronization therapy. J Am Coll Cardiol 2002;40:723-730, with permission from The American College of Cardiology Foundation.)*

among patients undergoing pacing therapy for conduction system disease.[14] It is in this population of patients in which it was found to be superior to fixed AV delay settings. An experience is currently being gathered in the CRT patient population. Other limitations relate to the assessment of electrical-mechanical intervals with Doppler echocardiography. Because the electrocardiographic signal is often of suboptimal quality on most currently available echocardiographic instrumentation, identifying the onset of the QRS complex when measuring the Q-A interval may be quite difficult, potentially resulting in significant intraobserver and interobserver variability. This problem may be eliminated if a prominent pacing spike can be identified. A more definitive solution would be to input the pulse generator's electrogram signal directly into the echocardiograph. The terminal end of the Q-A duration measurement, which involves the acquisition and identification of the termination of the mitral inflow A wave, can also prove to be problematic. Pulsed-wave Doppler sample volume positioning, filter and gain settings, and image quality can all significantly impact the quality of the Doppler signal and therefore the accuracy of the Q-A interval. The sonographer will often find that positioning the pulsed-wave sample volume toward the left atrium (as opposed to the standard position at the mitral leaflet tips) will optimize the mitral A-wave modal velocity signal, clarifying the terminal portion of the signal for more precise measurement of the end of the atrial contribution to filling (Figure 8–3).

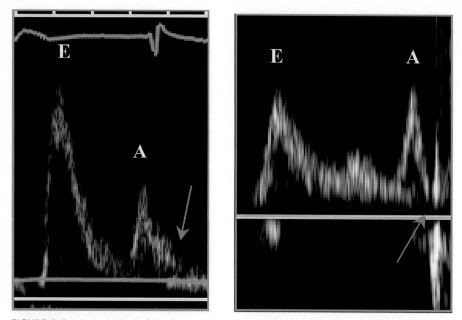

**FIGURE 8–3.** Measurement of the Q-A interval requires accurate identification of the termination of the A wave. Suboptimal instrument settings may lead to inaccurate measurements. *Left,* Despite a satisfactory pulsed Doppler mitral inflow signal, the termination of the A wave is unclear. *Right,* Improved mitral A wave signal (by adjusting the sample volume towards the left atrium) with clear termination of the A wave resulting from optimal gain adjustment, optimal sample volume position, and filter adjustments. *(Reprinted from Sogaard P, Egeblad H, Kim WY, et al: Tissue Doppler imaging predicts improved systolic performance and reversed left ventricular remodeling during long-term cardiac resynchronization therapy. J Am Coll Cardiol 2002;40:723-730, with permission from The American College of Cardiology Foundation.)*

Other limitations include the failure of the optimization protocol to take into account the relative importance of interatrial and interventricular conduction times; the lack of a simple, rapid, noninvasive, and reproducible method for estimating cardiac outputs; and the fact that the current method must be used with caution if atrial function is depressed (such as after cardioversion) or in those with high, left atrial pressures in the presence of congestive heart failure. Finally, it has been suggested that this method for AV delay optimization may be oversimplified, and others would argue that it is unnecessary. Some CRT device manufacturers have specific recommendations for AV optimization algorithms after implantation; others simply recommend a standard "out of the box" AV delay setting of between 80 and 120 msec.

In the event of suboptimal Doppler or electrocardiographic data or questionable calculated AV optimization data, or simply as a means of reassurance and confirmation that the hemodynamics have been "optimized," it is customary for the laboratory at my facility (The Cleveland Clinic Foundation) to make an assessment of LV diastolic filling and an estimation of LV and/or left atrial filling pressures. This can be performed routinely with minimal additional time or effort on the part of the technical staff by utilizing Doppler echocardiography and targeting a stage-1 diastolic filling pattern, which would imply normalized left atrial filling pressures in the setting of ventricular systolic dysfunction and a reasonably optimized AV delay. The additional data required for the estimation of filling pressures would include those from a pulsed-wave Doppler acquisition of pulmonary vein flow (Figure 8–4) and from Doppler tissue imaging of the lateral mitral anulus motion (Figure 8–5).

## AV Delay Optimization in Heart Failure and in the Cardiac Resynchronization Therapy Population

Although the importance of AV delay optimization for the AV conduction disease population requiring dual chamber pacing is unquestioned, the impact for the heart failure population that often manifests spontaneous conduction remains uncertain. Early reports suggested that AV synchronization in patients with short AV delays significantly improved the status of those with end-stage heart failure.[15,16] However, subsequent, more rigorous studies found no beneficial effects of AV synchronous pacing with optimized AV delay in patients with severe heart failure.[17] Some have speculated that the lack of improvement in patients with heart failure is

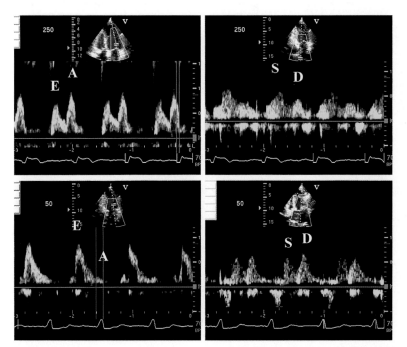

**FIGURE 8–4.** Mitral inflow and pulmonary vein flow signals, which, when this data is coupled and integrated, can be utilized to make an assessment of diastolic filling and an estimation of left ventricular filling pressures. The top panels show a stage I diastolic filling pattern at an atrioventricular (AV) delay of 250 msec with E:A reversal on mitral inflow sampling (*left*) and an S:D ratio of greater than 1 in the pulmonary vein flow (*right*). The bottom panels show a stage III diastolic filling pattern (restrictive physiology) at an AV delay of 50 msec with E:A of greater than 2 on mitral inflow sampling (*left*) and an S:D ratio of less than 1 in the pulmonary vein flow (*right*).

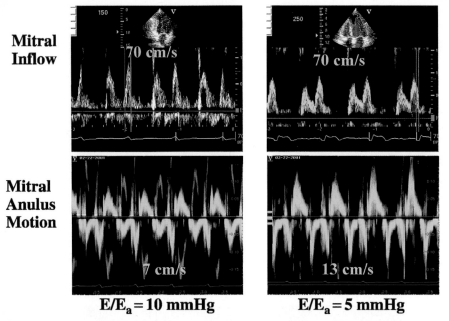

**Mitral Inflow**

**Mitral Anulus Motion**

$E/E_a = 10$ mmHg          $E/E_a = 5$ mmHg

**FIGURE 8–5.** Estimation of left atrial pressures by determining the ratio of the mitral inflow peak E wave velocity and peak velocity of the early diastolic mitral anulus motion ($E_a$) by Doppler tissue imaging ($E/E_a$) in the same patient at two different atrioventricular (AV) delay settings. At an AV delay of 150 msec, the estimated pulmonary capillary wedge pressure (PCWP) is 10 mmHg, whereas at an AV delay of 250 msec, the estimated PCWP is 5 mmHg.

due to the possibility that AV delay programming may influence both the AV mechanical sequence as well as the ventricular activation sequence. Furthermore, the importance of AV delay optimization is even less understood in the CRT patient population. It seems reasonable to speculate that optimization of AV delay is an important factor in patients undergoing CRT; however, only one study has systematically examined the impact of a patient-specific AV delay on hemodynamics. Auricchio et al. concluded that although the pacing chamber is paramount when it comes to relative importance, AV delay does positively impact hemodynamics.[18] In fact, given the relatively small incremental improvements in hemodynamics reported with optimized AV delays in patients undergoing DDD pacing, as compared to the potentially large improvements reported in ejection fraction (from trials such as the Multicenter InSync Randomized Clinical Evaluation [MIRACLE]) in patients undergoing CRT, it would stand to reason that other factors such as resynchronization of ventricular contraction (mechanical synchrony) may play a much larger role in overall improvement in hemodynamics as compared to AV synchrony alone.

As mentioned previously, AV delay optimization was initially described in the patient population undergoing pacing therapy for conduction disease. It is therefore important to recognize that although many of the patients who are candidates for CRT also have significant conduction disease, many others may have relatively normal AV conduction. Therefore when one attempts to optimize the AV delay in these patients, it is essential that biventricular pacing is maintained whether the atrium is sensed or paced while the AV delay optimization testing is performed. In patients with conduction disease, prolonged AV delays (i.e., 150–250 msec) may prove optimal, especially if significant atrial enlargement and hence interatrial conduction delay are present. Fortunately, many patients in this population also have chronotropic incompetence, thereby minimizing the likelihood of significant tachycardia, which would in turn be a limiting factor in prolonging the AV delay. We have found that diastolic filling patterns can be further improved by prolonging the AV delay beyond the estimated AV delay, as determined by the Ritter method. Conversely, in patients with normal AV nodal conduction, the AV delay may need to be set unusually short, particularly if the atrial lead position inappropriately senses a longer PR interval than is actually present. This situation might not allow for consistent biventricular pacing, thereby allowing intermittent intrinsic or fused beats to occur. In this case, hemodynamic performance of the heart would undoubtedly be compromised.

# Left Ventricular Resynchronization

## Importance of Mechanical Synchrony

Although AV delay optimization can clearly impact hemodynamics in patients undergoing CRT,[18] it has less influence on ventricular function than the optimal pacing site,[19] because the primary mechanism for improvement in ventricular mechanics is a more coordinated electrical-mechanical coupling within the ventricle and hence improved ejection fraction, cardiac output, and chamber efficiency.[19-22] This improved mechanical synchrony is the result of optimized regional timing of stimulation. To date, electrical data (QRS duration), hemodynamic data (i.e., dP/dt), and findings of selected imaging modalities have been proposed as surrogate markers to assess degree of dyssynchrony as well as the response to CRT, in an attempt to identify not only potential candidates but also parameters that may be used to assess the status of the ventricle following implantation.

The primary parameter used to determine candidacy (in addition to the presence of heart failure) has been QRS duration.[18,21] Data from the PATH-CHF study suggested that a QRS duration of more than 155 msec had the best positive and negative predictive accuracy for predicting hemodynamic improvement with biventricular pacing. Additionally, the wider the QRS and the greater the cardiodepression (as defined in this study as a dP/dt of less than 700), the greater the immediate response to therapy. However, QRS duration has proven unsatisfactory, because patients with narrow complexes may respond and some with wide complexes may not respond.[18,21] Finally, it is unclear whether the extent of QRS narrowing due to CRT can predict the extent of the response to therapy. Although most of the early seminal investigation utilized invasively derived hemodynamic data as measures for global response to interventions, this is impractical for routine clinical use.

Yet another factor that has delayed the development of a diagnostic modality that could accurately assess the results of resynchronization therapy postimplantation has been the nominal effect of CRT on traditional noninvasive measures of ventricular function, such as ejection fraction. This issue was highlighted in the MIRACLE trial results. At baseline there was no significant difference in ejection fraction between controls and the CRT group, whereas at 3 months the difference in ejection fraction was only 5% (30% for the control group versus 35% in the

CRT group).[2] This difference is within the recognized measurement error of echocardiographically derived ejection fraction measurements. Hence other parameters such as indices of ventricular synchrony have been sought as a surrogate measure of improved mechanics and thus improved function. Several methods have been proposed to evaluate improved synchrony of contraction in order to document immediate success as well as to "fine tune" or optimize the resynchronization therapy. Investigations are ongoing to determine which of these indices of synchronicity will prove most reliable and most practical for clinical practice. The importance of an objective assessment of mechanical synchrony cannot be overstated, because this parameter will ultimately prove to be the index by which the evaluation and programming of CRT is based. The following will be a review of those parameters that have been reported and appear to hold the most promise for widespread application.

### Noninvasive Assessment of Myocardial Strain

Mechanistic studies attempting to analyze asynchronous electrical activation of the ventricle and the impact on mechanical function have employed mapping of regional myocardial strain with magnetic resonance imaging (MRI) tagging to identify degrees of contractile dyssynchrony.[21,23,24] Ventricular pacing at the right ventricular (RV) apex, which causes an activation pattern similar to left bundle branch block (LBBB) conduction delay, induces uncoordinated LV contraction. In these studies, MRI-tagged imaging demonstrated and quantified the mechanical dyssynchrony, as seen in an RV apical pacing canine model[23,24] as well as in patients with dilated cardiomyopathy and LBBB conduction disturbances.[21] Although MRI is feasible for the identification and assessment of mechanical dyssynchrony, it is contraindicated for patients with pacemakers. An alternative noninvasive method for evaluating myocardial strain or tissue deformation is Doppler tissue imaging (DTI).[25] DTI allows real-time determination of strain rate as the time integral of regional Doppler velocity gradients and from which regional myocardial strain may be derived. Our group evaluated myocardial strain in 22 patients before and after CRT with DTI to assess myocardial synchrony as part of a substudy of the MIRACLE trial.[26] This study found evidence of significant dyssynchrony at baseline that improved following cardiac resynchronization, as shown by a significant improvement in the coefficient of variation of regional myocardial strain (Figure 8–6). Although promising, further study is necessary to determine the robustness of this Doppler echocardiographic parameter as a measure of synchrony in a clinical setting. Several other noninvasive methods have been proposed as measures of dyssynchrony, all of which have associated advantages and disadvantages.

### Septal-Posterior Wall-Motion Mechanical Delay (SPWMD)

This method has been reported by Pitzales and colleagues and utilizes standard M-mode echocardiography to take full advantage of the excellent temporal resolution, as well as the widespread familiarity and clinical availability of this technique.[27] Aligning the M-mode cursor perpendicular to the long axis of the ventricle at the base of the heart in the parasternal long axis view, one can determine the earliest point of activation in the basal septum as well as the latest point of

## LV Strain Coefficient of Variations

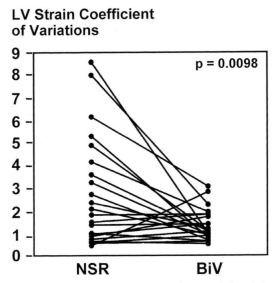

FIGURE 8–6. Left ventricular (*LV*) coefficient of variation of myocardial strain in patients before and following cardiac resynchronization therapy (CRT). The myocardial strain coefficient of variation was significantly decreased following CRT. BiV = Biventricular; NSR = normal sinus rhythm.

activation and movement anteriorly in the basal posterior wall (Figure 8–7). In patients with heart failure and an LBBB on the surface electrocardiogram, baseline SPWMD was a strong predictor of the occurrence of reverse remodeling following CRT. At 1 month following initiation of CRT, the septal to posterior wall motion delay decreased from an average of $192 \pm 92$ msec to $14 \pm 67$ msec ($P < 0.0001$). Not only did SPWMD have a higher specificity than QRS duration (63% versus 13%), with use of 130 msec and 150 msec as cutoffs, but the positive predictive value and accuracy were also significantly greater (80% and 85% versus 63% and 65%). The advantage of this method is its high temporal resolution, simplicity, and widespread availability. The disadvantage is that SPWMD is a regional index and limits interrogation to only two segments of a 16-segment ventricle.

### Regional Myocardial Velocities as Determined by Two-Dimensional Echocardiography with Tissue Doppler Imaging

Using the same theoretical bases as the septal to posterior wall motion delay concept, Yu and colleagues used DTI to measure segmental myocardial velocities and the time to peak myocardial sustained systolic velocity ($T_s$) over six basal and six midventricular segments. Prior to pacing there was a marked segmental variation in $T_s$, occurring earliest at the basal anterior septal segment ($148 \pm 25$ msec) and latest in the basal lateral segment ($216 \pm 52$ msec). After pacing the difference in $T_s$ between the two regions was eliminated ($191 \pm 32$ versus $213 \pm 44$ msec; $P = NS$)

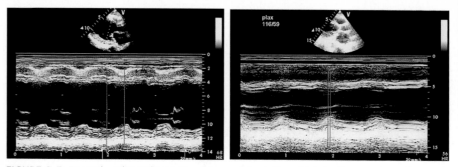

**FIGURE 8–7.** M-mode echocardiography at base of the left ventricle in the parasternal long axis view demonstrating septal-posterior wall-mechanical delay (SPWMD) before (*left*) and after (*right*) cardiac resynchronization therapy as described by Pitzalis et al. The measured SPWMD before implant was 360 msec and after implant was 20 msec.

(Figure 8–8). Limitations of this method include the accuracy of the local tissue velocity data, which can be impacted by translational motion of the heart as well as tethering effects from other regions. Additionally, this method can be very time consuming. Furthermore, although a more global method may, intuitively, seem better and possibly more comprehensive, the regional method using M-mode and focusing on the basal anterior septum and posterior wall segments may suffice in identifying this asynchrony in patients with heart failure and conduction delay and hence improvement following CRT. The relative advantages and disadvantages of these different methods have yet to be compared.

### Doppler Tissue Tracking

Another noninvasive method that has been proposed for identifying ventricular dyssynchrony and that utilizes the DTI modality is known as tissue tracking. As opposed to sampling regional or global myocardial velocities, tissue tracking simply quantifies myocardial displacement in the longitudinal direction. This method has been applied to the CRT population and was reported on by Sogaard and colleagues.[28] With use of color-coded myocardial displacement maps from the apical 4 chamber, apical 2, and apical long axis views, segmental displacement can be timed throughout the cardiac cycle. In the example shown in Figure 8–9, no myocardial displacement occurs in the base and midportion of the posterior wall during ventricular synchrony (depicted as a gray area), whereas motion toward the apex clearly is occurring in the anterior septum (depicted as bluish-green on the velocity map). In the bottom panel, in the frame depicting early diastole, the early diastolic displacement of the posterior wall toward the apex is seen (green). This phenomenon of early diastolic displacement involving the basal posterior and basal lateral wall has been termed *delayed longitudinal contraction* and has been correlated to an improvement in the change in ejection fraction following CRT. Additionally, this phenomenon has been found to be characteristic of patients with an LBBB conduction abnormality.

## Interventricular Timing

It is believed that sequential biventricular pacing (V-V timing) potentially maximizes stroke volume over simultaneous biventricular pacing during CRT.

## $S_M$ Sept. Before Lat. Wall

LBBB

After
Biventricular
Pacing

Basal Septum

Basal Lateral

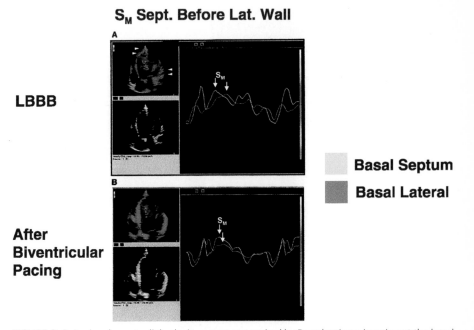

FIGURE 8–8. Regional myocardial velocity curves as acquired by Doppler tissue imaging at the basal septum (*Sept.; yellow*) and basal lateral (*Lat.; green*) walls. The top panel displays the time to peak velocity in the septum ($S_M$ *yellow line*) and lateral wall ($S_M$ *green line*) in a patient with left bundle branch block (*LBBB*). Note the difference in time delay from QRS onset to peak velocity (*arrows*). The bottom panel shows the same patient following cardiac resynchronization therapy as the time difference from QRS onset to peak systolic myocardial velocity between septum and lateral wall is essentially zero. (*Reproduced with permission from Yu CM, Chau E, Sanderson JE, et al: Tissue Doppler echocardiographic evidence of reverse remodeling and improved synchronicity by simultaneously delaying regional contraction after biventricular pacing therapy in heart failure. Circulation 2002;105:438-445.*)

Optimal V-V timing is believed to be approximately 40 msec, but in patients with heart failure and significant conduction delay undergoing CRT, simultaneous stimulation of the left ventricle and the right ventricle may not be appropriate. Therefore altering LV-RV stimulation by varying durations may further optimize LV resynchronization. Preliminary studies have demonstrated improvement in hemodynamics. It has been speculated that this in part may be the result of compensation for suboptimal lead position.[29]

Sogaard and colleagues used DTI with tissue tracking to identify candidates with the delayed longitudinal contraction and compared sequential versus simultaneous biventricular resynchronization.[30] They studied 21 patients with LBBB, a QRS duration of greater than 130 msec, and an NYHA functional class III or IV heart failure with DTI techniques specifically (tissue tracking and strain rate imaging) before and after implantation (CRT). Postimplantation studies were performed during simultaneous CRT at 12-, 20-, 40-, 60-, and 80-msec delay intervals with either LV or RV pre-excitation. The study population consisted of 11 patients with ischemic cardiomyopathy and 9 patients with idiopathic dilated cardiomyopathy, all of whom manifested an LBBB pattern electrocardiographically. As noted in prior studies,

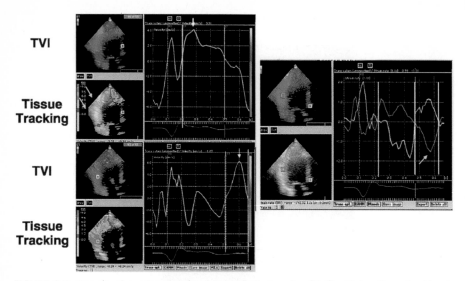

TVI

Tissue Tracking

TVI

Tissue Tracking

FIGURE 8–9. Doppler tissue imaging (or tissue velocity imaging [*TVI*]) utilizing tissue tracking to identify evidence of delayed longitudinal contraction. *Top left,* Apical long axis imaging with tissue tracking demonstrating lack of movement of the posterior wall toward the apex (*gray*) during systole. The anterior septum on the other hand moves apically as expected. This movement can be seen in graph form as well as the calipers, which highlight the segment of systole that is being examined. *Bottom left,* Still frame of the apical long axis view demonstrating movement of the base of the posterior wall toward the apex during early diastole. This segment represents delayed longitudinal contraction (DLC). *Right,* Myocardial strain mapping demonstrating negative (normal) strain values during early diastole at the base of the posterior wall. This would suggest that the segment that demonstrated DLC by tissue tracking is viable rather than scarred. *(Reproduced from Sogaard P, Egeblad H, Kim WY, et al: Tissue Doppler imaging predicts improved systolic performance and reversed left ventricular remodeling during long-term cardiac resynchronization therapy.* J Am Coll Cardiol *2002;40:723-730, with permission from* The American College of Cardiology Foundation.*)*

delayed longitudinal contraction was identified in the lateral and posterior walls of the left ventricle (Figure 8–10*A*). In contrast, patients with ischemic cardiomyopathy manifested delayed longitudinal contraction in the septum and inferior walls (Figure 8–10*B*). Echocardiographic parameters improved during sequential CRT, with LV preactivation being superior in 9 patients and RV preactivation proving superior in 11 patients. Compared to simultaneous CRT, optimum sequential CRT reduced the extent of segments with delayed longitudinal contraction in the base from $23.2 \pm 13\%$ to $11.1 \pm 7.2\%$ ($P < 0.05$). Ejection fraction increased from $29.7 \pm 5\%$ to $33.6 \pm 6\%$ ($P < 0.01$). Additionally, the diastolic filling time increased without any further AV delay optimization. Finally, the investigators reported that the location of delayed longitudinal contraction predicted the optimum sequential CRT as posterior lateral wall–delayed longitudinal contraction was associated with optimum sequential CRT via LV preactivation and septal and inferior wall–delayed longitudinal contraction was associated with optimum sequential CRT via RV preactivation. The optimum RV and LV preactivation intervals ranged between 12 and 20 msec. Preactivation of the lead opposite the one that demonstrated the optimum resynchronization caused a significant reduction in global systolic contraction amplitude in comparison with simultaneous CRT.

## IHD patient, systolic tracking, before pacing

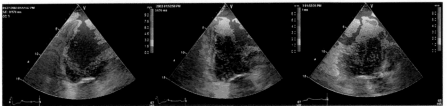

## IHD patient, diastolic tracking (DLC), before pacing

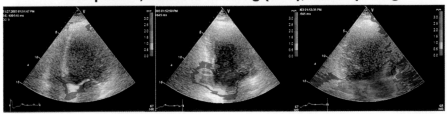

## IHD patient, systolic tracking, during pacing

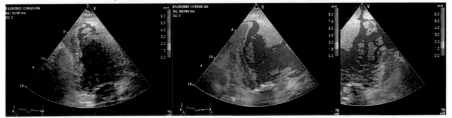

**FIGURE 8–10.** Tissue tracking images in a patient with ischemic heart disease (*IHD*) in the apical 4 chamber (*left*), apical 2 chamber (*center*) and apical long axis (*right*) views during systole before cardiac resynchronization therapy (CRT; *top*), diastole before CRT (*middle*), and systole after CRT (*bottom*). Movement toward the apex is demonstrated during systole as expected for the majority of the myocardial segments, including the mid- and apical septum and inferior, anterior, and lateral walls. The middle panel shows evidence of delayed longitudinal contraction (*DLC*) involving the basal septum, basal inferior septum, and basal anteroseptum. This is the territory of an old myocardial infarction. After CRT (*bottom*) the patient demonstrates increased displacement toward the apex (*purple* on the color map), especially at the basal segments involving the septum and inferior walls where DLC was identified before CRT. This pattern of DLC (involving the basal septum and basal inferior wall) would also be expected to be further optimized with right ventricular preactivation, in contrast to DLC involving the basal posterior and/or lateral wall, which might best respond to left ventricular preactivation with sequential preactivation.

# Recommendations for Evaluating CRT and Optimizing Results

### Considerations Prior to Attempting an Optimization Procedure in CRT Patients

Before embarking on an optimization protocol, one must recognize the current limitations of the procedure and not have unreasonable expectations of its potential. First, there are currently no data from controlled, prospective studies that support the utility of performing an optimization protocol. All reports are anecdotal, primarily describe issues as they relate to AV optimization, and have not yet proved superiority to fixed settings. Second, because most of the benefits from CRT will be achieved with placement of the LV lead and resultant ventricular resynchronization, little incremental benefit is likely to be derived from an AV optimization protocol in the majority of cases. However, screening all patients appears necessary in order to identify those who may derive benefit. Third, the primary goal of CRT should be to select appropriate candidates for the therapy and ensure the best practice when performing an implantation procedure. In other words, avoiding implantations in patients unlikely to derive benefit (on the basis of the current literature) and not tolerating suboptimal LV lead positions are guidelines that will prevent frustration following an implantation, because expecting to optimize these patients would likely prove futile. Selected patients in whom optimal lead position is desired might be considered for thoracotomy for epicardial lead placement. Once these issues have been resolved, one can proceed to an attempt at programming by first coordinating the electrophysiology technician and the sonographer to perform the testing under the supervision of a cardiologist.

### Proposed Protocol for Programming CRT

1. Optimize the AV delay utilizing the Ritter method. If the calculated AV delay is either unreliable (because of suboptimal Doppler data) or seemingly inappropriate for the physiology or if the acquisition of diagnostic Doppler data simply is not feasible, it is suggested that one should attempt to target an optimized diastolic filling pattern (stage-I diastolic filling).
2. Improve coordination of mechanical synchrony, utilizing one of the methods described previously, such as improved SPWMD, improved time to peak systolic velocity, or the absence or minimization of delayed longitudinal contraction by the tissue tracking method. Additionally, a global assessment of ventricular function and a regional wall motion assessment should be performed, using B-mode echocardiographic imaging. The primary utility of this assessment is to determine whether CRT achieved its anticipated response. If not, the options are limited, although in exceptional cases one might consider unconventional alternatives such as repositioning of the LV lead, epicardial lead placement if improved positioning is believed to be feasible, LV pacing alone, or even reversion to intrinsic conduction if pacing appears detrimental to function. Although the assessment of mechanical synchrony is feasible with any one of the indices of synchrony mentioned, the more practical issue of how best to respond to the data has yet to be determined.
3. If the CRT device has the capability of modifying sequential RV-LV timing, one can utilize DTI with tissue tracking as described by Sogaard et al. to test interventricular synchrony. Additionally, the difference between the QRS onset to the onset of pulmonic flow and QRS to aortic flow onset can be used as a parameter to assess interventricular timing. As is the case with the assessment of mechanical synchrony, further investigation is necessary to prove efficacy.
4. Re-assessment of these parameters in 3–6 months is advisable.

# Conclusion

Our understanding of the mechanisms of improvement in ventricular function has evolved considerably over the years, from an early belief that resolution of mitral regurgitation was a prime factor in the reverse remodeling process to the current wisdom, which is recognition of the impact of mechanical synchrony as the primary mechanism for improvement. Because our understanding of the mechanisms of improvement are still evolving, programming of CRT can be considered only a goal of optimal management at present. Ongoing investigation will determine the most appropriate and practical methods for analysis of mechanical synchrony and global function, as well as the optimal timing intervals for selected patient profiles.

## REFERENCES

1. Cazeau S, Leclercq C, Lavergne T, et al: Investigators. ftMSiCS: Effects of multisite bi-ventricular pacing in patients with heart failure and intra-ventricular conduction delay. *N Engl J Med* 2001;344:873-880.
2. Abraham W, Fisher WG, Smith AL, et al., for the MIRACLE Study Group: Cardiac resynchronization in heart failure. *N Engl J Med* 2002;346:1845-1853.
3. Stelbrink C, Breithardt OA, Franke A: Impact of cardiac resynchronization therapy using hemodynamically optimized pacing on LV remodeling in patients with congestive heart failure and ventricular conduction disturbances. *J Am Coll Cardiol* 2001;38:1957-1965.
4. Saxon L, De Marco T, Schefer J, et al: Effects of long term biventricular stimulation for resynchronization on echocardiographic measures of remodeling. *Circulation* 2002;105:1304-1310.
5. Leclercq C, Kass DA: Retiming the failing heart: Principles and current clinical status of cardiac resynchronization. *J Am Coll Cardiol* 2002;39:194-201.
6. Bradley DJ, Bradely EA, Baughman KL, et al: Cardiac resynchronization and death from progressive heart failure: A meta-analysis of randomized controlled trials. *JAMA* 2003;289:730-740.
7. Investigators TDT: Dual-chamber pacing or ventricular backup pacing in patients with an implantable defibrillator. *JAMA* 2002;288:3115-3123.
8. Ronaszeki A: Hemodynamic consequences of the timing of atrial contraction during complete AV block. *Acta Biomedica Lovaniensia* 1989:15.
9. Carlton RA, Rassovoy M, Graettinger JS: The importance and timing of left atrial systole. *Chemical Science* 1969;30:151-159.
10. Rey JL, Slama MA, Triboulloy C, et al: Etiude par echo-Doppler des variations hemodynamics entre modes double stimulation et detection de loreillette chez des patients porteurs d 'un stimulateur double chamber. *Arch Mal Coevr* 1990;83:961-966.
11. Ritter P, Dib JC, Lelievre T, et al: Quick determination of the optimal AV delay at rest in patients paced in DDD mode for complete AV block [abstract]. *Eur J CPE* 1994;4(2)A163.
12. Ritter P, Padeletti L, Gillio-Meina L, et al: Determination of the optimal atrioventricular delay in DDD pacing: comparison between echo and peak endocardial acceleration measurements. *Europace* 1999;1:126-130.
13. Tei C, Ling LH, Hodge DO, et al: New index of combined systolic and diastolic myocardial performance: A simple and reproducible measure of cardiac function - A study in normals and dilated cardiomyopathy. *J Cardiol* 1995;26:357-366.
14. Kindermann M, Frohlig G, Doerr T, Schieffer H: Optimizing the AV delay in DDD pacemaker patients with high degree AV block: mitral valve doppler versus impedance cardiography. *PACE* 1997;20:2453-2462.
15. Meshanur, Hochleitner M, Hortnagl H, et al: Usefulness of physiological chamber pacing in drug resistant idiopathic dilated cardiomyopathy. *Am J Cardiol* 1990;66:198-202.
16. Nishimura RA, Hayes DL, Holmes DR, et al: Mechanisms of hemodynamic improvement by dual chamber pacing for severe left ventricular dysfunction: an acute Doppler and catheterization study. *J Am Coll Cardiol* 1995;25:281-288.
17. Linde C, Gadler F, Edner M, et al: Results of atrioventricular synchronous pacing with optimized delay in patients with severe congestive heart failure. *Am J Cardiol* 1995;75:919-923.

18. Auricchio A, Stellbrink C, Block M, et al: Effect of pacing chamber and atrio-ventricular delay on acute systolic function of paced patients with congestive heart failure: the Pacing Therapies for Congestive Heart Failure Study Group: The Guidant Congestive Heart Failure Research Group. *Circulation* 1999;99:2993-3001.

19. Kass DA, Chen CH, Curry C, et al: Improved left ventricular mechanics from acute VDD pacing in patients with dilated cardiomyopathy and ventricular conduction delay. *Circulation* 1999;99: 1567-1573.

20. Yu CM, Chau E, Sanderson JE, et al: Tissue Doppler echocardiographic evidence of reverse remodeling and improved synchronicity by simultaneously delaying regional contraction after biventricular pacing therapy in heart failure. *Circulation* 2002;105:438-445.

21. Nelson GS, Curry CW, Wyman BT, et al: Predictors of systolic augmentation from left ventricular preexcitation in patients with dilated cardiomyopathy and intraventricular conduction delay. *Circulation* 2000;101:2703-2709.

22. Sogaard P, Kim WY, Jensen HK, et al: Impact of acute biventricular pacing on left ventricular performance and volumes in patients with severe heart failure: a tissue Doppler and three-dimensional echocardiographic study. *Cardiology* 2001;95:173-182.

23. Prinzen FW, Hunter WC, Wyman BT, McVeigh ER: Mapping of regional myocardial strain and work during ventricular pacing: Experimental study using magnetic resonance imaging. *J Am Coll Cardiol* 1999;33:1735-1742.

24. Wyman BT, Hunter WC, Prinzen FW, McVeigh ER: Mapping propagation of mechanical activation in the paced heart with MRI tagging. *Am J Physiology* 1999;276:881-891.

25. Edvardsen T, Gerber BL, Garot J, et al: Quantitative assessment of intrinsic regional myocardial deformat. *Circulation* 2002;106:50-56.

26. Popovic Z, Grimm RA, Perlic G, et al: Noninvasive assessment of cardiac resynchronization therapy for congestive heart failure using myocardial strain and left ventricular peak power as parameters of myocardial synchrony and function. *J Cardiovasc Electrophysiol* 2002;13:1203-1208.

27. Pitzalis MV, Iacoviello A, Romito R, et al: Cardiac resynchronization therapy tailored by echo-cardiographic evaluation of ventricular asynchrony. *J Am Coll Cardiol* 2002;40:1615-1622.

28. Sogaard P, Egeblad H, Kim WY, et al: Tissue Doppler imaging predicts improved systolic performance and reversed left ventricular remodeling during long-term cardiac resynchronization therapy. *J Am Coll Cardiol* 2002;40:723-730.

29. Greenberg J, Delurgio DBM, Mera F: Left ventricular lead location in biventricular pacing with variable RV-LV Timing does not affect optimal stroke volume. *NASPE* 2002:151.

30. Sogaard P, Egeblad H, Pedersen AK, et al: Sequential versus simultaneous biventricular resynchronization for severe heart failure: evaluation by tissue Doppler imaging. *Circulation.* 2002;106:2078-2084.

# Index

Page numbers followed by a *t* indicate tables; page numbers followed by an *f* indicate figures.